Handbook of Neonatal Intensive Care

Handbook of Neonatal Intensive Care

Fourth edition

Henry Halliday MD FRCPE FRCP FRCPCH,
Garth McClure MB FRCPE FRCPCH,
Mark Reid MB FRCPG FRCPI FRCPCH,

Edited by
Angela Bell MD FRCP FRCPCH
Richard Tubman BSc MD MRCP FRCPCH

WB Saunders Company Ltd
London Philadelphia Toronto Sydney Tokyo

W.B. Saunders Company Ltd 24–28 Oval Road London NW1 7DX

The Curtis Centre
Independence Square West
Philadelphia, PA 19106-3399, USA

Harcourt Brace & Company
55 Horner Avenue
Toronto, Ontario M8Z 4X6, Canada

Harcourt Brace & Company, Australia
30-52 Smidmore Street
Marrickville, NSW 2204, Australia

Harcourt Brace & Company, Japan
Ichibancho Central Building, 22–1 Ichibancho
Chiyoda-ku, Tokyo 102, Japan

W.B. SAUNDERS
An imprint of Harcourt Brace & Company Limited
© Harcourt Brace & Company Limited 1998

First published 1981
Fourth edition 1998

A catalogue record for this book is available from the British Library

ISBN 0-7020-1772-8

Typeset by Saxon Graphics Ltd, Derby, UK
Printed in Great Britain by WBC Book Manufacturers Ltd, Bridgend, UK

Contents

vi   *Contents*

Contributors

Angela Bell MD, FRCP, FRCPCH
Consultant Paediatrician, Ulster Hospital Dundonald, Belfast, Northern Ireland

Henry L Halliday MD, FRCPE, FRCP, FRCPCH
Consultant Neonatologist, Royal Maternity Hospital, and Honorary Professor, Department of Child Health, Queen's University of Belfast, Belfast, Northern Ireland

B Garth McClure MB, FRCPE, FRCPCH
Consultant Paediatrician, Royal Maternity Hospital, and Professor of Neonatal Medicine, Queen's University of Belfast, Belfast, Northern Ireland

Mark Reid, MB, FRCPG, FRCPI, FRCPCH
Consultant Paediatrician, Royal Maternity Hospital, Belfast, Northern Ireland

Carol Simpson, RGN, RM, ENB COURSE 405
Family Care Midwife, St Michael's Hospital, Bristol, England

Fiona Stewart, MA, MRCP, FRCPCH, DCH
Consultant Clinical Geneticist, Belfast City Hospital, Belfast, Northern Ireland

Richard Tubman BSc, MD, MRCP, FRCPCH
Consultant Neonatologist, Jubilee Maternity Hospital and Mater Hospital, Belfast, Northern Ireland

David Wilson, MD, MRCP (UK), FRCPCH
Senior Lecturer in Paediatric Gastroenterology and Nutrition, Department of Child Life and Health, University of Edinburgh, Scotland

Preface

In the 17 years since the first edition of this book, neonatal medicine has changed radically, and it has been clear for some time that a fourth edition is overdue. However, since the first edition the authors have become somewhat older, and certainly wiser, so the major task of revising this book has been undertaken by our two younger colleagues Dr Angela Bell and Dr Richard Tubman, with the further assistance of Dr Fiona Stewart (Chapter 1), Dr David Wilson (Chapter 11) and Carol Simpson (Nursing points).

They have made a remarkable change to the book which has been extensively reformatted, and is as up-to-date as possible. Neonatology is now based on a much more solid footing than previously. Two major advances have lead to this improvement: a better understanding of basic science (particularly fetal and neonatal physiology), and collaborative clinical trials to determine effective interventions in perinatal medicine. We would hope that in the next edition all our recommendations will be derived from evidence-based medicine.

Our thanks are due to the many medical and nursing colleagues who continue on a daily and nightly basis to provide care for sick babies. We also wish to thank the parents and the children we have looked after over many years and about whom this book has been written. Finally, we would like to thank Samantha Jamison for retaining her pleasant demeanour while typing and retyping this manuscript.

Henry L Halliday
Garth McClure
Mark Reid

Abbreviations

AChE	acetylcholinesterase
ADH	antidiuretic hormone
AFP	α-fetoprotein
AGA	appropriate for gestational age
AP	anteroposterior
APH	antepartum haemorrhage
ARDS	acute respiratory distress syndrome
ASD	atrial septal defect
BPD	bronchopulmonary dysplasia
BPP	biophysical profile
CAVH	continuous arteriovenous haemofiltration
CFTR	cystic fibrosis transmembrane receptor
CDH	congenital dislocation of the hip
CHD	congenital heart disease
CLD	chronic lung disease
CPAP	continuous positive airway pressure
CPIP	chronic pulmonary insufficiency of prematurity
CPR	cardiopulmonary resuscitation
CRP	C-reactive protein
CSF	cerebrospinal fluid
CT	computed tomography
CVB	chorionic villous biopsy
DIC	disseminated intravascular coagulation
DNA	deoxyribonucleic acid
DPPC	dipalmitoylphosphatidylcholine
EBM	expressed breast milk
ECG	electrocardiography
ECM	external cardiac massage
ECMO	extra-corporeal membrane oxygenation
ELBW	extremely low birth weight
ESR	erythrocyte sedimentation rate

ET	endotracheal tube
FAS	fetal alcohol syndrome
FHR	fetal heart rate
FiO_2	fraction of inspired oxygen concentration
FRC	functional residual capacity
G6PD	glucose 6-phosphate dehydrogenase
GBS	group B β-haemolytic streptococci
Hb	haemoglobin
HBV	hepatitis B virus
hCG	human chorionic gonadotrophin
Hct	haematocrit
HCV	hepatitis C virus
HDN	haemorrhagic disease of the newborn
HFJV	high-frequency jet ventilation
HFOV	high-frequency oscillatory ventilation
HIE	hypoxic-ischaemic encephalopathy
HIV	human immunodeficiency virus
HSV	herpes simplex virus
ICP	intracranial pressure
IDM	infant of diabetic mother
IMV	intermittent mandatory ventilation
IPPV	intermittent positive pressure ventilation
ITP	idiopathic thrombocytopenic purpura
IUFT	intrauterine fetal transfusion
IUGR	intrauterine growth retardation
IVH	intraventricular haemorrhage
IVIG	intravenous immunoglobulin
LATS	long-acting thyroid stimulator
LBW	low birth weight
LGA	large for gestational age
MAP	mean airway pressure
MAS	meconium aspiration syndrome
MCUG	micturating cystourethrogram
MRI	magnetic resonance imaging
MRSA	methicillin-resistant *Staphylococcus aureus*
MSUD	maple syrup urine disease
NEC	necrotizing enterocolitis
NICU	neonatal intensive care unit

NSE	neurone-specific enolase
NST	non-stress test
NTE	neutral thermal environment
OFC	occipitofrontal circumference
OTC	ornithine transcarbamylase
PCKD	polycystic kidney disease
PCV	packed cell volume
PDA	patent ductus arteriosus
PEEP	positive end-expiratory pressure
PG	phosphatidylglycerol
PGE	prostaglandin E
PI	phosphatidyl inositol
PIE	pulmonary interstitial emphysema
PIP	peak inspiratory pressure
PKU	phenylketonuria
PN	parenteral nutrition
PPHN	persistent pulmonary hypertension of the newborn
PTV	patient-triggered ventilation
PVL	periventricular leucomalacia
RDS	respiratory distress syndrome
ROP	retinopathy of prematurity
SGA	small for gestational age
SIDS	sudden infant death syndrome
SLE	systemic lupus erythematosus
SVT	supraventricular tachycardia
TAPVR	total anomalous pulmonary venous return
TGA	transposition of the great arteries
TPN	total parenteral nutrition
TSH	thyroid stimulating hormone
TTN	transient tachypnoea of the newborn
USS	ultrasound scan
VLBW	very low birth weight
VSD	ventricular septal defect
VUR	vesicoureteric reflux

1 Prenatal Diagnosis

Prenatal diagnosis has become an increasingly important part of obstetric care over the past 20 years with many conditions now being detected antenatally. In cases where the pregnancy is to continue, the availability of prenatal diagnosis may help in planning optimal management for infants with an abnormality. Its benefits are limited, however unless there is good communication between those involved in the care of the baby before birth and those likely to be involved after birth, such as the neonatologist, paediatric surgeon or paediatric cardiologist. It is important to remember that this can be a very stressful time for parents, and where possible they should be kept informed of plans for the baby and be given realistic opinion on the possible outcomes. In the case of a baby likely to require surgery, a meeting with the surgeon and a visit to the infant surgical unit may help prepare the parents for the events following the baby's birth.

Women undergoing prenatal diagnosis fall into two groups: those in whom it is part of their routine antenatal care and those who are at special risk of fetal abnormality and require more specialized investigations and also more support.

Pregnancies at increased risk of fetal abnormality include:

- Older maternal age
- Previous affected child
- Affected parent
- Family history of genetic disorder
- Parent(s) known carrier of gene disorder or chromosome rearrangement
- High-risk ethnic group.

Fetal anomaly scan

Although many women have an early ultrasound scan to confirm viability and gestation, it is the scan performed at 18–20 weeks that is used to look for congenital malformations. A wide range of abnormalities can be detected at this stage, such as anencephaly (Fig 1.1), spina bifida (Fig 1.2), renal agenesis and cystic hygroma. It is important to realize that some abnormalities such as congenital heart defects may be missed at this stage.

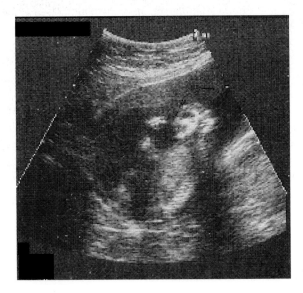

Figure 1.1. **Ultrasound scan showing anencephaly.**

Abnormalities which may be detected on fetal anomaly scan include:

- Anencephaly (Fig. 1.1)/neural tube defects, e.g. spina bifida (Fig. 1.2)
- Renal agenesis
- Polycystic kidneys
- Hydronephrosis
- Hydrocephalus

- Short limbs
- Diaphragmatic hernia
- Cystic hygroma.

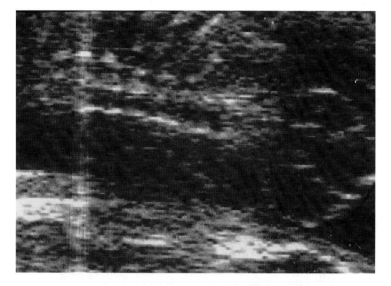

Figure 1.2. Ultrasound scan showing spina bifida. A large cystic lesion can be seen arising from the lumbar spine.

✚ Neural tube defects

Although ultrasonography will detect many cases of neural tube defect, some will be missed. For this reason many centres also offer screening with serum α-fetoprotein (AFP) at 16–18 weeks. AFP is a glycoprotein produced by the fetus which passes into the amniotic fluid and thence into the maternal circulation. Levels of AFP are significantly increased with an open neural tube defect compared to normal levels in relation to gestational age. Most laboratories give results as Multiples of the Median (MoM) and a value >2.0 MoM warrants further detailed ultrasonography and possibly amniocentesis.

Causes of raised maternal serum AFP include:

- Multiple pregnancy
- More advanced gestation
- Threatened abortion
- Open neural tube defect/anencephaly
- Abdominal wall defect
- Oesophageal/gastrointestinal atresia
- Cystic hygroma
- Congenital nephrotic syndrome (massively elevated)
- Placental abnormality, e.g. haemangioma or retroplacental clot
- Maternal factors, e.g. lupus, erythematosus, liver tumour.

In women undergoing amniocentesis, amniotic fluid AFP can be measured. If raised, the presence of an acetylcholinesterase (AChE) band on electrophoresis should alert the obstetrician to the possibility of a neural tube defect.

Down's syndrome

Traditionally, prenatal diagnosis for Down's syndrome has been offered on the basis of maternal age either by chorionic villous biopsy (CVB) or amniocentesis. An individual female's risk of having a baby with Down's syndrome increases throughout her reproductive lifetime. However, as the number of women having babies in their 40s is small compared to those in their twenties, the majority of babies with Down's syndrome are born to younger mothers. About 70% of babies with Down's syndrome have mothers aged under 35 years who usually are not offered CVB or amniocentesis.

Serum screening

Serum screening was designed to try to identify those women who are at a higher risk of having a baby with Down's syndrome than maternal age alone would suggest. It is based on the fact that on average women carrying babies with Down's syndrome have lower serum levels of AFP and oestriol and higher levels of human chorionic gonadotrophin (hCG). The test is often referred to as the triple test. A woman opting for serum screening has a sample of blood taken at 15 weeks' gestation (confirmed by ultrasonography). The three assays are performed and these results together with maternal age and gestation are used to calculate an altered risk of the baby having Down's syndrome. When the risk is <1/250 the woman is told she is at low risk of a Down's baby and no further action is usually recommended. If the result is >1/250, the mother is at high risk of having a baby with Down's syndrome and is offered an amniocentesis. The test identifies about 60% of Down's syndrome babies as 'high risk'. This compares favourably with screening on the basis of maternal age alone which will detect at best about 30% of Down's syndrome babies. However, paediatricians should be aware that there will be a number of women who, having received a low-risk result from their serum screen, go on to have a baby with Down's syndrome. If these women have not been adequately counselled about the limitations of serum screening they are often very confused and angry.

> **!** Serum screening for Down's syndrome is not 100% sensitive. Parents should be clearly counselled in this regard.

Amniocentesis

Amniocentesis is a well-established technique for determining a fetal karyotype. It may also be used in more specialized investigations. With an experienced operator it can be performed from 12 weeks' gestation onwards. Under ultrasound guidance a needle is inserted into the amniotic sac and 5–10 ml of amniotic fluid is aspirated. The amniocytes are cultured for 2–3 weeks and are then stained to obtain a fetal karyotype. Although this procedure is most commonly performed to detect Down's syndrome, other chromosome abnormalities such as Edward's syndrome, Patau's syndrome and Klinefelter's syndrome may also be detected. The risk of the procedure causing an abortion is about 1–2%. Amniocentesis may be performed much later in pregnancy when a congenital abnormality, e.g. tracheo-oesophageal fistula, is detected on scan.

Chorionic villous biopsy (CVB)

This is a newer technique than amniocentesis. It is usually performed between 10 and 12 weeks' gestation. Under ultrasound guidance a needle is passed through the mother's abdominal wall to the chorionic plate and a chorionic villous sample is removed. Short-term culture will provide a karyotype within 48 hours which should detect a trisomy. However, as the quality of the preparation may be poor, back-up conventional culture is needed to detect more subtle chromosome abnormalities. The risk of abortion is about 2–3%. Like amniocentesis, CVB may also be used for more specialized investigations.

Molecular diagnosis

Many conditions in which there is an identifiable genetic defect can be diagnosed prenatally. Examples include cystic fibrosis where there is a mutation in the CFTR gene and Duchenne muscular dystrophy in families where there is an identifiable deletion in the dystrophin gene (about 80% of cases). Fetal cells are obtained either by amniocentesis or CVB. If amniocentesis is used the amniocytes must be cultured before DNA is extracted, whereas with CVB it can be extracted almost directly. DNA analysis is then performed. This technique may also be used for rapid fetal sexing by looking for the presence of Y-chromosome material.

Conditions for which molecular prenatal diagnosis is available include:

- Cystic fibrosis
- Duchenne muscular dystrophy
- Becker muscular dystrophy
- Spinal muscular atrophy

- Huntington's disease
- Fragile X syndrome
- Myotonic dystrophy

Inborn errors of metabolism

Metabolic disorders for which prenatal diagnosis is now available

- Hurler's syndrome
- Hunter's syndrome
- San Filippo's syndrome
- I-Cell disease
- Tay-Sachs disease
- Metachromatic leucodystrophy
- Cystinosis.

It is vital to make sure that there is a confirmed biochemical diagnosis in the suspected index case. Many of the assays are only carried out in certain specialized laboratories and so a certain amount of forward planning may be required. The majority of enzyme assays can be performed either on samples obtained by CVB or by amniocentesis. Some disorders such as ornithine transcarbamylase deficiency (OTCD) require a fetal liver biopsy — a highly specialized invasive technique only performed in a few fetal medicine units.

All prenatal diagnosis is vulnerable to error. Therefore, even if a fetus is felt to be unaffected prenatally it is vital that confirmatory enzyme studies are performed after birth.

Other techniques

Cordocentesis

A needle is inserted transabdominally into the umbilical cord and a sample of fetal blood is obtained. As this is a more specialized technique with greater risk to the fetus than amniocentesis or CVB, it is usually reserved for later in pregnancy when a more rapid result is required.

Fetoscopy

An invasive technique used when prenatal diagnosis requires direct visualization of the fetus or if a skin biopsy is required, e.g. epidermolysis bullosa. The indications for this procedure have declined with improvements in ultrasonography and advances in molecular genetics.

Fetal liver biopsy

A very specialized procedure required for the diagnosis of a very few metabolic disorders.

Chromosome abnormalities

The trisomy syndromes are the commonest (Table 1.1). Incidence tends to increase logarithmically with maternal age after 37 years (Table 1.2). Other chromosomal abnormalities include cri du chat syndrome and sex chromosome abnormali-

Table 1.1. Trisomy syndromes

	Down's	Edward's	Patau's
Trisomy:	21	18	13
Incidence:	1/600	1/2000	1/5000
Features:	Flat head, epicanthic folds, Brushfield's spots, low-set ears, small nose, prominent fissured tongue, broad short neck, simian crease, clinodactyly, ventricular septal defect (VSD) or endocardial cushion defects	Long narrow head, extended neck, short palpebral fissures, micrognathia, flexed overlapping fingers, rocker bottom feet, renal anomalies, VSD, atrial septal defect (ASD)	Holoprosencephaly, micro-ophthalmia, low-set ears, bilateral cleft lip and palate, flexed overlapping fingers, omphalocele, renal anomalies, VSD, persistent ductus arteriosus, dextrocardia

Table 1.2. Incidence of Down's syndrome by maternal age

Maternal age (years)	Incidence
20	1/1200
25	1/1100
30	1/1000
35	1/400
40	1/100
45	1/40

ties such as Turner's or Klinefelter's syndrome. More sophisticated methods of chromosome analysis, e.g. banding, have led to minor abnormalities being identified as the explanation for babies with abnormal facial features.

Nursing points

Baby

- The place of delivery should be carefully chosen to ensure the needs of the baby can be met. *In utero* transfer is advised whenever possible.

Family

- Before undertaking any tests, the parents should be fully informed of the possible outcomes and options available to them.
- In the event of an abnormality being detected, counselling should be offered. The parents are likely to experience feelings of grief and bereavement. Siblings, grandparents and members of the extended family may also need support.
- The opportunity to visit the neonatal intensive care unit (NICU) should be offered to parents before the birth. They may benefit from more than one visit.
- Parents should be introduced to the staff and given the opportunity to discuss the treatment their baby may need. This should include immediate care at birth and subsequent treatment on the NICU.
- Contact numbers for local and national support groups should be offered. An introduction to the parents of a baby with a similar condition may be of benefit after a few weeks.

Equipment

- Parents should be shown some of the equipment which will be used to care for their baby and a typical room in the NICU.
- A brief explanation of the equipment should be given, but care must be taken not to frighten or overload the family with information.

Staff

- Neonatal staff should liaise with obstetricians to ensure that adequate cots, staff and equipment are available for the baby at the time of delivery.

References and further reading

Bonthron D, FitzPatrick D, Porteous M, Trainer A (1998). *Clinical Genetics: A Case Based Approach.* Edinburgh: WB Saunders.

Cleary MA, Wraith JE (1991). Antenatal diagnosis of inborn errors of metabolism. *Arch Dis Child* **66**: 816.

Harper PS (1993). *Practical Genetic Counselling*, 4th edn. London: Butterworth Heinemann.

Kingston HM (1997). *ABC of Clinical Genetics*, 2nd edn. London: BMJ Publishing Group.

Whittle MJ, Connor JH (eds) (1995). *Prenatal Diagnosis in Obstetric Practice*, 2nd edn. London: Blackwell Scientific Publications.

2 Examination of the Normal Newborn

All newborn babies should be examined before discharge from hospital. A first examination is carried out soon after birth to assess adaptation to normal extrauterine life, and to exclude major malformations requiring urgent surgical correction.

A second complete examination is performed at 2–5 days of age as a screening procedure to look for congenital abnormalities, to ensure feeding is established and to reassure the parents. The timing of this examination, which remains controversial, varies between units because of the trend of earlier discharge of mothers and infants from hospital.

Delivery room examination

This examination should be performed shortly after birth by the midwife, obstetrician or paediatrician. A note should be made of any relevant history and the Apgar scores. It is useful if examination findings are recorded on a set proforma (e.g. Fig. 2.1). Normal findings may simply be indicated by a tick but any abnormalities should be clearly described with plans for management.

The baby should also be measured: birth weight in grams, and crown–heel length and occipitofrontal circumference (OFC) in centimetres. These measurements should be plotted on appropriate percentile charts (see Appendix VIII).

Second complete examination

This examination should be performed by a suitably trained doctor in the presence of the mother to allow discussion of the baby's progress. Findings and plans should be recorded on a proforma as before.

POSTURE	HEART RATE		....
COLOUR including cyanosis jaundice, pallor	MURMUR YES/NO		....
SKIN	FEMORAL PULSES		....
NUTRITION Subcut Tissue	UMBILICUS including 2 arts.		....
OEDEMA	ABDOMEN including liver, spleen, kidneys		....
SKULL including sutures fontanelle	GENITALIA		
FACIES	ANUS		
EARS	SPINE		DESCRIPTION OF ABNORMALITIES
EYES	ARMS/HANDS including palmar creases		
NOSE/NASAL AIRWAY	HIPS		
MOUTH/PALATE	LEGS/FEET		
NECK including clavicles	BEHAVIOUR/ACTIVITY		
CHEST	MUSCLE TONE		
RESPIRATION Rate/min.	MOVEMENTS		
AIR ENTRY	CRY		
	REFLEXES specify		

CONCLUSION   NORMAL = ✓   ABNORMAL = ✗   NOT EXAMINED = O

NORMAL HEALTHY INFANT

MOTHER SEEN AFTER EXAMINATION   If not specify

Examined by Dr.
Status:
Date .... Time ....

Figure 2.1. **Example of a proforma for neonatal examination.**

Order of examination depends on the baby and taking advantage of the opportunity to examine the heart, for example, whenever the baby is in a quiet state.

Skin

Look for:
≺ Pallor
≺ Jaundice
≺ Cyanosis
≺ Rash and abnormal skin lesions.

Heart and lungs

➤ Record heart rate and respiration rate. Normal heart rate should be between 110 and 160 beats/minute and respiration rate <50 breaths/min.

➤ Listen for murmurs, accentuated second pulmonary heart sound, splitting of the second heart sound or crepitations.

➤ Cardiac murmurs persisting beyond 48 hours of age require investigation.

➤ Check for presence of femoral pulses which are best felt by partially abducting the thigh and placing the finger halfway between the pubic tubercle and the anterior superior iliac spine.

Head and face

➤ Measure occipitofrontal circumference, check size and tension of anterior fontanelle and palpate suture lines.

➤ Examine the eyes for conjunctivitis, cataracts, aniridia and coloboma. Use an ophthalmoscope to look for a retinal red reflex.

➤ Look at the ears for accessory auricles, malformation or low-set position.

➤ Check the mouth for the presence of cleft palate, neonatal teeth and oral thrush.

Abdomen

➤ Palpate for hepatosplenomegaly, abdominal distension, renal masses or imperforate anus.

➤ Check the umbilical stump for signs of infection, single umbilical artery (see p. 319) or small omphalocele.

External genitalia

➤ In the female, look for enlargement of the clitoris or increased pigmentation.

➤ In the male, look for hypospadias, undescended testes and hydrocele.

Limbs

➤ Check for dislocation of the hips using Ortolani–Barlow manoeuvre. With the baby lying on his back, adduct and flex the hips. The examiner's hands should be placed with the thumbs inside the thighs opposite the lesser trochanters and the tips of the middle fingers over the greater trochanters. A gentle attempt is made to push each femoral head backwards and forwards into or out of the acetabulum testing for a *dislocatable hip*. The flexed hips should then be abducted and a *dislocated hip* can be diagnosed if there is a definite movement of the femoral head into the acetabulum, often referred to as a 'clunk'.

➤ If abduction is limited, the hip may be abnormal and further investigation with ultrasound is indicated. Ultrasound screening of high-risk groups may be justified.

➤ If in doubt refer to a consultant paediatrician or orthopaedic surgeon.

➤ Examine for deformities of the feet such as talipes equinovarus or metatarsus adductus. Look for extra digits.

Risk of congenital dislocation of the hip (CDH) is increased if:

- Breech presentation
- Oligohydramnios
- Positive family history
- Female
- Small for gestational age (SGA)
- Other abnormalities, e.g. spina bifida
- Italian.

Back

Look for:

◄ Clues to spina bifida occulta such as midline swelling, dimple, hairy patches.
◄ Dermal sinus.

CNS

➤ Influenced by sleep state. Try to observe in quiet, awake state. Abnormal postures include neck retraction, frog-like posture, hyperextension or hyperflexion of limbs, and asymmetry.

➤ Check muscle tone for increase or decrease and asymmetry.

➤ Check tendon reflexes for absence, exaggeration or asymmetry.

➤ Look for abnormal involuntary movements, e.g. jitteriness, seizures or asymmetry.

➤ Listen for a high-pitched, weak or unusual cry.

➤ Check primitive reflexes (Moro or startle, sucking, rooting and tonic neck).

➤ Assess visual fixation and reaction to sound.

Blood screening

At 5–7 days capillary blood is taken to screen for phenylketonuria, homocystinuria, congenital hypothyroidism and other inborn errors of metabolism (see also Ch. 20). Some units screen routinely for other conditions such as cystic fibrosis and galactosaemia. The baby should be on full milk feeds at the time of the screening test.

Vitamin K prophylaxis

Until recently 0.5–1 mg of vitamin K was given intramuscularly or orally to all newborns or to selected high-risk groups (preterm and breast-fed babies primarily). A controversial case-control study implied a two-fold increase in the risk of childhood cancer in babies given intramuscular rather than oral or no vitamin K. Other studies have not confirmed this finding. In the UK there remains uncertainty about the best policy. Vitamin K prophylaxis should be given either intramuscularly or orally at birth depending on the mother's wishes. If administered orally, breast-fed babies must be given further doses to protect against late-onset vitamin K deficiency bleeding. The American Academy of Pediatrics continues to recommend that 0.5–1.0 mg intramuscular vitamin K should be administered to all newborn babies.

Nursing points

Baby

- The baby should be given to the parents as soon as possible following delivery. Early contact is a very important factor in the development of their future relationship.
- Many mothers enjoy a period of skin-to-skin contact with their baby following delivery. To reduce heat losses, dry and wrap the baby as soon as possible and cover the mother and baby.
- The midwife's examination of the baby will include recording:
    - Temperature
    - Respiration rate
    - Heart rate
    - Weight
    - Occipitofrontal head circumference
    - Apgar scores
    - Whether the baby has passed urine and meconium
    - Any birth marks
    - Any birth injuries, facial congestion, fetal scalp electrode or blood sampling sites
    - Any abnormalities
    - Security of cord clamp or ligatures.
- Accurate recording of the baby's condition and behaviour following birth are important as baseline observations, particularly in the event of any deterioration occurring, e.g. respiratory distress syndrome.
- The baby should be offered a feed within the first hour of delivery. This is particularly important in preterm and SGA babies who have low energy reserves. It also assists with establishing breast feeding.
- Vitamin K should be given by the appropriate route and recorded in the notes.

Family

- The parents should be given time alone with their baby following delivery.

- The parents' informed consent must be sought before giving vitamin K. The advised route of administration should also be discussed.

Equipment

- Ensure the cord clamp or ligature is securely fastened.
- Two namebands, checked by the parents or two members of staff, must be securely attached to the baby's limbs before he leaves the delivery room.
- Warm clothes and blankets should be available for the newborn baby. The temperature of the incubator must be within the appropriate range for the size and gestation of the baby.

Staff

- To help establish successful breast feeding the midwives and neonatal nurses must give adequate time, assistance and support to the mother during early feeds. All new staff should receive training about breast feeding to ensure consistency and adequate support is given to parents.

References and further reading

American Academy of Pediatrics: Vitamin K Ad Hoc Task Force (1993). Controversies concerning vitamin K and the newborn. *Pediatrics* **91**: 1001.

Cartilidge PHT (1992). Routine examination of babies — is it necessary? *Arch Dis Child* **67**: 1421–2.

Zipursky A (editorial) (1996). Vitamin K at birth. *Br Med J* **313**: 179.

3 High-Risk Pregnancy

A high-risk pregnancy is one that is complicated by maternal illness, obstetric or fetal disorder or drug therapy. In such circumstances it is imperative that the condition is identified as early in pregnancy as possible so that fetal growth and well-being may be monitored, a full discussion between all concerned may take place, the delivery may be planned and a skilled obstetrician and paediatrician are present at delivery. Full co-operation and communication between all health professionals concerned is mandatory in these cases.

Causes of a high-risk pregnancy include:

Maternal:
- Age: elderly primigravida (>35 years) or <17 years
- Hypertension and pre-eclampsia
- Diabetes mellitus
- Rhesus isoimmunization
- Drug therapy: steroids, β-adrenergic drugs, excessive narcotics, magnesium sulphate
- Maternal infection: rubella, herpes simplex, syphilis, HIV or chorioamnionitis
- Previous birth of a child with a hereditary disease, respiratory disorder or neonatal death
- Maternal illness (see p. 24).

Labour and delivery:
- Antepartum or intrapartum haemorrhage
- Prolonged rupture of membranes (>24 hours)
- Forceps or vacuum delivery for fetal distress
- Abnormal presentation (breech, brow, face or transverse)
- Emergency caesarean section
- Prolapsed cord

- Maternal hypotension (especially epidural or bleeding)
- Fetal distress: abnormal fetal heart rate, scalp pH <7.25, meconium staining

Fetal:
- Multiple births
- Premature delivery (<37 weeks) or post-term (>42 weeks)
- Growth retardation
- Immature lecithin/sphingomyelin ratio (L/S <2, absent phosphatidylglycerol)
- Polyhydramnios (oesophageal atresia, etc.)
- Oligohydramnios (Potter's syndrome of renal agenesis)
- Other fetal malformations.

Assessment of fetal wellbeing

Various methods are used in the antepartum and intrapartum period to assess the wellbeing of the fetus.

Antepartum assessment

Main indication is increased risk of uteroplacental insufficiency. The most commonly used tests are the non-stress test (NST) and biophysical profile (BPP). Use of the contraction stress test has decreased in popularity.

The *non-stress test* is based on the assumption that the heart rate of a normal healthy fetus will accelerate temporarily with fetal movement. Continuous fetal heart rate monitoring is performed and the trace observed for accelerations of at least 15 beats/min and lasting 15 s. Loss of reactivity may reflect metabolic consequences of hypoxaemia.

Biophysical profile assesses the fetus in a resting state with the following observations:

≺ NST
≺ Fetal breathing movements
≺ Fetal movements (3 or more body or limb movements in 30 mins)

≺ Fetal tone (observe episodes of extension with return to flexion)
≺ Quantification of amniotic fluid volume.

The NST acts as a screening test in most units and if the trace is non-reactive it is followed by BPP.

Intrapartum assessment

Monitoring of fetal wellbeing during labour is performed using the following methods:

Assessment of amniotic fluid
Fetal heart rate monitoring: intermittent auscultation, continuous electronic monitoring
Fetal blood sampling

Amniotic fluid assessment

Assessment of volume and colour of amniotic fluid is important in the management of labour. The presence of a reduced volume of amniotic fluid is associated with an increased incidence of fetal heart decelerations and thus a greater chance of fetal distress being diagnosed. Passage of meconium into the amniotic fluid during labour is a traditional marker of fetal distress. Passage of meconium before 34 weeks' gestation is unusual but may occur if the fetus is infected (see p. 164). Many labours with meconium present will have a normal outcome. Presence of meconium, however, is an indication for further assessment of the fetus using fetal heart rate monitoring.

Fetal heart rate (FHR) monitoring

Intermittent auscultation with a fetal stethoscope is considered adequate in low-risk pregnancies. If bradycardia (<120/min) or tachycardia (>160/min) is noted, then continuous monitoring should be employed.

The cardiotacogram (CTG) is composed of a continuous recording of FHR and uterine contraction activity.

The FHR is decribed by:

≺ baseline heart rate: normal 120–160/min

≺ Variability
≺ Decelerations: early, late, variable, prolonged.

Lack of acceleration, frequent and prolonged deceleration and prolonged bradycardia are all associated with a fall in pH.

 Staff attending mothers in the delivery suite should be proficient in interpreting FHR traces.

If FHR pattern is abnormal, scalp pH should be measured to assess the degree of acidosis.

Fetal scalp pH measurement

Can be difficult to perform but is an invaluable method of assessing fetal acidosis. Not to be regarded as a definitive test as babies (particularly SGA) have been found to suffer from hypoxaemia in the presence of a normal pH.

 Any unit which performs continuous FHR should have the facility to perform fetal scalp pH measurement.

Preterm labour

Defined as onset of labour after 20 and before 37 completed weeks of pregnancy. Diagnosed by assessment of regular uterine contractions accompanied by dilatation of the cervix. The aetiology of some preterm labours is known but in most cases a specific cause is not found.

Factors involved in aetiology of preterm labour include:

- Cervical incompetence
- Uterine malformations
- Infection (e.g. chorioamnionitis)
- Antepartum haemorrhage
- Multiple pregnancy
- Polyhydramnios
- Intrauterine growth retardation (IUGR)

- Hypertension
- Diabetes
- Associated factors: low socio-economic status, smoking, maternal undernutrition.

Management

➤ Confirm diagnosis by careful cervical assessment to establish cervical effacement and dilatation. Absence of fetal breathing occurs during the second stage of labour and may be useful in diagnosis.

➤ Establish presence or absence of premature rupture of the membranes and test for an infective aetiology — vaginal, cervical and urine culture.

➤ Confirm dates from early ultrasound scan and maternal history.

➤ Ultrasound estimation of fetal size, presentation and fetal breathing.

➤ Tocolytic agents, e.g. β-sympathomimetics such as ritodrine, should be considered. May be used to suppress uterine contractions for 48–72 hours to allow administration of corticosteroids and plan appropriate delivery. Long-term treatment does not improve neonatal outcome. Side effects include maternal tachycardia, flushing and hyperglycaemia.

➤ Corticosteroids are recommended from 24–34 weeks' gestation to enhance lung maturation. Steroids may also be effective outside this range of gestational age and are currently being studied. Recommended course is betamethasone 12 mg 12 hourly for 48 hours, often repeated weekly. There are few contraindications.

➤ Counsel parents on expected plans and outcome.

➤ Mode of delivery varies with presentation and gestational age. At <26 weeks most would advise vaginal delivery with expert assessment of the baby after birth. Between 26 and 32 weeks' gestation with vertex presentation there is no advantage of elective caesarean unless there are other indications such as fetal distress. However, if there is breech presentation, mode of delivery is controversial. There is a major risk of trauma to the baby whether delivery is by vaginal route or by caesarean, although many advocate elective caesarean. After 32 weeks management is as for a term delivery.

Prolonged premature rupture of membranes (>24 hours)

Obstetric management

Depends on:
≺ Gestational age
≺ Evidence of infection.

In an immature fetus (<34 weeks' gestation) it is best not to induce labour unless there are signs of infection. Corticosteroids are indicated provided there are no signs of infection. Conservative management at term is also considered superior.

Neonatal management

➤ Admit baby to the neonatal unit if preterm, needs resuscitation, shows signs of early respiratory distress or sepsis.

➤ If the baby is well and of normal gestation at birth he may be transferred to the postnatal ward.

➤ If a stable preterm baby is born, screen for infection and observe.

➤ If the baby is ill, a full sepsis screen should be performed including lumbar puncture and antibiotics commenced intravenously. Recommended doses are given in Appendix II.

Multiple pregnancy

The incidence of higher multiple births (i.e. triplets and above) is increasing due to an increase in fertility treatment. Multiple pregnancies are the commonest reason for the birth of babies at high risk and account for about 5% of all high-risk pregnancies.

Problems which may be encountered are:

Malpresentation

Preterm labour

Growth retardation

Risk of fetal abnormality

Twin-to-twin transfusion

Need for resuscitation — additional assistance will be required.

Maternal illnesses

Maternal conditions that can complicate pregnancy include:

- Diabetes mellitus
- Thyrotoxicosis
- Phenylketonuria
- Idiopathic thrombocytopenic purpura
- Systemic lupus erythematosus
- Myasthenia gravis, myotonic dystrophy
- Substance abuse
- Haemoglobinopathies, sickle cell anaemia
- Other endocrine disorders: Cushing's, Addison's, Simmond's, hyperparathyroidism, adrenal hyperplasia
- Cardiac disease: congenital, ischaemic, rheumatic
- Malignant disease
- Epilepsy
- Renal failure
- Psychiatric illness
- Open tuberculosis
- Other: ulcerative colitis

✚ *Diabetes mellitus*

Good maternal control in pregnancy reduces fetal hyperinsuli-naemia and risk of neonatal macrosomia and hypoglycaemia.

Good control is indicated by maternal postprandial blood glucose <7 mmol/l or fasting <5 mmol/l. Long-term (6–8 weeks) diabetic control may be assessed by glycosylated haemoglobin (HbA1c) <7%.

Good pre-pregnancy control lowers congenital malformation rates:
   HbA1 >10% at booking — 24% major malformations
   HbA1 <8% at booking — 3% major malformations

Indications for admission of the infant of a diabetic mother (IDM) to the neonatal unit:

≺ Preterm — gestational age <36 weeks
≺ Obvious congenital abnormality, e.g. cardiac, central nervous system or skeletal
≺ Respiratory distress persisting >1 hour
≺ Cyanosis in room air
≺ Hypoglycaemia persisting after first feed (<1.5 mmol/l — see below)
≺ Severe asphyxia (Apgar score <5 at 5 min) or traumatic delivery
≺ Subsequent problems developing on postnatal ward, e.g. hypoglycaemia, hypocalcaemia, severe jaundice.

Most IDMs can be admitted to postnatal wards with their mothers. Asymptomatic hypoglycaemia occurs in 50% of babies but doubt exists as to whether it is harmful. Hypoglycaemia occurs early (Fig. 3.1) so check glucose strip at birth and at 30 min (see pp. 194–196). Babies on the postnatal wards should be fed early, beginning within the first hour and 3 hourly thereafter until blood glucose levels are stable (Fig. 3.1). Blood glucose should be checked with reagent strips at birth, every half hour for the first 2 hours and then 3 hourly for 24–48 hours. Levels <2.6 mmol/l indicate hypoglycaemia and necessitate an immediate feed and recheck within an hour. If blood glucose falls <2.6 mmol/l a blood sample should be sent to laboratory for confirmation and the paediatrician informed. Persistent levels <2.6 mmol/l or the development of symptoms warrant intravenous fluids (see p. 197).

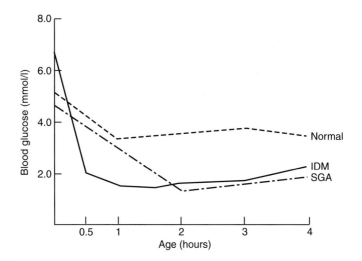

Figure 3.1. Changes in blood sugar after birth in three groups of infants: normal, infants of diabetic mothers (IDM) and small for gestational age (SGA) infants.

Other problems of IDM include:

Birth complications: asphyxia, shoulder dystocia

Increased incidence of respiratory distress syndrome (RDS)

Congenital malformations:

Renal — agenesis, cystic, duplex

CNS — neural tube defect, hydrocephalus, holoprosencephaly

Heart — truncus, transposition, Fallot's, VSD

Skeletal — sacral dysgenesis

Transient tachypnoea of the newborn

Increased jaundice and hypocalcaemia

Polycythaemia

Hypertrophic cardiomyopathy

Other: renal vein thrombosis, small left colon

 Any IDM with heart failure should have an echocardiogram performed before any treatment is started to distinguish a cardiac malformation from hypertrophic cardiomyopathy as the latter should not be treated with digoxin.

➕ *Thyrotoxicosis*

The long-acting thyroid stimulator (LATS), an IgG antibody, crosses the placenta and may cause temporary neonatal thyrotoxicosis. Arises in mothers who have Graves' disease or have been treated for it in the past.

This presents with:

➢ Tachycardia, congestive heart failure
➢ Weight loss
➢ Hyperthermia
➢ Goitre, exophthalmos
➢ Jitteriness, seizures
➢ Diarrhoea, vomiting.

Onset of symptoms may be delayed because of the effects of maternal antithyroid drugs on the fetus.

Measure LATS, T4 and TSH in cord blood and observe baby closely.

Management

➤ Treatment of symptoms:
    β-Blocker, e.g. propranolol 2 mg/kg/day, 8 hourly
    Digoxin and diuretics for heart failure
➤ Anti-thyroid preparations:
    Carbimazole 0.5–1 mg/kg/day, 8 hourly
    Potassium iodide, 10%, 8 mg/kg/day, 8 hourly

LATS half-life about 6 weeks and therapy not usually needed beyond this. No long-term effects on infant but developmental follow-up needed.

➕ *Phenylketonuria (PKU)*

Fetal damage occurs if maternal PKU is not controlled by diet. Common effects are:
    Abortion
    Microcephaly

Mental retardation
Congenital heart disease
Intrauterine growth retardation

Women with PKU should start a strict low phenylalanine diet before conception aiming for blood levels of 60–180 μmol/l.

Idiopathic thrombocytopenic purpura (ITP)

This is an uncommon but important condition. Mothers with ITP or systemic lupus erythematosus (SLE) may have IgG antiplatelet antibodies which cross to the fetus and result in thrombocytopenia in approx. 50% of cases. The severity of thrombocytopenia in newborn is usually proportional to that of the mother at time of delivery, but mothers previously treated by splenectomy may have normal platelet counts but give birth to affected infants.

Petechiae and bruising are common; bleeding may occur from umbilicus, nose, gastrointestinal and genitourinary tracts, injection sites or into the brain. Risk of haemorrhage is maximal in the first 3 days after birth or when platelet count is below $20\,000/mm^3$.

Management

➤ Platelet transfusions have short-lived benefit if severe bleeding occurs.

➤ Steroids (prednisolone 2 mg/kg) may protect against severe haemorrhage even though platelet count does not increase.

➤ Infusion of immunoglobulins (1 g/kg) increases platelet count by acting as a blocking antibody.

The neonatal illness is self-limiting and platelet count becomes normal by 6 weeks; discharge from hospital if platelet count is $>50\,000/mm^3$.

For other causes of neonatal thrombocytopenia see p. 355.

> **!** Differentiate autoimmune from alloimmune thrombocytopenia which has a worse prognosis (see p. 355).

✚ *Systemic lupus erythematosus (SLE)*

Associated with an increased risk of abortion, stillbirth and preterm delivery, especially if renal involvement is present. The baby may also show complications of maternal drug therapy or thrombocytopenia, anaemia, leucopenia, and skin rashes, especially of the face. Endocardial fibroelastosis and heart block can occur.

The baby rarely develops SLE but may have LE cells transiently. Usually no treatment is needed.

✚ *Myasthenia gravis*

One-quarter of babies may be affected with temporary myasthenia. May present with respiratory difficulty, feeding problems and hypotonia which may have delayed onset.

Symptoms are relieved by test dose of edrophonium (Tensilon) 1 mg intramuscularly. Maintenance with neostigmine 1–5 mg orally with feeds.

✚ *Myotonic dystrophy*

Babies of affected mothers may be stillborn, premature or suffer severe birth asphyxia or respiratory failure. Affected babies may have hypotonia and a myopathic facies but do not show myotonia.

Long-term outcome is variable with some babies improving while others have developmental delay or remain ventilator-dependent. On occasions the neonatal illness precedes the diagnosis of the mother.

✚ *Drug addiction*

Drug addiction is widespread in most Western countries, particularly in the major cities. In the USA, crack cocaine is now the major drug problem and is very common among inner-city residents.

Heroin addiction is associated with repeated maternal infections (including septicaemia, hepatitis and AIDS), fatal over-doses, poor attendances at antenatal clinics and poor nutrition.

Complications include:
Pre-eclampsia
Preterm delivery
IUGR

Cocaine use may lead to prematurity, IUGR, microcephaly. It also causes destructive lesions in the brain of the fetus due to cerebral infarction secondary to vasospasm.

Early neonatal withdrawal symptoms (24–48 h after birth) are:

◄ Tremors
◄ High pitched cry
◄ Regurgitation of feeds
◄ Irritability
◄ Sneezing
◄ Increased tone
◄ Loose stools
◄ Sweating
◄ Tachypnoea

Late withdrawal symptoms are:

◄ Vomiting
◄ Diarrhoea
◄ Dehydration
◄ Circulatory collapse
◄ Seizures.

Management

➤ Serology for syphilis, serum hepatitis and HIV (after consent) should be performed in the neonate.

➤ Treatment of drug withdrawal depends on symptoms:

Irritability:

chlorpromazine 1.5–3 mg/kg/day

> chloral hydrate (sedation) 50 mg/kg/day
>
> swaddling may be helpful

Vomiting:

> Chlorpromazine 1.5–3 mg/kg/day

Seizures:

> Phenobarbitone (anti-convulsant) 5–8 mg/kg/day

Chlorpromazine is particulary useful as acts as a sedative and an anti-emetic. Seizures should be treated as in Ch. 16. May require treatment for several weeks.

➤ Detailed assessment of the social circumstances should be performed prior to discharge of the baby.

Naloxone may precipitate an acute withdrawal reaction when resuscitating a baby of an opiate-dependent mother and should not be used in such situations.

> **!** Breast feeding is contraindicated as variable drug levels in breast milk may lead to unpredictable withdrawal effects in the baby (Table 3.1 and p. 182), and there may be a risk of transmission of HIV.

Alcohol addiction

Incidence of fetal alcohol syndrome (FAS) is about 1:750 births and 40% of mothers who drink heavily give birth to babies with FAS. Some risk occurs with 2 units/day but substantial risk with 5 or more units/day.

Characteristic features of FAS are:
- Growth retardation – prenatal and postnatal
- Hirsutism
- Microcephaly
- Eye abnormalities
- Elongated upper lip, absent philtrum
- Developmental delay, lowered intelligence
- Congenital heart lesions
- Rarely, renal anomalies.

Babies born to alcoholic mothers may also develop similar withdrawal symptoms to those born to drug-dependent mothers (fetal alcohol effects) and may need sedation.

Table 3.1. **Drugs affecting the fetus and newborn**

Drug	Effect
Alcohol	Fetal alcohol syndrome. Withdrawal: seizures, hyperactivity
Aminoglycosides	Ototoxic, nephrotoxic
'Aminopterin'	Abortion, skeletal abnormalities
Amphetamines	Generalized arteritis, developmental delay
Androgens	Virilization
	? Congenital anomalies
Aspirin	Platelet dysfunction, risk of kernicterus, prostaglandin inhibition
Azathioprine	Reduced immunocompetence
Barbiturates	Multiple abnormalities, withdrawal, haemorrhage
Cannabis	Chromosome breakage, skeletal anomalies
Carbamazepine	Neural tube defects
Cigarettes	Stillbirth, reduced birth weight and head growth, ? hyperactivity, ? heart defects (PDA)
Chlorpropamide	Fetal death, prolonged hypoglycaemia
Cocaine	IUGR, CNS anomalies
Corticosteroids	? Teratogenic
Cytotoxic drugs	Multiple abnormalities
Danazol	Virilization
Dicoumarol	Fetal death, haemorrhage, abnormal facies, retardation
Diazepam	Hypotonia, hypothermia, apnoea. Withdrawal: irritability, ? cleft lip and palate
Diazoxide	Hyperglycaemia, ? diabetes, genital anomalies, hypertrichosis
Diethylstilboestrol	Vaginal carcinoma and adenosis Genital anomalies in male infants
Glutethimide	SGA, irritability, hyperthermia, diarrhoea
Hydralazine	? Cleft palate
Indomethacin	Prolonged labour, premature ductus closure, pulmonary hypertension
Iodine	Goitre, altered thyroid function

Drug	Effect
Isoniazid	Pyridoxine deficiency
Isotretinoin	Abortion, multiple anomalies
Lithium	Respiratory distress, lethargy, congenital heart disease, goitre
Lysergic acid diethylamide (LSD)	Probably teratogenic
Magnesium sulphate	Respiratory depression, hypotonia, seizures
Narcotics (morphine, methadone, heroin, codeine, pentazocine)	Apnoea, hypothermia, withdrawal
Nitrofurantoin	Haemolysis
Oestrogens	Later vaginal adenosis and adenocarcinoma, uterine abnormalities in females; hypospadias, possible subfertility in males
Oxytocin	Increased bilirubin, hyponatraemia
Paradione	Fetal death and multiple abnormalities
Paraldehyde	Apnoea, cerebral and respiratory depression
Phenobarbitone	? Teratogenic, haemorrhagic disease
Phenothiazines	Apnoea, hypotonia or hyperactivity, withdrawal, extrapyramidal signs, ? chromosome breakage
Phenytoin	Cleft lip and palate, congenital heart disease, skeletal anomalies, haemorrhage, ? retardation
Primidone	Teratogenic
Progestogens	Virilization
Propranolol	Prolonged labour, bradycardia, hypoglycaemia, respiratory depression
Pyrimethamine	Do not combine with sulpha drugs or dapsone
Quinidine	Fetal death, thrombocytopenia, retinal haemorrhage
Quinine	CNS and skeletal anomalies, thrombocytopenia, deafness, small optic nerve
Radioiodine	Hypothyroidism
Reserpine	Nasal stuffiness, bradycardia, hypothermia
Retinoids	*see* isotretinoin
Ritodrine	Fetal tachycardia, hyperglycaemia

continued overleaf

Table 3.1. (continued)

Drug	Effect
Salicylates	Fetal death, haemorrhage, prolonged labour, premature ductus closure, pulmonary hypertension
Scopolamine	Apnoea at birth especially in preterm
Steroids	SGA, adrenal and immunosuppression, surfactant induction, DNA reduction
Streptomycin	Deafness
Sulphonamides	Kernicterus, thrombocytopenia
Tetracyclines	Multiple anomalies, bone and teeth
Thalidomide	Phocomelia, heart defects, gut defects
Thiazides	Thrombocytopenia, hypokalaemia, haemolysis
Tridione	As for Paradione
Tolbutamide	Thrombocytopenia, prolonged hypoglycaemia
Vaccines	Avoid live viral and attenuated bacterial vaccines, i.e. BCG, measles, mumps, Sabin polio, rubella, smallpox, yellow fever
Valproate	? Multiple anomalies, neural tube defects
Vitamin A (in excess)	Raised intracranial pressure, dry skin, hair loss, brittle bone, irritability
Vitamin K (water soluble)	Jaundice
Vitamin B_6 (pyridoxine)	Withdrawal seizures
Vitamin D (in excess)	Hypercalcaemia, may cause syndrome of elfin facies, aortic stenosis, retardation
Warfarin	Haemorrhage, nasal hypoplasia, stippled epiphyses, CNS defects, microcephaly

✚ *Epilepsy*

The risk of fetal anomalies is increased to approx. 1 in 10 in mothers with epilepsy and may be higher if multiple therapy is used.

Anomalies have been reported with most available anticonvulsants (Table 3.1). The commonest are cleft lip and heart defects but neural tube defects can also occur.

Babies are at greater risk of haemorrhagic disease of the newborn.

Management

➤ Pre-pregnancy counselling should be arranged in case anti-convulsants can be discontinued.

➤ AFP levels should be measured at 18 weeks and careful ultrasound scan performed.

➤ Vitamin K_1 supplements should be given in the week before delivery to increase fetal levels.

➤ Vitamin K_1 should also be given to the baby after birth.

Breast feeding is generally not contraindicated.

Nursing points

Baby

● A neonatal nurse should be present at delivery to assist the paediatrician. Ideally this should be someone who will be involved in the subsequent care of the baby.

● Vitamin K should be administered, with the parents' informed consent, via the appropriate route following delivery.

● Anticipation of potential problems, depending on the maternal condition, may help early recognition and treatment of symptoms. Note any drugs taken by the mother, particularly in late pregnancy or labour.

Family

● Some preparation of the parents is possible antenatally by:

➤ Explaining events at delivery, e.g. the baby may be resuscitated or intubated immediately, the number of people likely to be present

➤ Showing them around NICU

➤ Introducing them to NICU staff

➤ Discussing the potential problems and treatment of their baby

➤ Explaining some of the equipment on the NICU.

Equipment

● Resuscitation equipment must be checked prior to delivery. This includes the resuscitaire, heater, transport incubator and its ventilator, and emergency drugs.

- On admission to the NICU, photographs of the baby should be taken for the parents, preferably with as little equipment visible as possible.

Staff

- Neonatal staff should be involved in all antenatal meetings to plan the care of high-risk mothers and their babies.

References and further reading

American Academy of Pediatrics: Committee on Substance Abuse and Committee on Children with Disabilities (1993). Fetal alcohol syndrome and fetal alcohol effects. *Pediatrics* **91**: 1004.

Baker L, Thornton PS, Stanley CA (1991). Management of hyperinsulinism in infants. *J Pediatr* **119**: 755.

British National Formulary (1993). *Prescribing in Pregnancy*. London: British Medical Association and the Pharmaceutical Society of Great Britain.

Dornan JC, Halliday HL, McClure G (1988). High-risk pregnancy. In *Perinatal Medicine* (eds, McClure G, Halliday HL, Thompson W). London: Baillière Tindall.

Halliday HL, Traub AI (1988). Metabolic and endocrine disorders. In: *Perinatal Medicine* (eds, McClure G, Halliday HL, Thompson W). London: Baillière Tindall.

James DK, Steer PJ, Weiner CP, Gonik B (1994). *High Risk Pregnancy: Management Options*. London: WB Saunders.

Lang RM (1979). The nursing management of neonates born of diabetic mothers. *Pract Diabetes* **2**: 16.

Lissauer T (1989). Impact of AIDS on neonatal care. *Arch Dis Child* **64**: 4.

McCurdy CM, Seeds JW (1993). Route of delivery of infants with congenital anomalies. *Clin Perinatol* **20**: 81.

Meadow R (1991). Anticonvulsants in pregnancy. *Arch Dis Child* **66**: 62.

O'Brien MD, Gilmour-White S (1993). Epilepsy and pregnancy. *Br Med J* **307**: 492.

Rylance G, Houtman P (1988). Drugs and the neonate. *Hospital Update* **June**: 1726.

Pacifici GM, Nottoli R (1995). Placental transfer of drugs administered to the mother. *Clin Pharmacokinet* **28**: 235.

Shiono PH, Klebanoff MA (1993). A review of risk scoring for preterm birth. *Clin Perinatol* **20**: 107.

Volpe JJ (1992). Effect of cocaine use on the fetus. *N Engl J Med* **327**: 399.

4 Resuscitation of the Newborn

Effective resuscitation of infants is extremely important because of the serious consequences of asphyxia:

- Cerebral hypoxia, oedema and necrosis
- Seizures (from raised intracranial pressure or cerebral necrosis)
- Increased incidence of intraventricular haemorrhage in preterm
- Renal failure: tubular necrosis
- Shock lung and/or respiratory distress syndrome, pulmonary haemorrhage
- Heart failure, 'hypoxic cardiomyopathy'
- Disseminated intravascular coagulopathy
- Pulmonary hypertension/persistent fetal circulation
- Bowel perforation and necrotizing entercolitis
- Adrenal haemorrhage
- Metabolic disturbances: hypocalcaemia, hyponatraemia (inappropriate ADH), hypoglycaemia or hyperglycaemia, disordered temperature control, metabolic acidosis.

 Resuscitation should be performed by the most experienced person available.

The goals of resuscitation are:
Clearing the airway
Expansion and ventilation of the lungs
Ensuring adequate cardiac output
Minimizing oxygen consumption by preventing heat loss

The ability of the newborn to withstand asphyxia depends on:
Systemic arterial pressure
Cardiac glycogen stores

In asphyxia, shunting of blood occurs through the foramen ovale and the ductus venosus and this helps to maintain circulation to brain, heart and adrenals.

Fig. 4.1 demonstrates changes in respiration, heart rate and blood pressure following acute asphyxia. Primary apnoea occurs soon after the onset of asphyxia. During the phase of primary apnoea, circulation is not greatly compromised so that heart rate remains above 100/min and blood pressure is maintained. Primary apnoea is followed by repeated single gasps which increase in rate after 4–5 min before the last gasp occurs. After the last gasp, secondary or terminal apnoea occurs and the infant is pale and shocked with a heart rate <100/min and poor tone. This whole sequence of asphyxia probably extends over 10–15 min, after which time irreversible brain damage is likely to result. The duration of asphyxia may be estimated retrospectively as approximately half the time taken from the onset of respiration to the attainment of regular spontaneous breathing.

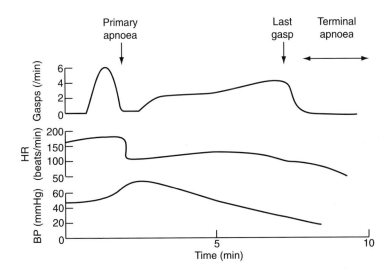

Figure 4.1. Changes in respiration, heart rate (HR) and blood pressure during asphyxia. If resuscitation is delayed after the last gasp, irreversible brain damage will occur. From Dawes (1968) with kind permission of Year Book Medical Publishers.

Many conditions other than asphyxia can lead to delayed onset of respiration after birth. All require prompt resuscitation.

Causes of delayed onset of respiration:

- Asphyxia
- Trauma
- Sepsis — Group B steptococcus, listeria
- Drugs — opiates leading to depression of CNS function
- Immaturity
- Severe RDS in immature baby
- Muscle disease
- Anaemia
- Congenital abnormalities — diaphragmatic hernia, obstruction of upper airway.

Anticipation of resuscitation

The need for resuscitation can be anticipated in approximately 70% of deliveries. Planned attendance by personnel skilled in advanced neonatal resuscitation at deliveries regarded as 'high risk' is essential for effective resuscitation. Each unit should have a policy outlining which deliveries require such personnel to attend.

Conditions which may require neonatal resuscitation at delivery:

- Fetal distress:
    persistent late decelerations
    severe variable decelerations with poor baseline variability
    meconium stained liquor
    scalp pH <7.25
    cord prolapse
- Forceps or ventouse (except simple 'lift out')
- Emergency caesarean section
- Vaginal breech delivery
- Antepartum haemorrhage
- Low birth weight
    preterm
    growth retardation

- Multiple pregnancy
- Prolonged, unusual or difficult labour
- Serious fetal abnormality such as hydrops fetalis, diaphragmatic hernia
- Concerns of attending staff.

Equipment

Equipment for resuscitation should be readily available and in working order. All equipment should be checked on a daily basis by staff responsible for the delivery suite (Table 4.1).

Prior to each delivery the person responsible for resuscitation should re-check the equipment and ensure:

Radiant heater is turned on and warm towels are available

Room temperature is appropriate at 24°C

Suction apparatus is working at 100 cmH$_2$O

O$_2$ supply is working with blow-off valve set at 30 cmH$_2$O

Other preparation such as drawing up of drugs or preparing appropriate ET tubes should be performed in advance of delivery if resuscitation is anticipated from the maternal history.

On arrival in delivery suite the person responsible for resuscitation should clarify the maternal history in order to anticipate the needs of the infant after birth. This is also an opportunity to meet the parents and discuss any potential problems.

Assessment of the infant

Rapid assessment of the infant after birth is needed to decide on appropriate resuscitation. The infant should be placed below a radiant heater and dried with warm towels while this assessment is performed.

The Apgar scoring system of newborn assessment at birth was developed as a rapid means of assessment of babies depressed by maternal analgesic drugs but is now universally applied to assess condition of babies at 1 and 5 min after birth (Table 4.2).

Table 4.1.   **Equipment required for neonatal resuscitation**

Resuscitation table:
  radiant heat source
  light
  stop clock
  stethoscope

Piped air/oxygen supply:
  flow up to 10 l/min
  variable O_2 concentration
  blow-off valve set at 30–40 cm H_2O

Vacuum supply for suction:
  negative pressure up to 200 cm H_2O
  suction catheters size 5,6,8 FG
  bulb suction available as standby

Ventilator bag and transparent neonatal face masks sizes 0,1 and 2

Oropharyngeal airways sizes 000, 00 and 0

Neonatal laryngoscope with straight blades sizes 0, 1 and 2

Endotracheal tubes (ET) and adapters sizes 2.5, 3.0 and 3.5 mm
Introducers for ET tubes

Drugs:
  Naloxone 20μg/ml and 400μg/ml
  4.2% sodium bicarbonate (for dilution)
  10% dextrose in water
  0.9% sodium chloride
  Adrenaline 1: 1000 and 1: 10 000
  Plasma or plasma sustitutes, e.g. albumin

Umbilical venous catheterization tray

Equipment for IV therapy, blood sampling or temporary thoracentesis:

  IV cannulae
  butterfly needles, injection needles
  3-way taps and extension sets
  alcohol wipes, syringes, specimen containers
  adhesive tape, disposable scissors
  blood sugar test strips

Table 4.2 **Apgar scoring system**

Signs	0	1	2
Heart rate	0	<100	>100
Colour	Blue or pale	Blue at peripheries	Pink
Respiration	0	Weak, gasping	Strong and regular
Responses to suction	0	Slight	Cries
Tone	0	Fair	Active

Asphyxia is only one of many causes of a low Apgar score and other factors which cause delayed onset of respiration (p. 40) and congenital heart disease should be taken into account. Although used as an indicator of the need and extent of resuscitation, intervention should *not* be delayed to assess the Apgar score.

A mnemonic for Apgar score is:

A Appearance, i.e. colour
P Pulse, i.e. heart rate
G Grimace, i.e. response to suction
A Activity, i.e. tone
R Respiration

The Apgar score should be assessed at 1 and 5 min after birth of the infant. The score should be assessed by a person not involved in resuscitation of the infant if possible. If the score is <7 at 5 min, it is valuable to continue assessment every 5 min until 20 min have elapsed or 2 successive scores of > 7 are obtained.

If Apgar score at 1 min is:

>7: No further resuscitation is likely to be needed
5–6: Infant is likely to respond to bag and mask ventilation
<4: Vigorous resuscitation including intubation and/or
   external cardiac massage may be required

Sometimes an infant will appear well at birth but later become apnoeic with worsening of the Apgar score.

Causes of worsening Apgar score at 5 min are:

- Excessive maternal analgesia during labour
- Respiratory obstruction: mucus and blood, choanal atresia, Pierre Robin syndrome
- Intrauterine infection (pneumonia)
- Excessive suctioning of the pharynx leading to reflex bradycardia
- Ineffective or poor response to resuscitation.

Resuscitation techniques

Maintenance of temperature

It is important to keep the infant warm by preventing heat loss from evaporation and radiation, otherwise a fall in temperature may occur (1°C every 5 mins). Cooling results in:

- Increased metabolic rate
- Increased oxygen consumption
- Hypoglycaemia
- Acidosis
- Worsening RDS
- Persistent fetal circulation

Careful drying of the baby and use of a radiant warmer are vital in preterm and severely asphyxiated babies.

Suctioning

Suctioning of the nose and/or oropharynx is not necessary in the majority of infants. It may be indicated if there are copious secretions or blood in the mouth and should be performed by gently sucking out the mouth after inserting a catheter not more than 5 cm from the lips. Suctioning is essential in the presence of meconium and should be performed thoroughly before delivery of the shoulders in a cephalic presentation and immediately after delivery of the head in a breech presentation. If thick meconium is present further suctioning with direct visualization of the larynx should be performed (see p. 99).

> **!** Avoid overvigorous suction. It can cause vagal stimulation resulting in reflex bradycardia and worsening of the infant's condition.

Ventilation

Spontaneous

Normal infants will usually take their first breath within seconds of birth with regular respirations within 1 min and do not usually require any intervention.

If the infant has shallow, irregular respirations but has a heart rate >100/min he should be allowed to breathe oxygen spontaneously while applying gentle tactile stimulation.

Currently 100% O_2 is used for resuscitation. However, preterm babies may have a reduction in cerebral blood flow if allowed to become hyperoxic. Therefore, if air/oxygen mixing facilities are available, it may be more appropriate to use 40% oxygen initially for resuscitation and to increase this as necessary using oxygen saturation monitoring.

Bag and mask ventilation (p. 97)

Indications:

≺ Persistently poor respiratory effort despite O_2 administration and tactile stimulation
≺ Apnoea with cyanosis
≺ Poor respiratory effort with heart rate <100/min.

Before applying bag and mask ventilation, ensure infant is on a flat surface with head in 'sniffing' position, avoiding hyperextension of the neck. Clear airway gently before placing a transparent face mask over infant's mouth and nose, ensuring it does not press on the eyes or overhang the chin. Maintain a tight seal and ventilate the infant at a rate of 40 breaths/min. For initial lung inflation, a pressure of at least 30–40 cm H_2O applied for 1 sec may be required, with pressures of 15–20 cm of H_2O for subsequent breaths. The majority of infants will respond to this procedure without further intervention.

Endotracheal intubation (p. 99)

Indications:

≺ Bag and mask ventilation ineffective
≺ Heart rate <60–80/min despite adequate mask ventilation
≺ Terminal apnoea at birth, i.e. apnoea, pale, flaccid
≺ Thick meconium staining and baby not vigorous
≺ Diaphragmatic hernia
≺ Extreme immaturity

Intubation is the preferred method of ventilation if resuscitation is required in the presence of thick meconium staining or if meconium is visualized below the cords. Do *not* wash out the lungs as this liquefies the meconium allowing it to pass distally.

Extremely immature infants fare better if their respiration is assisted early in postnatal life before severe RDS presents. These infants should be given surfactant soon after birth.

Oral intubation is preferred compared to nasal intubation in emergency situations because it can be performed more rapidly. Ventilate the infant at a rate of 40/min as above.

External cardiac massage (ECM)

Indications:

≺ Absent heart beat at birth unless maceration, extreme immaturity or gross congenital anomaly
≺ Heart rate <60–80/min with effective ventilation.

Both thumbs are placed over the middle to lower thirds of the sternum (Fig. 4.2). Perform chest compressions at a rate of 120/min to a depth of 2–3 cm. Assisted ventilation should be continued during ECM with 3 compressions per assisted breath. Efficient ECM can only provide 50% of normal cardiac output. For optimal performance two operators are needed.

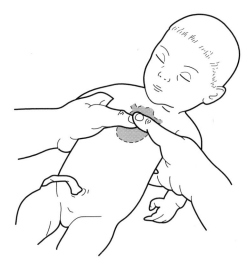

Figure 4.2. Neonatal cardiac massage. Thumbs should be placed over the middle third of the sternum.

Drugs

Drugs are rarely needed in the immediate resuscitation of infants. They should only be administered after ventilation has been established. Umbilical vein is the route used for emergency administration of drugs in the delivery suite because of rapid delivery to the central circulation.

Correction of acidosis

The adverse effects of acidosis are:

- Decreased myocardial contractility
- Increased pulmonary vascular resistance with right-to-left shunting
- Decreased cellular metabolism especially within the brain

Correct the primary cause of the acidosis. Respiratory acidosis should be corrected by establishing ventilation. Metabolic acidosis resulting from hypoxia or hypovolaemia should be corrected by ventilation and/or volume expansion.

The administration of alkali (sodium bicarbonate) is controversial although it is still commonly included in resuscitation guidelines.

Risks of sodium bicarbonate therapy include:

- Transient rise in $PaCO_2$ and fall in PaO_2
- Reduction in cerebral blood flow
- Increased incidence of intracranial haemorrhage

Sodium bicarbonate is indicated for persistent bradycardia with evidence of metabolic acidosis in spite of adequate ventilation.

Dosage: Give 1–2 mmol/kg slowly intravenously, i.e. 4 ml/kg of 4.2% sodium bicarbonate (8.4% solution can be diluted with an equal part of 5% dextrose).

Volume expansion

Rarely needed during resuscitation. Indicated in the presence of clear signs of hypovolaemia in the presence of acute blood loss, including feto-maternal haemorrhage.

Clinical signs of hypovolaemia are:

≺ Pale and limp appearance
≺ Tachycardia (not always present)
≺ Poor capillary filling
≺ Low blood pressure.

Risks of volume expanders include:
    Patent ductus arteriosus
    Intracranial haemorrhage.

 Avoid volume administration in babies who may appear 'shocked' due to myocardial insufficiency after asphyxia because of the danger of compromising the circulation further.

Dosage: 10 ml/kg of plasma or plasma substitute, such as 5% albumin, given slowly intravenously. Repeat aliquots to a maximum of 30 ml/kg should be given until the infant has a satisfactory response.

Naloxone hydrochloride (Narcan)

Indicated if respiratory depression is thought to be due to narcotic administration to the mother within 6 hours of delivery.

Dosage: Give naloxone 100µg/kg intramuscularly promptly in association with assisted ventilation. Intramuscular naloxone takes effect rapidly, within a few minutes, and is the preferred route of administration. When given intravenously the effect can diminish very quickly and therefore repeat doses by intramuscular route may be required.

 Avoid giving naloxone to babies of narcotic-dependent mothers as acute withdrawal may be precipitated.

Adrenaline

Indicated for bradycardia that persists after adequate ventilation and cardiac massage.

Dosage: Adrenaline 0.1 ml/kg of 1: 10 000 intravenously or 1: 1000 intratracheally. Risks of intracardiac injection preclude this route of administration. Repeat doses may be given after 3 mins.

Calcium gluconate

Administration of calcium gluconate (10%) is no longer recommended for resuscitation of the newborn.

Failure to respond to resuscitation

If the infant does not make any initial response to resuscitation certain conditions should be considered:

- Technical problem:
    oxygen not connected
    blow-off valve set incorrectly
    ET in incorrect position
- Pneumothorax
- Severe underlying lung disease:
    pulmonary hypoplasia

respiratory distress syndrome
congenital pneumonia
- Congenital abnormality
  diaphragmatic hernia
- Maternal sedation
- Severe anaemia
- Congenital heart disease
- Profound asphyxia.

Management

➤ Check equipment and auscultate the chest for air entry and to assess ET position or for presence of a pneumothorax.

➤ If air entry is equal, higher pressure may be required to ventilate non-compliant lungs if severe lung disease is present.

➤ If an infant is pink, well perfused with a good heart rate but refuses to breathe, consider maternal opioid sedation or muscle disease.

➤ Although adrenaline is more likely to work after correction of acidosis, it is reasonable to try giving one dose via the ET as it sometimes has an immediate effect.

➤ If the baby does not respond, give sodium bicarbonate i.v. and then repeat the dose of adrenaline.

➤ If an infant remains cyanosed despite adequate ventilation consider congenital heart disease or persistent fetal circulation.

A resuscitation plan is useful and should be readily available beside resuscitation cots (Figs 4.3 and 4.4).

Unfortunately, the situation will occasionally occur when a baby will not respond to complete resuscitative efforts.

Perinatal cardiac arrest

If an infant has never shown signs of life, management is far from simple. The difficulty lies in the estimation of how long the circulation has ceased and whether the resulting hypoxaemic and

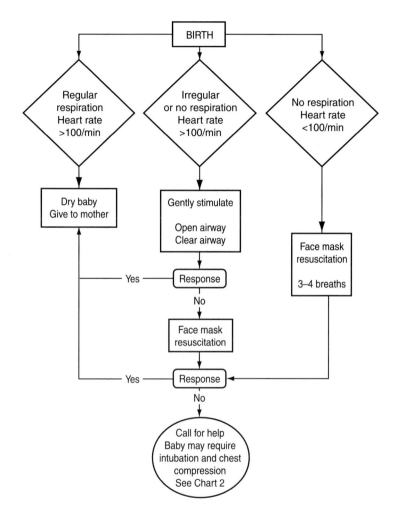

Note: If there is particulate meconium and the baby is unresponsive, proceed at once to Chart 2 (Figure 4.4).

Figure 4.3. Resuscitation Chart 1. From BPA/RCOG 1997 with kind permission.

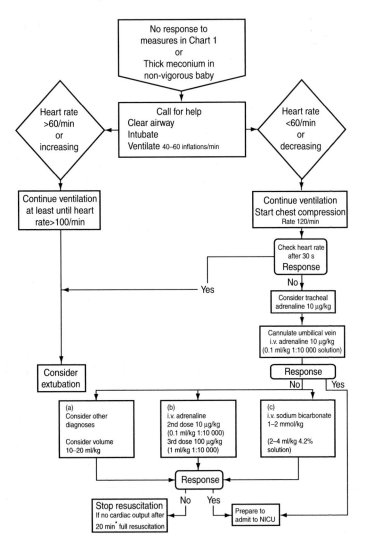

Figure 4.4. Resuscitation Chart 2. From BPA/RCOG 1997 with kind permission.

ischaemic damage to vital organs, especially the brain, is reversible.

Management

➤ Intubate and ventilate while performing cardiac massage unless gross congenital abnormality or maceration are present.

➤ If spontaneous heart beat is not regained within 3 min, then 0.3 ml/kg 1: 10 000 adrenaline should be given by endotracheal tube. Infants responding to this therapy by showing regular, spontaneous heart beat within 10 min and developing spontaneous respirations within 30 min, usually have a good prognosis.

➤ If the infant shows no response, *call senior colleague.*

Half of infants failing to regain regular, spontaneous respirations within 30 min after the return of spontaneous heart beat will die within 1 week and the remainder will survive with gross handicaps, although there are occasional exceptions.

Nursing points

Baby

• Apgar scores must be recorded in the notes at 1 and 5 min, and if low every 5 min until normal.
• Following each complicated delivery a sample of cord blood and the whole placenta must be sent for examination. The results may aid diagnosis and prompt treatment of the baby.
• Accurate recording of observations, condition of baby, timing of events and drugs administered is vital.

Family

• Parents should be prepared in advance if their baby is likely to require resuscitation.
• Parents should be supported throughout the resuscitation, and kept informed of the baby's progress as appropriate.
• A full explanation of events should be given to parents at the earliest possible opportunity.

Equipment

- Resuscitation equipment should be available in every delivery room, and for every baby on the NICU. This includes:
    Suction equipment and tubes
    Oxygen and air supply
    Resuscitation bag and mask
    Facilities to intubate and ventilate if necessary
    Overhead heater
    Emergency drugs.
- It is the responsibility of each nurse to check the resuscitation equipment for babies in their care at the beginning of each shift.
- All ventilated babies should have resuscitation equipment, an endotracheal tube pre-cut to the appropriate length, laryngoscope, introducer and stethoscope by their incubator.

Staff

- A paediatrician and neonatal nurse should be present at all high-risk deliveries.
- All midwives and neonatal nurses should attend regular updates on neonatal resuscitation skills.

References and further reading

American Academy of Pediatrics, Committee on the Fetus and Newborn and American College of Obstetricians and Gynecologists, Committee on Obstetric Practice (1996). Use and abuse of the Apgar score. *Pediatrics* **98**: 141.

American Academy of Paediatrics, American College of Obstetrics and Gynecology (1997). *Guidelines for Perinatal Care*, 4th edn. Elk Grove Village, Illinois: AAP/ACOG.

British Paediatric Association, Royal College of Obstetrics and Gynaecology. (1997). *Resuscitation of Babies at Birth*. London: BMJ Publishing Group.

Dawes GS (1968). *Fetal and Neonatal Physiology*. Chicago: Year Book Medical Publishers.

Hein HA (1993). The use of sodium bicarbonate in neonatal resuscitation: help or harm. *Pediatrics* **91**: 496.

5 Transitional Care, Admission and Transport

Transitional care

Infants who are obviously ill or distressed at birth should be admitted to the neonatal unit. There are some infants who at birth may be somewhat distressed, but with good resuscitation improve so that they require observation for a while before deciding whether to admit them either to the neonatal unit or the postnatal ward. This transitional care is best provided in the labour ward. The infant having transitional care should be placed naked in an incubator so that he may be observed and kept warm. Should central cyanosis be apparent, oxygen therapy should be given into the incubator, and measured with an oxygen analyser. Some transitional care units use pulse oximeters to measure oxygen saturation. If >40% oxygen is required at this time to abolish cyanosis, the infant should be admitted at once to the neonatal unit.

Transitional care includes:

➤ Close observation of the infant
➤ Recording of vital signs (temperature, heart rate, respiration rate, oxygen saturation)
➤ Measurement of packed cell volume
➤ Capillary blood glucose testing.

Infants who have mild or moderate asphyxia (Apgar score >5 at 5 min) but are normal by 1 hour of age, may be safely admitted to the postnatal ward, but their progress should be reviewed at 4 and 24 hours. Those that continue to have respiratory distress and require oxygen at 1 hour of age should be admitted to the neonatal unit.

Admission

Indications for admission to the neonatal unit include:

➤ Birth weight <1750 g or gestational age <34 weeks
➤ Babies needing >40% oxygen to abolish cyanosis
➤ Persisting respiratory distress; grunting, indrawing and tachypnoea (>60/min) after 1 hour
➤ Babies with malformations requiring assessment and surgery
➤ Babies who have suffered from severe birth asphyxia:
   Apgar scores <3 at 1 min or <5 at 5 min,
   needing intensive resuscitation
   meconium found below the cords
➤ Infant of diabetic mother with complications (see p. 26)
➤ Severe erythroblastosis (see Ch. 13)
➤ Seizures.

Medical staff working in the neonatal unit should be aware of the local admission policy.

Admission procedure

➤ Forewarn neonatal unit of impending admission — get necessary staff and equipment ready.

➤ Keep baby warm — servo-controlled radiant warmer or servo-controlled incubator

➤ Give enough warmed, humidified oxygen if cyanosis is present — start with about 40%.

➤ Attach electrodes for monitors — heart rate, respiration, transcutaneous PO_2 or pulse oximeter.

➤ Brief examination of infant — respiratory system, cardiovascular system, abdomen, central nervous system, weight, length and head circumference, gestational age — but do not remove from oxygen or allow to cool. Avoid excessive handling.

➤ Simple investigations — capillary blood glucose, haematocrit, blood gases, cultures, blood pressure. Chest X-ray after umbilical arterial catheter and endotracheal tube have been inserted if these are indicated (see Ch. 7).

➤ Senior medical staff should be informed early about admission of any severely ill baby.

➤ Clear and comprehensive documentation is essential.

Transportation

Ill infants born outside the referral centre may need to be transported for intensive care. Transportation of an ill and potentially unstable infant is not an ideal situation and, by anticipation of problems in high-risk pregnancies (see Ch. 3), prior transport of the mother for her delivery in the perinatal centre is to be preferred. However, about 30% of preterm labours cannot be predicted antenatally and some of these babies will be born outside perinatal centres. Their immediate resuscitation and stabilization may be critical as regards outcome. Not all transfers in the UK are successful and babies who cannot secure a place in a neonatal intensive care unit have an increased mortality rate.

Transportation of an ill baby is potentially hazardous and should only be undertaken by skilled personnel. Doctors and nurses involved must have a high degree of expertise since they may have to cope with seriously ill babies in unfamiliar circumstances. Any complication that can happen in the intensive care unit can occur in the back of an ambulance. Where possible, a dedicated transport team should be employed to collect a sick baby from the referring unit. Studies have shown that using a dedicated team reduces the frequency of complications during transport and reduces mortality. Adequate training and regular updating of all personnel concerned is vital. Facilities required for transportation are listed in Table 5.1.

Suggested indications for transfer of the newborn include:

◄ Very low birth weight infant (<1500 g) unless obviously small for gestational age, i.e. >32 weeks

◄ Severe RDS at any weight:
  PaO_2 <8 kPa (60 mmHg) in 60% oxygen

early apnoea or shock
acidosis (pH <7.15)

≺ Moderate RDS if <2000 g:
PaO_2 <8 kPa (60 mmHg) in 40% oxygen
apnoea or shock
pH <7.20

≺ Severe meconium aspiration syndrome: meconium below cords at birth and any subsequent respiratory distress, >40% oxygen needed, presence of complicating air leak, e.g. pneumothorax

≺ Requirement for urgent cardiological investigation

≺ Malformation requiring urgent assessment or surgery.

Table 5.1. **Facilities required for transportation**

Suitably equipped ambulance with short response time
Experienced medical and nursing staff available at all times

Transport incubator:
    battery and mains
    adequate heat supply
    easy access — portholes for intravenous infusions
    reliable air and oxygen supply

Lightweight, reliable monitors:
    axillary temperature
    heart rate
    respiration
    transcutaneous PO_2 or pulse oximeter

Syringe pumps for controlled fluid administration
Reliable, flexible and safe mechanical ventilator
Glucometer and reagent strips for measurement of glucose

Equipment for:
    peripheral and umbilical vessel catheterization
    endotracheal intubation
    chest drainage

Drugs and intravenous fluids (Table 4.1)
Other equipment (Table 4.1)

In future high frequency oscillatory ventilation (HFOV) and inhaled nitric oxide (INO) may be standard interventions during transportation.

Preparation for transportation

 Stabilization of the infant prior to transport is the most important aspect of the transfer procedure.

Before transportation, the transport team must assess and stabilize the baby's condition:

➤ Adequate airway or correctly positioned endotracheal tube
➤ Optimal blood gases
➤ Correction of acidosis
➤ Assisted ventilation at effective settings
➤ Adequate venous access for required infusions
➤ Arterial cannulation — well secured and visible
➤ Blood glucose in normal range
➤ Check blood pressure and correct if low
➤ Temperature.

Explanation to and reassurance of parents is very important. They should be given a Polaroid photograph of their baby. Obtain consent from parents for procedures (e.g. cardiac catheterization, surgery).

Copies of all relevant case notes (particularly the antenatal details and any treatment to date), radiographs, and a specimen of mother's blood for cross-matching should accompany the baby. It may be appropriate to send the placenta to the regional perinatal centre for histology.

The baby must be monitored carefully during transportation, with the same attention to detail as in the neonatal unit.

Specific problems

There are a number of special considerations to be taken into account before transfer can proceed:

➤ Significant RDS: intubate, administer surfactant and stabilize blood gases before transportation.

➤ Ventilated babies should receive sedation — extra care must be taken if the baby is already paralysed.

➤ Pneumothorax: insert chest drain and attach to Heimlich flutter valve before transportation

➤ Heart failure: begin digoxin and diuretics.

➤ Babies who have suspected or proven ductus-dependent cardiac lesions should have a PGE_2 infusion erected.

➤ Seizures: perform capillary blood glucose stix and lumbar puncture, if meningitis suspected, before transportation. Give anticonvulsants as indicated (see p. 267).

➤ Open lesions, e.g. myelomeningocele, omphalocele: cover with a sterile polythene bag (polybag) or clingfilm.

➤ Gastroschisis and intestinal obstruction: place nasogastric tube with free drainage and give intravenous fluids. Plasma volume expansion may be necessary.

➤ Oesophageal atresia: place nasogastric tube for continuous low-suction or frequent intermittent drainage.

➤ Babies being transferred to a specialist ECMO centre are often transported by its transport team.

Return to referring hospital

The transfer of infants back to the hospital of birth will depend upon:

Resolution of the major clinical problems

Capability of referring hospital to provide continuing care

Experience has shown that half of all transported infants qualify for transfer back to the referring hospitals after about 7–10 days. This has three main advantages:

Frees intensive care cots in perinatal centre

Moves the infant closer to parents' home so that visiting is easier

Encourages referring obstetricians and paediatricians to seek intensive care again

It is important for referring and returning hospitals to liaise closely with each other and to maintain good working relationships. If the baby has been in the perinatal centre for a prolonged period of time, parents often become apprehensive about the transfer and it may take time for them to get used to the staff in the referring hospital. Preparation prior to the transfer may alleviate some of their anxiety.

Discharge

This is determined in part by the availability of community services: community midwifery, health visiting, general practitioner and community paediatrics. The proposed date of discharge should be discussed with the parents in advance so that they can get prepared. Details of feeding, medication, vaccination schedules and follow-up visits should be given.

In general, a baby who is feeding well, can maintain body temperature in a cot and whose parents are confident and competent in providing care, can be discharged no matter what his weight. Some babies with weights of 1600 g have been safely discharged from hospital, although clearly smaller babies require close follow-up in the early days after discharge.

Babies with continuing problems such as congenital anomalies, apnoeic attacks, chronic lung disease or neurological sequelae can be successfully discharged but may need additional care, including tube feeding, domiciliary oxygen or home monitoring. In these situations the neonatal liaison nurse has an important supportive role.

Infant follow-up is discussed in Ch. 23.

Nursing points

Baby

- Ensure the baby is stable prior to transportation and update the receiving NICU on the condition of the baby.
- Check the baby's two namebands with the parents prior to leaving.

Family

- All parents should be able to see, hold or touch their baby for a while before transfer.
- Ensure parents are given the telephone number and directions to the destination hospital before transferring the baby.
- Contact numbers for the family should be obtained in case of an emergency.
- Families may require assistance with accommodation or travel costs if their baby is transferred a long way from their home.
- Where possible follow-up of the baby should be at a local clinic or hospital.

Equipment

- The transport incubator should be checked daily to ensure it is fully equipped and functioning.
- An instant camera should be kept with the transport incubator and photographs of the baby left with the parents on transfer.
- Copies of all maternal and neonatal notes and relevant radiographs should be transferred with the baby.

Staff

- Transitional care wards reduce the number of admissions to NICU and the separation of many mothers and babies. Staffing levels need to be higher than in normal postnatal wards.
- Staff should keep the referring hospital informed of the baby's progress and arrange transfer back as soon as possible.
- A pre-discharge meeting involving family, hospital and community staff is useful to plan care and support for the family.

References and further reading

Bristow A (1997). Interhospital transfer of neonates by air. In: Mir NA (ed.) *Manual of Neonatal Transport*. Manchester: E Petch, pp. 45–53.

British Association of Perinatal Medicine Working Group (1989). Referrals for neonatal medical care in the United Kingdom over one year. *Br Med J* 1989; **298**: 169.

Harding JE, Morton SM (1993). Adverse effects of neonatal transport between level III centers. *J Pediatr* **29**: 146.

Leslie AJ, Stephenson TJ (1997). Audit of neonatal intensive care transport — closing the loop. *Acta Pediatr* **86**: 1253.

Madar RJ, Milligan DWA (1994). Neonatal transport: safety and security. *Arch Dis Child* **71**: F147.

Roper HP, Chiswick ML, Sims DG (1988). Referrals to a regional neonatal intensive care unit. *Arch Dis Child* **63**: 403.

Shenai JP (1993). Neonatal transport. Outreach educational program. *Pediatr Clin N Am* **40**: 275.

Taskforce on Interhospital Transport (1993). Team composition, selection and training. In: *Guidelines for Air and Ground Transport of Neonatal and Pediatric Patients*. American Academy of Pediatrics, pp. 35–45.

6 The Low Birth Weight Infant

A low birth weight (LBW) infant is one whose birth weight is 2500 g or less. Subgroups of very low birth weight (VLBW, ≤1500 g) and extremely low birth weight (ELBW, ≤1000 g) have special problems.

Growth charts of weight against gestation (see Appendix VIII) are used to determine whether an infant is appropriately grown (AGA) or not. SGA babies lie below the 10th percentile of weight for gestation and large-for-gestational-age infants (LGA) lie above the 90th percentile. Infants are post-term if they are born beyond the 42nd week of pregnancy (see Ch. 7).

Low birth weight may be due to:

- short gestation (preterm, defined as < 37 weeks)
- growth retardation (small for gestational age (SGA), defined as < 10th percentile)
- both

The two main groups of LBW infants have different problems so early accurate assessment is necessary.

Assessment involves:

➤ Estimation of gestational age:

menstrual history
early antenatal ultrasound scan
Dubowitz or Ballard assessment (Appendices VIIA–D)

Below 28 weeks, gestational age assessment using external characteristics is unreliable. Gestational age is a better predictor of outcome than birth weight for infants of over 800 g.

➤ Growth: plot weight, length and head circumference against gestational age (Appendix VIII).

The preterm infant

Characteristically the preterm infant shows:

◄ Inactive, extended posture
◄ Feeble cry
◄ Irregular respirations
◄ Translucent skin, thick vernix, few skin creases
◄ Prominent lanugo
◄ Poor breast development
◄ Soft or poorly formed nails
◄ Immature external genitalia.

Physiological handicaps

Most organ systems are functionally immature and this results in a variety of physiological handicaps.

Temperature instability

The preterm baby has difficulty in maintaining body temperature because of:

● Increased heat loss
● Reduced subcutaneous fat
● Large surface area to body weight ratio
● Reduced heat production because of inadequate brown fat and inability to shiver.

Respiratory difficulties

◄ Deficiency of pulmonary surfactant leading to respiratory distress syndrome (see Ch. 10)
◄ Risk of aspiration because of poor gag and cough reflexes, uncoordinated suck and swallow

≺ Pliable thorax and weak respiratory musculature result in less efficient ventilation
≺ Periodic breathing and apnoea (see p. 253) because of immaturity of the respiratory centre in the medulla.

 The more immature the baby, the earlier should be the intervention. Nasal prong CPAP and/or surfactant replacement should be considered soon after birth, especially in ELBW babies with respiratory distress.

Gastrointestinal and nutritional problems

≺ Poor sucking and swallowing reflexes especially at <34 weeks' gestation
≺ Decreased intestinal motility leading to abdominal distension
≺ Decreased gastric volume and increased gastric emptying time
≺ Reduced digestion and absorption of fats, fat-soluble vitamins and certain minerals
≺ Lactase in intestinal brush border is deficient before term, but enzyme activity is rapidly induced by feeding
≺ Body stores of calcium, phosphorus, proteins, vitamins A, C and E, trace elements and iron are less than in the term infant and deficiencies may occur with growth.

Hepatic immaturity

≺ Impaired conjugation and excretion of bilirubin
≺ Deficiency of vitamin K-dependent clotting factors.

Renal immaturity

≺ Inability to excrete large solute loads; a relatively dilute urine is produced
≺ Fluid and electrolyte balance may be difficult

≺ Metabolic acidosis may result from accumulation of inorganic acids
≺ Renal elimination of drugs, e.g. aminoglycosides, may be impaired.

Immunological disturbances

≺ Reduced ability to combat infection as a result of absent or reduced placental transmission of immunoglobulins
≺ Relative inability to produce antibodies
≺ Impaired phagocytosis and reduced inflammatory response (see Ch. 14)

Neurological immaturity

≺ Immature sucking and swallowing reflexes
≺ Decreased intestinal motility
≺ Recurrent apnoea and bradycardia (paradoxical response to hypoxia and hypercapnia)
≺ Intraventricular haemorrhage — most common in smaller babies. Increased susceptibility to intraventricular haemorrhage is due to relatively unsupported but highly vascular periventricular area which may be subject to perinatal stresses such as hypercapnia and hypertension (p. 270)
≺ Poor regulation of cerebral perfusion. Periventricular leucomalacia (PVL), a cystic lesion of brain, may be caused by ischaemia and/or venous infarction (see Ch. 16).

The very low birth weight baby

Infants ≤1500 g (<30–32 weeks' gestation) comprise only 1–2% of liveborn population, but account for 70% of all neonatal deaths not due to congenital anomalies. Table 6.1 shows survival of infants of birthweight ≤1500 g admitted to the Royal Maternity Hospital, Belfast, 1994–95. These results can only be achieved in centres where neonatal intensive care is available. Table 6.2 shows survival and morbidity rates for ELBW and VLBW babies born in Northern Ireland over the same period.

Table 6.1. Survival of VLBW infants

Gestational age (weeks)	Average birth weight (g)	Expected birth weight (g)	Survival to discharge (%)
23	550	650	33
24	600	725	38
25	700	850	54
26	850	930	88
27	950	1050	81
28	1100	1200	92
29	1200	1350	86
30	1300	1530	100
31	1400	1720	100
32	1500	1920	99

Table 6.2. Survival and morbidity of VLBW and ELBW infants born in Northern Ireland, 1994–95[*]

	Birth weight	
	≤1000 g	≤1500 g
Survival to discharge	82%	86%
Respiratory distress syndrome	69%	54%
Needed IPPV	82%	65%
Needed CPAP alone	7%	8%
Pneumothorax	15%	11%
Intraventricular haemorrhage (IVH) (all grades)	55%	23%
Patent ductus arteriosus	46%	35%
Necrotizing enterocolitis	9%	8%
Chronic lung disease	18%	17%
Retinopathy of prematurity:		
All stages	42%	31%
Stage IV/V	3%	1%

[*] Reproduction with kind permission of the Northern Ireland Neonatal Audit Group.
Figures include babies with congenital abnormalities.

Problems and their management

The problems of the preterm infant are mainly seen in the smaller babies who withstand intervention least well.

Asphyxia and resuscitation

Prenatal management is designed to detect and correct fetal distress and to minimize trauma. Expert delivery and neonatal resuscitation is especially important for the LBW infant.

 Experienced staff should attend the delivery of a very immature baby.

An increasing proportion of immature infants are being born by elective caesarean section, especially those that are breech presentations, but this may also be traumatic if the lower uterine segment is poorly formed.

Asphyxia in the preterm infant is poorly tolerated and increases morbidity in the immediate and late postnatal period. Asphyxia inhibits surfactant production increasing the severity of RDS and risk of subsequent IVH. One study has shown improved survival of VLBW infants who were electively intubated at birth for resuscitation, but this was not a randomized controlled trial.

There are major practical and ethical problems with the most immature babies (<24 weeks). During labour the parents should be spoken to sympathetically, but realistically, about the prognosis of their baby. A decision about management may be made at this time. When the baby is born, a poor outcome may be expected if the baby is depressed, has firmly fused eyelids, marked bruising or birth weight <500 g.

If it is decided to attempt to treat the baby, endotracheal intubation should be performed and surfactant given as soon as possible, unless the baby is very active and has regular respiratory activity, when nasal CPAP may be attempted. When doubts arise there should be full discussion with a senior doctor.

Temperature

VLBW infants should be stabilized under a radiant warmer and then placed in a servo controlled incubator to reduce high insensible water losses. The incubator temperature may need to be kept at 37–39°C with high humidity during the first hours of life. A heat shield or bubble wrap may be used to reduce heat losses.

More mature infants should be placed in a neutral thermal environment where oxygen consumption is minimal (see Ch. 8). A servo-controlled incubator or radiant heater should be employed to maintain skin temperature at 36.5°C. Woollen hats help to prevent heat loss.

When the preterm infant reaches about 1600 g, he is usually able to maintain temperature out of an incubator.

Handling

All preterm babies tolerate handling very poorly but many procedures are necessary, so handling should be as deft as possible during the initial phase of resuscitation and stabilization. Thereafter, handling should be kept to a minimum.

 Small sick babies should be handled as little as possible.

Respiratory distress

Respiratory problems and their sequelae are the major causes of death and their management may be very difficult. Diagnosis and treatment should be carried out rapidly. Respiratory assistance from birth is often needed for babies weighing <1000 g.

Oxygen therapy is often required, although preterm infants should not be placed routinely in oxygen. Hypoxaemia is the only true indication for oxygen therapy. If cyanosis is present, the infant should be placed initially in the minimum oxygen concentration that is required to abolish cyanosis. When oxygen therapy is being used, the ambient oxygen level must be continuously recorded.

If an infant requires oxygen 30 min after birth to maintain normal colour, it is essential that arterial oxygen tension be measured. This may be performed using intermittent radial artery puncture, umbilical or radial arterial catheterization or transcutaneous oxygen monitoring if the infant is not shocked (see Ch. 9). The inspired oxygen concentration should be adjusted to keep arterial oxygen tension in the range 6–9 kPa (50–70 mmHg), in order to reduce the risks of retinopathy of prematurity (ROP) and to avoid hypoxic brain damage.

Surfactant replacement for surfactant deficiency has improved the outcome of these immature babies (see Ch. 10).

Apnoea

Infants of <34 weeks' gestation or <1750 g birth weight have an increased risk of apnoea and bradycardia, which is often present from 3 days to at least 2 weeks of age. Over 90% of babies <1000 g and 60% from 1000 to 1500 g have apnoea. Heart and respiration rate monitors must be used on all infants <32 weeks' gestation until apnoea-free for at least 1 week. Always look for predisposing factors, especially infection. Start with simple therapies first, but drugs and assisted ventilation are frequently needed (see p. 255).

Fluids and nutrition (see also Ch. 11).

The quantity and route of administration will depend upon the size, age and condition of the infant.

For small or distressed infants:

➤ Intravenous 5 or 10% dextrose at a rate of 80–100 ml/kg/day is used during the first 24 hours.

➤ If radiant warmers or phototherapy are used, insensible water losses may increase by 50–100% and an extra 30–60 ml/kg/day is needed.

➤ The very immature baby with thin shiny skin may have massive insensible water losses, particularly if nursed under a radiant warmer, and have fluid requirements up to 250–300 ml/kg/day for first 3 days. Electrolytes are usually not needed during this time.

➤ In the very immature infant, glycosuria or hyperglycaemia (capillary glucose >8 mmol/l) may occur, so the concentration of dextrose should be reduced. An insulin infusion may be necessary.

Enteral feeds should be introduced as soon as possible after birth. The intravenous dextrose should be supplemented with amino acids after 24 hours of life, according to the local parenteral nutrition protocol (see Ch. 11).

For infants <34 weeks' gestation who are not distressed, tube feeding may be required because of the risk of aspiration as a result of uncoordinated suck and swallow. Orogastric tube feeds may be given either intermittently or continuously; intermittent (bolus) feeding has some advantages since normal enterohumoral responses may be stimulated, but immature babies may tolerate better the smaller quantities of milk used in continuous feeding. The orogastric route is preferred by many as nasogastric intubation causes an increase in airway resistance and may lead to apnoea.

The feeds should begin with quantities of 1–3 ml/kg/h and increase cautiously every 12 hours, depending upon the amount of gastric aspirate. After starting feeding watch for abdominal distension, increasing gastric aspirates and reducing substances or blood in stool. Some babies have poor gastric emptying, which may result in large gastric aspirates and vomiting. When this is troublesome, transpyloric (orojejunal) feeding using a silastic feeding tube may reduce risk of reflux and aspiration.

Expressed breast milk (EBM) is probably the best food for smaller or asphyxiated infants (see Ch. 11). Banked human milk must be pasteurized and donors screened for HIV. Preterm babies fed on EBM do not grow as rapidly as babies fed on proprietary formulae but other benefits such as anti-infective properties of breast milk outweigh this disadvantage.

Breast milk feeds are deficient in protein, iron, phosphorus, sodium and chloride and supplementation may be necessary. EBM given to preterm babies should be supplemented with breast milk fortifier (see p. 182, Ch. 11).

Fluid requirements increase daily to a maximum of 150–200 ml/kg/day depending on environmental and renal losses.

Minimal energy and protein requirements for growth are 460

kJ/kg/day (110 kcal/kg/day) and 2–3 g/kg/day, respectively. Expected weight gain is 1–1.5% of body weight/day, i.e. for a 750 g infant, 7.5–10 g daily.

Electrolyte problems

Acid–base and electrolyte balance should be carefully controlled. Hypernatraemia is common in the first few days due to high insensible water losses; additional electrolytes are usually not needed for the first 2–3 days. Hyponatraemia often follows due to inappropriate ADH secretion in the acute phase of RDS, and increased renal sodium losses in the recovery phase of RDS. These should be treated with fluid restriction and increased sodium supplements (up to 6–8 mmol/kg/day) respectively.

Later, metabolic acidosis may occur because the kidney is unable to excrete an increased acid load related to a high protein intake. Other causes of metabolic acidosis include sepsis, hypovolaemia, PDA, anaemia, necrotizing enterocolitis and intraventricular haemorrhage.

✚ Intraventricular haemorrhage (IVH)

IVH and periventricular leucomalacia are not uncommon in very immature babies. The main problem appears to be an alteration in cerebral blood flow which may be increased by any major upset, e.g. pneumothorax. Regular ultrasound scans should be performed to detect and monitor progress and help with prognosis (see Ch. 16). The role of drugs such as ethamsylate, indomethacin or phenobarbitone in the prevention of IVH remains unclear; there is now reasonable evidence of the benefits of indomethacin but long-term follow-up studies are not complete.

✚ Patent ductus arteriosus (PDA)

This may be present but clinically silent in first few days. By around the third day, the pulmonary vascular resistance falls, increasing the L→R shunt, and a systolic or continuous murmur becomes audible. 'Run-off' from the aorta to pulmonary artery results in a widening of the pulse pressure with bounding pulses, and pulmonary congestion ensues. An ominous clinical sign is apnoea because this may mean decreased cerebral blood flow. Echocardiography is used to confirm the diagnosis (see p. 287).

Initial treatment is conservative, consisting of fluid restriction and diuretics. Haemoglobin should be maintained above 14 g/dl (PCV 45%). Treatment with indomethacin should be considered early in the immature baby, unless there are contraindications to its use (see p. 288).

Infection (see Ch. 14)

Infection is common in LBW babies, especially those receiving intensive care. The main reasons for this are handling, invasive procedures and poor resistance to infection. Infection may be the cause of premature delivery. After culture of blood, gastric aspirate and superficial swabbing, antibiotics should be started if infant has any symptoms or mother is ill and febrile, or Gram stain of gastric aspirate shows organisms or pus cells.

✚ Necrotizing enterocolitis

Factors predisposing to this condition are extreme immaturity, birth asphyxia, hypotension, polycythaemia, hypothermia, exchange transfusion, patent ductus arteriosus and possibly umbilical artery catheterization and early milk feeding. Milk feeds should be introduced carefully in these situations. Any distension of the bowel with increased gastric aspirate means that feeding should be reduced, at least temporarily.

Surgery is reserved for infants with evidence of perforation, i.e. free peritoneal air or cellulitis of anterior abdominal wall. Drainage of peritoneal cavity is an alternative to laparotomy and enterostomy, particularly in the very unstable immature baby.

✚ Chronic pulmonary disease

This probably encompasses a number of separate entities with different aetiologies but bronchopulmonary dysplasia and Wilson–Mikity syndrome are perhaps the best known (see Ch. 10).

✚ Retinopathy of prematurity (ROP)

This is seen with increasing frequency in the very immature baby. Oxygen is only one of many possible factors in the aetiology. It is important to routinely screen for ROP at 5–6 weeks of life to detect changes that might benefit from laser treatment or cryotherapy (see p. 88).

✚ Anaemia

Onset is earlier and severity greater than in the more mature baby. Reasons for this are a lower initial haemoglobin (12–14 g/dl), decreased red cell survival and greater losses from blood sampling. The growth rate is relatively faster and the 900 g infant may treble his birth weight in 10 weeks and exhaust iron stores. Therapy with iron, vitamin E and erythropoietin are discussed in Ch. 21.

Parent–infant bonding

Being the parent of a 23–25 week premature baby is an emotionally draining experience. The baby may seem to pass from one crisis to another and it may be several weeks before the mother realizes that her infant may survive. Parents should be encouraged to visit their infant and touch him. Visits by siblings and grandparents should also be encouraged. Photographs should be provided, especially if parents live far away and are unable to visit often or use parental accommodation within the hospital. The parents should be allowed, where possible, to take part in the baby's care, e.g. by providing expressed breast milk and clothing of their choice.

Infrequent visiting may be an early warning sign of future parenting problems and all visits by the parents should be documented by nursing staff (see Ch. 22).

The small-for-gestational-age (SGA) baby

There are two broad types of SGA baby, each exhibiting different intrauterine growth curves.

Asymmetrical growth retardation

This is due to intrauterine 'malnutrition' and shows relative sparing of length and head circumference compared with body weight.

Causes include:

- Placental insufficiency
- Pre-eclampsia
- Hypertension
- Renal disease
- Long-standing diabetes mellitus
- Smoking
- Altitude
- Multiple pregnancy.

Symmetrical growth retardation

All three growth measurements are reduced.

Causes include:

- Constitutional
- Early intrauterine infection
- Chromosomal abnormality
- Skeletal abnormality
- Fetal alcohol syndrome.

Problems

SGA infants have higher rates of morbidity than infants who are appropriate for gestational age, partly because of the greater incidence of congenital abnormalities and congenital infection.

Other major problems in these babies include:

- ≺ Hypoglycaemia (poor hepatic glycogen stores)
- ≺ Polycythaemia (caused by chronic intrauterine hypoxia)
- ≺ Coagulation disorders (hepatic disturbance)
- ≺ Pulmonary haemorrhage (promoted by hypothermia, hypoglycaemia and coagulation disorders).

Management

➤ At birth give vitamin K and assess for congenital malformations and intrauterine infection.

➤ Measure capillary glucose and packed cell volume (haematocrit) on all SGA infants on admission to the neonatal unit.

➤ If blood glucose <2.6 mmol/l (45 mg/dl) treat for hypoglycaemia. About 60% of preterm SGA infants and 30% of term SGA infants will develop hypoglycaemia.

➤ Maintain blood sugar above 2.6 mmol/l (45 mg/dl) with intravenous 10% dextrose by infusion (not as bolus, as this will stimulate insulin production).

➤ Polycythaemia may occur and is defined as venous packed cell volume of over 65%. Partial exchange transfusion with plasma or 5% albumin should be considered for all infants with venous packed cell volume over 70%, or for symptomatic infants with packed cell volume over 65% (see pp. 351).

➤ For infants whose birthweight is below the 3rd percentile measure coagulation (prothrombin time and partial thromboplastin time) and give fresh frozen plasma 10 ml/kg if prothrombin time is >20 s and partial thromboplastin time >70 s.

Long-term follow-up is indicated for both the preterm and the SGA infant (see Ch. 23).

Nursing points

Baby

● All neonatal staff should take care to avoid iatrogenic injuries to neonates:
　careful positioning of babies to prevent postural problems developing
　reduction of noise and light levels in the NICU
　skin is thin and friable: care is needed when attaching and removing leads and in choice of strapping or tape used, close monitoring of infusion sites for early signs of extravasation.

● Intervention should be kept to a minimum; the benefits of procedures must outweigh their costs.

- SGA babies have poor glycogen stores in the liver. Blood glucose test strips should be performed at least 3 hourly to detect hypoglycaemia.
- Small babies have a large surface area and little subcutaneous fat. Close attention is needed to maintaining their temperature.
- Regular recordings of weight and occipitofrontal head circumference should be plotted on the appropriate percentile chart.

Family

- The family should be involved in the care of the baby whenever possible. Siblings have an important role to play.
- Keep parents informed of the condition of their baby and of any changes, or planned changes, to care.
- It is important that neonatal staff are honest with parents about the prognosis for their baby.

Equipment

- Servo-controlled incubators and continuous monitoring of heart rate, respiration rate and blood pressure reduce the need for frequent handling.
- Dressing the baby in warm clothing not only aids temperature control but may also enhance the appearance of a very small baby to his family.
- Equipment must be regularly changed and cleaned to reduce infection risks.

Staff

- Good communication between staff is vital to ensure consistency of information given to the family.

References and further reading

Amiel-Tison C (1968). Neurological evaluation of the maturity of newborn infants. *Arch Dis Child* **43**: 89.

Ballard JL, Khoury JC, Wedig K, *et al* (1991). New Ballard score, expanded to include extremely premature infants. *J Pediatr* **119**: 417.

Dornan JC, Halliday HL (1988). Preterm birth. In: *Perinatal Medicine* (eds, McClure G, Halliday HL, Thompson W). London: Bailliere Tindall.

Dubowitz LM, Dubowitz V, Goldberg C (1970). Clinical assessment of gestational age in the newborn infant. *J Pediatr* **77**: 1.

Halliday HL, McClure G, Ritchie JWK (1988). Intrauterine growth retardation. In: *Perinatal Medicine* (eds, McClure G, Halliday HL, Thompson W). London: Bailliere Tindall.

Keen DV, Pearse RG (1988). Weight, length, and head circumference curves for boys and girls of between 20 and 42 weeks' gestation. *Arch Dis Child* **63**: 1170.

Polin RA, Fox WW (eds) (1992). *Fetal and Neonatal Physiology*, Vols 1 and 2. Philadelphia: WB Saunders.

Taeusch WH, Ballard RA, Avery ME (eds) (1991). *Schaffer and Avery's Diseases of the Newborn*, 6th edn. Philadelphia: WB Saunders.

Whitelaw A, Cooke RWI (1988). The very immature infant: less than 28 weeks' gestation. *British Medical Bulletin*, Vol. 44. Edinburgh: Churchill Livingstone for British Council.

Wilcox M, Gardosi J, Mongelli M, Ray C, Johnson I (1993). Birth weight from pregnancies dated by ultrasonography in a multicultural British population. *Br Med J* **307**: 588.

7 The Big Baby

Large for gestational age (LGA): babies whose birth weight >90th percentile for gestational age (see Appendix VIII).

Post-term (prolonged pregnancy): babies whose gestational age exceeds 42 weeks.

Postmaturity: This refers to the appearance of the baby from a prolonged pregnancy who shows signs of growth retardation: dry, cracked, meconium-stained skin, alert (old man) appearance and signs of recent weight loss.

Causes of big babies:

- Constitutionally large
- Maternal diabetes mellitus or gestational diabetes
- Severe erythroblastosis
- Other causes of hydrops (see below)
- Prolonged pregnancy
- Transposition of the great arteries
- Beckwith's syndrome
- Nesidioblastosis
- Sotos, Marshall and Weaver syndromes

About 1.6% of babies weigh >4.5 kg and the incidence has increased over the past decade. Less than 50% are diagnosed before birth. Big babies may have problems related to their size, to prolonged pregnancy or associated with the underlying causes.

Problems

Obstetric trauma

Shoulder dystocia — Erb's palsy, fractured clavicle

Fractured skull or long bones
Subdural haemorrhage
Bruising

Prolonged pregnancy

Birth asphyxia
Meconium aspiration
Hypoglycaemia
Polycythaemia
Coagulation defects

Other

Congenital anomalies
Jaundice (from bruising)

Causes of Hydrops Fetalis:

- Rhesus isoimmunization

- Homozygous α-thalassaemia

- Chronic fetomaternal haemorrhage

- Cardiac failure:
   congenital heart disease
   supraventricular tachycardia

- Hypoproteinaemia:
   congenital nephrotic syndrome
   renal vein thrombosis
   congenital hepatitis

- Intrauterine infection:
   syphilis
   TORCH
   parvovirus

- Other:
   umbilical vein thrombosis
   fetal neuroblastoma
   placental chorioangioma

- Skeletal dysplasia.

Nursing points

Baby

- Observations required for big babies will depend on their condition. For example:

  Infants of diabetic mothers are at greatest risk of hypoglycaemia between 2 and 8 hours of age. Early and regular feeding is important. 3-hourly blood glucose monitoring should be carried out during this period.

  Babies with Beckwith's syndrome need careful attention to their airway as they may develop respiratory embarrassment due to their large tongue.

- Gestational age of the baby should be remembered when planning care as large babies may be perceived as stronger or more mature than they actually are.

Family

- Parents of big babies often feel they look out of place on the NICU, even if they are preterm. Careful explanation of their condition is needed.

Equipment

- Large babies are often nursed in open incubators or cots, making them more accessible to staff and parents. They may still benefit from minimal handling.

Staff

- Communication between the hospital and community staff must ensure information regarding admission to the NICU is shared.
- Parents may need extra support or still consider their baby vulnerable on discharge home.

References and further reading

Nocon JJ, McKenzie DK, Thomas LJ, Hansell RS (1993). Shoulder dystocia: an analysis of risks and obstetric maneuvers. *Am J Obstet Gynecol* **168:** 1732.

Stevenson DK, Hopper AO, Cohen RS *et al* (1982). Macrosomia: causes and consequences. *J Pediatr* **100:** 515.

8 Basic Principles of Neonatal Intensive Care

Basic principles of neonatal intensive care are to support physiological processes by:

Anticipation
Prevention
Detection
Early correction
Minimal disturbance

The aim of neonatal intensive care is to provide life support and vital-signs monitoring in a controlled, stable environment, with minimal upset to the ill infant. This environment should be clean, warm and friendly. Every effort should be made to accommodate parents and their needs and to involve them in the care of their baby.

Hygienic environment

Nosocomial infection is transmitted by the hands of staff members and by use of communal equipment. The hands of the medical and nursing attendants, and all equipment that is used to treat the newborn, should be scrupulously clean. Hands and forearms should be washed after removing rings and watches and rolling up sleeves before and after handling each infant. The risk of cross-infection is increased with overcrowding of infants in the unit and at times of staff shortage.

Staff or visitors with or recovering from an infectious illness, such as respiratory infection, gastroenteritis, active herpes simplex lesions (before crusting) or boils, should be excluded from the nursery. Mothers with infected wounds or with pathogens in vaginal swab should be admitted after careful hand washing. Infected infants should be isolated. Invasive techniques such as intravascular cannulation (see Ch. 9) should be carried out under full aseptic conditions.

Temperature control

Temperature balance is precarious in babies.

Heat production is limited because of:

- Reduced physical activity
- Absence of shivering
- Reduced non-shivering thermogenesis due to poor stores of brown fat

Heat losses are increased because of:

- Large surface area to body ratio
- Reduced subcutaneous fat for insulation
- Limited central control of body temperature.

The newborn is able to maintain body temperature over quite a narrow range so it is important to reduce energy consumption by nursing in a neutral thermal environment (NTE). The NTE is defined as that range of environmental temperature over which heat production, oxygen consumption and nutritional requirements for growth are minimal provided body temperature is normal. The NTE will vary according to the maturity of the infant and whether he is nursed clothed in an incubator or naked under a radiant warmer. For the first 12–24 hours, it is common practice to treat babies under a radiant warmer as this allows easy access with minimal environmental disruption. The servo-control should be set to maintain skin temperature at 36.5°C.

When a baby is treated in an incubator, the guidelines in Table 8.1 should be followed regarding its temperature.

The incubator temperature should be lowered by 1°C each week, and at about 1600 g weight the baby can be moved into an open cot. Rapid lowering of environmental temperature should be avoided as this can lead to apnoea.

Table 8.1. Neutral thermal environment (NTE) during first 3 days

Birth weight (g)	Incubator temperature (°C)
1000	35
1500	34
2000	33.5
2500	33.2
3000	33
4000	32.5

After Scopes and Ahmed (1966), and Hey and Katz (1970).

Disadvantages of servo-control include:
   Loss of thermal instability as an indication of sepsis
   Overheating — detachment of probe

Avoid radiant heater after 12–24 hours because prolonged use leads to:

   Increased insensible water losses
   Electrolyte upsets, increased bilirubin levels
   Tendency to overhandle the infants

Measures to reduce heat loss in babies include:

➤ Maintainenance of room temperature of the neonatal unit at 24–25°C and draught free.

➤ Use of a woollen hat reduces radiant heat loss from the baby's relatively large head.

➤ Dressing the baby, provided it does not interfere with observation and monitoring.

➤ High incubator humidity should be used in very immature babies of 28 weeks and less.

➤ Use of heat shields and double-walled incubators minimizes radiant heat loss.

Hypothermia (<35.5°C) should be avoided as it causes:

- Increased oxygen consumption
- Vasoconstriction and acidosis
- Increased free fatty acid production (may displace bilirubin from albumin)
- Hypoglycaemia
- Coagulation disorders
- Persistent fetal circulation
- Decreased surfactant production.

Hyperthermia should be avoided in the immature infant as it may cause:

- Apnoea or tachypnoea
- Tachycardia
- Restlessness.

The usual cause of hyperthermia is overheating of the environment but it may occur as a result of loss of temperature control in neonatal sepsis, brain injury or drug therapy.

Sweating does not occur but the baby may lie in an extended 'sun-bathing' posture.

Oxygen therapy

The primary aim of oxygen therapy is to maintain oxygen saturation measured by pulse oximetry at 89–95% (depending upon the baby and the oximeter) or at normal or 'safe' arterial oxygen tensions:

Mature infant	7–10 kPa	(53–75 mmHg)
Immature infant (<1500 g)	6–9 kPa	(45–68 mmHg)

Oxygen is a dangerous drug and should not be used without a specific indication such as cyanosis, respiratory distress or a low PaO_2. Oxygen free radical disease in the newborn is a concept with growing support. In the preterm newborn it has been associated with retinopathy of prematurity and bronchopulmonary dysplasia. Atelectasis can also occur after nitrogen washout (resorption atelectasis).

The inspired oxygen concentration (FiO_2) must be constantly measured and the oxygen must be warmed and humidified before entering the incubator or headbox. Record amount of oxygen as a concentration (%) not a flow in l/min.

 Maintain constant oxygen concentrations at all times – care must be taken during suctioning or feeding to ensure that hypoxaemia does not occur.

Episodes of hypoxaemia have been shown to correlate with both retinopathy of prematurity and outcome.

⊞ Retinopathy of prematurity (ROP)

The aetiology of ROP is complex and many factors have been implicated.

Aetiological factors in ROP:

- Gestational age and low birth weight
- Genetic factors
- Multiple births
- Congenital anomalies
- Blood transfusions
- Vitamin E deficiency
- Vitamin A deficiency
- Hypoxia and hyperoxia
- Hyper- and hypocarbia
- Acidosis and alkalosis
- Infections
- Drugs: indomethacin, dexamethasone, theophylline
- Bright light
- Antepartum haemorrhage
- β-blockers in pregnancy
- Periventricular haemorrhage/periventricular leucomalacia.

Oxygen therapy has been identified as a major factor but the time and duration of high oxygen tension required to cause ROP are unknown.

In ROP, marked retinal vascoconstriction occurs which may be followed by new vascular proliferation if there has been retinal ischaemia. This in turn leads to fibrosis, scarring and retinal detachment (Table 8.2).

Table 8.2. **International classification of retinopathy of prematurity**

Stage No.	Characteristic
1	Demarcation line
2	Ridge
3	Ridge with extraretinal fibrovascular proliferation
4	Subtotal retinal detachment
	(a) extrafoveal
	(b) retinal detachment including fovea
5	Total retinal detachment
	Funnel: Anterior Posterior
	open open
	narrow narrow
	open narrow
	narrow open

All babies of <32 weeks or <1250 g should have their eyes examined by an ophthalmologist before discharge or transfer back to the referring hospital. The earliest changes of ROP are not seen until 6 weeks after birth and repeat examinations are necessary for oxygen-dependent babies. The incidence of ROP in the UK is lower than that reported from the USA (10–20% versus 30–40%) and the difference may be partly due to classification. There is disputed evidence that large prophylactic doses of vitamin E (100 mg) may reduce the incidence of ROP. The most important recent advance has been the demonstration that cryotherapy prevents progression of ROP and improves long-term visual outcome. Laser therapy is now more widely used than cryotherapy. These treatments are begun when stage 3 plus disease is found.

> **!** Retinopathy of prematurity is related to high arterial oxygen tensions, not high environmental oxygen concentrations. There is no safe lower limit of oxygen concentration for a preterm infant.

Monitoring

To ensure a constant environment for the ill infant undergoing neonatal intensive care, various measurements are monitored either continuously or intermittently:

- Heart rate and variability (continuously)
- Respiration rate and pattern (continuously)
- Temperature: skin temperature (continuously) and core temperature (axillary or rectal) intermittently, about 4-hourly
- Blood gases: arterial (intermittently, about 4-hourly), transcutaneously or by pulse oximetry (continuously)
- Glucose strip test/blood glucose (intermittently, about 4-hourly)
- Electrolytes and urea (intermittently, at least once daily)
- Calcium (intermittently, at least once daily)
- Bilirubin (intermittently, usually at least 12-hourly for the first 5 days)
- Packed cell volume (intermittently, at least daily)
- Blood pressure (6-hourly or continuously)
- For babies having parenteral nutrition see p. 190.

Cardiorespiratory monitors should be used to monitor heart rate and respiration rate continuously in all ill infants undergoing intensive care. This continuous monitoring detects and records any attacks of apnoea and bradycardia that occur in the spontaneously breathing infant. Periodic respiration will also be detected. Reduced long-term heart rate variability (<5 beats/min) is highly predictive of the severity and outcome of respiratory distress syndrome. Persistent reduction in long-term variability is associated with increased mortality of all babies undergoing intensive care.

Most blood gases are sampled from indwelling umbilical or radial arterial catheters (see Ch. 9). When arterial cannulation is contraindicated or has failed, measure arterial blood gases by intermittent arterial puncture of the radial artery (see Ch. 9).

The introduction of transcutaneous oxygen tension monitoring and pulse oximetry has been of great benefit. Carbon dioxide tensions however cannot be measured as reliably and tissue pH measurement is not yet perfected.

Blood gases

Transcutaneous oxygen monitoring

Measures oxygen tension using a skin electrode heated to 42–44°C to obtain adequate capillary blood flow to the skin.

Accuracy is *improved* at:
  High PaO_2 levels
  Higher electrode temperatures

Accuracy is *reduced* by:
  Hypotension or poor perfusion
  Age >30 days

The monitor should be recalibrated every 8 hours and the electrode site changed at least every 4 hours to reduce the risk of contact burns (see Ch. 9).

Pulse oximetry

Measures oxyhaemoglobin saturation using an infrared light and a photodetector positioned over an artery (see Ch. 9). Does not require heating therefore there is no risk of contact burns but there is a risk of pressure necrosis if velcro is too tight. Requires a knowledge of the oxygen–haemoglobin dissociation curve (Fig. 10.1).

 In a baby with saturation >92% the pulse oximeter will be less sensitive in identifying an unacceptably high PaO_2.

Accuracy is *reduced* by:
  Hypotension, or poor perfusion
  Movement artefact
  Exposure to direct high intensity light
  Methaemoglobinaemia

 Transcutaneous oxygen and pulse oximetry should not replace direct measurement of arterial oxygen tension. Correlate with PaO_2 measurements every 8–12 hours.

In some infants with chronic respiratory disease, arterialized capillary blood is used to measure blood gases (see Ch. 9). With proper warming of the heel and a free flow of blood the values for pH, $PaCO_2$ and PaO_2 obtained reflect fairly closely those of arterial blood (Table 8.3).

Up to PaO_2 7 kPa (53 mmHg), there is one-to-one relationship between arterial and arterialized capillary blood.

Normal blood gas values in the newborn are shown in Table 8.3. pH and $PaCO_2$ are slightly lower than the normal values in adults. Fig. 8.1 shows the change in blood gas values over the first 3 days of life. Table 8.4 shows typical blood gas values in situations of acidosis and alkalosis.

Table 8.3. Normal blood gas values

	pH	$PaCO_2$ kPa (mmHg)	PaO_2 kPa (mmHg)	Base excess	Standard bicarbonate (mmol/l)
Arterial	7.30–7.40	4.5–5 (34–38)	7–11 (53–83)	0 to –2	20–22
Capillary	7.28–7.38	4.5–5 (34–38)	5–7 (38–53)	–2 to –4	16–22
Venous	7.25–7.30	5–6.5 (38–49)	3.5–5.5 (27–42)	–4 to –6	13–20
Arterialized Capillary	7.30–7.40	4.5–5 (34–38)	7 (53)	0 to –2	20–22

Table 8.4. Abnormal arterial blood gas values

	pH	PaCO$_2$ kPa (mmHg)	PaO$_2$ kPa (mmHg)	Base excess	Standard bicarbonate (mmol/l)
Respiratory acidosis (with hypoxaemia)	7.25	7.5 (56)	5 (38)	–2	23
Metabolic acidosis	7.25	4.5 (34)	9 (68)	–11	15
Mixed acidosis (with hypoxaemia)	7.20	7 (53)	6 (45)	–7	19
Respiratory alkalosis	7.50	3.5 (26)	12 (90)	–2	22
Metabolic alkalosis	7.50	5 (38)	9 (68)	+6	30

Causes of respiratory acidosis are:

- Alveolar hypoventilation: e.g. RDS, respiratory depression, asphyxia, pneumonia, pneumothorax
- Alveolar – capillary block: e.g. RDS, pneumonia

Causes of metabolic acidosis are:

- Hypoxia and shock
- Infection
- Patent ductus arteriosus and cardiac failure
- Excessive protein intake, parenteral nutrition or starvation
- Hyperchloraemia (p. 206)
- Diarrhoea
- Renal failure, renal tubular acidosis, amino acidurias, organic acidurias, congenital lactic acidosis.

In severe respiratory distress syndrome, asphyxia and pneumonia, there is usually a mixed metabolic and respiratory acidosis.

Treatment of respiratory acidosis is by improvement of alveolar

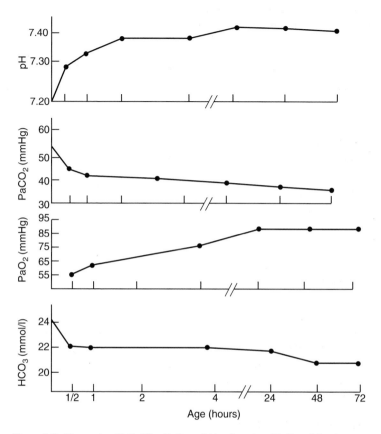

Figure 8.1. Change in pH, PaCO₂, PaO₂ and bicarbonate with time following birth. After Klaus and Fanaroff (1979).

ventilation with assisted ventilation. In metabolic acidosis the underlying cause should be sought and corrected. If shock is present, a blood or plasma transfusion should be given. Bicarbonate solutions are administered to correct metabolic acidosis where the pH is <7.25 and the base excess >−10, provided shock is not present (correct shock first).

Causes of metabolic alkalosis are:

- Hypochloraemia (p. 206)
- Excessive bicarbonate therapy

- Hypokalaemia (p. 206)
- Post-hypercarbia
- Phosphate excess
- Post-exchange transfusion.

In neonatal intensive care, respiratory alkalosis is more common than metabolic alkalosis and is usually due to over-zealous mechanical ventilation. The ventilator settings should be reduced (see Ch. 9) as marked respiratory alkalosis (pH >7.50, $PaCO_2$ <2.5 kPa (19 mmHg)) may be hazardous as it is associated with severe reduction in both cerebral blood flow and cardiac output.

Continuous EEG monitoring

Continuous EEG monitoring is now considered important in the high-risk newborn for the detection of seizures, especially in the paralysed infant and in prediction of eventual outcome.

Two methods of providing a cot-side display of EEG are available:

Cerebral function monitor (CFM) records amplitude integrated EEG

Density spectral array records frequency distribution and power using power spectral analysis

Indications:

◁ Infants with asphyxia

◁ Suspect seizures: includes infants with atypical symptoms such as apnoea in a term infant

◁ Prematures with severe RDS — requiring ventilation.

◁ Very ill infants, e.g. septicaemia, meningitis, hypotension and hypoglycaemia.

Nursing points

Baby

- Care should centre around the needs of individual babies, not a system whereby procedures are performed routinely and their necessity not questioned.

- Care must be taken to ensure babies do not sustain injuries or problems as a result of care given, e.g. reflex bradycardia from over-vigorous suctioning, infection from poor hygiene or tissue damage from extravasation of infusions.

Family

- NICU should be as welcoming as possible to families; consideration needs to be given to the decor, furnishings, layout and routines. Facilities for making tea and coffee, a quiet room away from the main unit and a play area for siblings are important.
- The needs of families from all cultures, beliefs and religions should be considered. A translator may be required to ensure parents fully understand events, to enable them to ask questions and explain their wishes.
- A team-nursing approach allows continuity of care and enables families to identify closely with a small number of staff.
- Explanation of all equipment used should be given to parents.
- The importance of strict hand washing and hygiene must be emphasized to all visitors.
- Parents should be taught how to position their baby correctly in cots and incubators, to prevent postural defects developing.

Equipment

- Non-invasive, continuous monitoring should be used wherever possible.
- NICU policies should give guidelines about how frequently equipment needs changing and cleaning.

Staff

- Recommended staffing levels relevant to the number of intensive and special care cots on NICU should be adhered to. The Royal College of Paediatrics and Child Health lays down guidelines for NICUs in the UK.
- Each NICU should have an orientation course for new staff and ongoing education opportunities.

References and further reading

Commmittee for the Classification of ROP (1984). The International classification of ROP. *Pediatrics* **74:** 127.

Cryotherapy for Retinopathy of Prematurity Co-operative Group (1990). Multicentre trial of cryotherapy for retinopathy of prematurity: one year outcome – structure and function. *Arch Ophthalmol* **108:** 1408.

Hey, EN, Katz G (1970). The optimal thermal environment for naked babies. *Arch Dis Child* **45:** 328.

Klaus M (1972). Respiratory function and pulmonary disease in the newborn. In *Pediatrics* 15 edn. (ed., Barnett H), pp. 1255–61. New York: Appleton-Century-Crofts.

Scopes JW, Ahmed I (1966). Range of critical temperatures in sick and premature newborn babies. *Arch Dis Child* **41:** 417.

Speidel BD (1978). Adverse effects of routine procedures on preterm infants. *Lancet* **i:** 864.

9 Procedures in Neonatal Intensive Care

Ill infants may deteriorate with even minimal handling. Balance cost-to-benefit ratio in all situations before performing a procedure.

Before performing any procedure on an infant:
    Ensure the procedure is necessary
    Prepare equipment needed in advance
    Decide if local/systemic analgesia is required

During any procedure ensure that the baby is kept warm and monitor for deleterious effects.

 Do not undertake a procedure unless you have performed it satisfactorily under supervision on several occasions.

Bag and mask ventilation

Most commonly used method of emergency assisted ventilation.

Resuscitation bags are of two types.

Anaesthetic bags

Contain an inflatable gas reservoir which is refilled between breaths. This type of bag and mask is often necessary for resuscitation as others generate insufficient pressures.

Advantages:
    Ability to generate high pressure
    Can provide high oxygen concentrations

Disadvantages:
> More difficult to use
> Delivery of high pressure with risk of pneumothorax

Self-inflating bags

Are independent of an external oxygen or compressed air source.

Advantages:
> Simplicity of use
> Function if oxygen supply fails

Disadvantages:
> Unable to generate high pressures needed if lungs very non-compliant
> Cannot deliver end-expiratory pressure

Technique

➤ Place infant on firm surface, briefly aspirate airway if secretions present.

➤ Place infants head in 'sniffing' position avoiding over-extension

➤ Choose mask of correct size — preferably clear, soft and circular.

➤ Place mask firmly over mouth and nose, ensuring it does not press on the eyes or overhang the chin.

➤ Allow 4–5 l/min flow

➤ Set blow-off valve (anaesthetic bag only).

➤ Insufflate lungs at rate of 30–40 breaths/min.

This should result in:
> Good chest wall movement
> Good air entry on auscultation
> Improved colour

If air entry is poor and little chest movement:

➤ Insufficient pressure: tighten blow-off valve slightly.

➤ Airway blocked: inspect with laryngoscope and aspirate.

➤ Correct position of neck: avoid flexion or over-extension.

If still no improvement, intubate (see below).

Intubation of the trachea

Indications:

≺ Resuscitation

≺ Removal of meconium or thick secretions from airway

≺ Apnoea

≺ Respiratory failure.

Intubation may be performed by the oral or nasal route. Both methods have advantages and disadvantages (Table 9.1).

Table 9.1. Advantages and disadvantages of oral and nasal routes

	Oral intubation	Nasal intubation
Advantages	Speed in emergency	Ease of stabilization
Disadvantages	Difficult to stabilize	More difficult skill to acquire
	Trauma to palate	Trauma to nasal septum

Oral intubation should therefore be used for resuscitation and emergencies, whereas many units prefer nasal intubation for prolonged mechanical ventilation.

Technique

➤ Check equipment

laryngoscope — straight blade: size 1 term; size 0 preterm
suction apparatus
bag and mask, and bag and tube connector.

➤ Select and prepare appropriate size of tube (Table 9.2). For oral intubation an introducer is sometimes needed. Curve distal end ensuring tip of introducer does not protrude beyond the end of the tube. If using a curved, shouldered Cole's type tube an introducer is not necessary. For nasal intubation cut tube to appropriate length (Table 9.2) and smear tip with lubricating jelly.

➤ Place infant on firm surface (in incubator or under radiant warmer) with head raised into 'sniffing position'.

➤ Pre-ventilate by bag and mask for 30 s.

➤ Gently insert laryngoscope, held in left hand into the baby's mouth keeping in midline.

➤ Gently pull tongue and epiglottis forwards by lifting the blade and cords should come into view — do *not* rotate blade to use as a lever as this will damage the gingival margin. Gentle pressure on the larynx with the fourth finger of the left hand may be needed to bring cords into view.

➤ Aspirate airway if necessary

➤ Pass tube into right side of mouth and advance gently through cords to about 2 cm below glottis, or if using a Cole's tube, as far as the shoulder. For nasal intubation pass tube through nose; keep tip angled medially and along floor of nose. When tube is visible in pharynx, use Magill forceps to direct it through the cords.

➤ Gently insufflate lungs and auscultate chest to check tube position.

Table 9.2. Tube sizes for neonatal intubation

Infant's weight (g)	Tube diameter (mm)	Distance from anterior nares to mid trachea (cm)*
500–750	2.5	7.5
750–1250	2.5–3.0	8.5
1250–2000	3.0–3.5	9.5
2000–2500	3.5	10.5
2500–4000	3.5–4.0	11.0–12.0

* Allow 2 cm extra for tube fixation. Tube should be 1 cm above carina which is usually visible on X-ray.
After Coldiron (1968).

Tube is in *correct* position if:
   Chest moves both sides
   Air entry good on auscultation
   Heart rate increases
   Colour improves

If tube is too far in, it will usually pass into right main bronchus reducing air entry and chest movement on the left.

 Do not make repeated attempts at intubation. Maintain infant with bag and mask ventilation and seek help from senior staff.

Fixation of endotracheal tube

Following intubation the endotracheal tube should be fixed securely to prevent accidental extubation.

Methods of fixation include:
   Oral plate
   Plastic holder
   Cotton tapes
   Strong elastoplast

If using elastoplast paint tincture of benzoin on tube and infant's skin before applying tape to ensure proper adherence of tape.

After fixation of endotracheal tube perform chest X-ray to ensure tip of tube is placed satisfactorily, approximately 1–2 cm above the carina.

 Method of endotracheal tube fixation should allow full movement of infant's head.

Care of endotracheal tube

This is one of the most important nursing procedures in neonatal intensive care.

Endotracheal tubes should be aspirated as dictated by the infant's condition. Infants with pneumonia may require aspiration more frequently than those with RDS, who do not usually need tube care for at least 24 hours after birth.

Technique

➤ Prepare equipment:
  sterile suction catheter of appropriate size
  sterile glove
  sterile normal saline
  suction apparatus.

➤ Instill 0.25–0.5 ml sterile saline into endotracheal tube if needed to facilitate removal of secretions

➤ Manually ventilate the infant for 30 s and reconnect to ventilator — increasing FiO_2 if clinically indicated by oximetry or transcutaneous monitor.

➤ Pass suction catheter down endotracheal tube to measured length using aseptic technique.

➤ Occlude suction hole and using continuous suction withdraw catheter steadily. The whole procedure should not take longer than 5–10 s.

➤ Reventilate infant and assess if further suction is required.

Continuous positive airway pressure (CPAP)

The effects of CPAP are to increase functional residual capacity (FRC) and induce more regular breathing. Work of breathing is usually lessened but may be increased if resistance in system is high. Although compliance, minute volume and tidal volume are decreased, PaO_2 rises as a result of decreased intrapulmonary shunting. Sometimes $PaCO_2$ is increased, especially if CPAP pressures above 8–10 cmH_2O are used.

Indications:

◄ Respiratory distress syndrome
◄ Recurrent apnoea

≺ Post extubation
≺ Pulmonary oedema.

CPAP may be applied by several methods:
    Endotracheal tube
    Nasal prongs
    Nasopharyngeal tube

Advantage of nasal-prong and nasopharyngeal CPAP is ease of application for low and medium pressure CPAP. Their *disadvantages* include difficulty in achieving pressure >8 cm H_2O, gastric distension and instability in large active infants.

Advantages of endotracheal CPAP are stability of the system, use of higher pressures if needed and the ability to change to IPPV instantly. *Disadvantages* are it is more difficult to apply and complications include those associated with intubation, such as tube blockage and infection.

> **!** CPAP should only be undertaken in neonatal units where IPPV can be used if respiratory failure develops.

Mechanical ventilation

Ventilators

Positive pressure ventilators may be either pressure controlled or volume controlled.

Pressure-controlled ventilators deliver a volume of gas at a constant pressure to the lung during the set inspiration. This type of ventilator is the most commonly used and has the advantage of achieving peak inspiratory pressure (PIP) rapidly with improved patient–ventilator synchrony.

Volume-controlled ventilators deliver the same preset tidal volume with each breath inflating the lungs only at the peak of inspiration. They are less commonly used but with improved inbuilt monitoring are now finding a role.

Settings

Flow rate: Normal setting of 6–12 l/min.

Start at 5–7 l/min and increase to achieve higher pressure settings.

Always use minimum required to achieve PIP as high flow increases airway resistance and may overdistend the lung.

FiO_2: Select FiO_2 0.05 higher than before ventilation.

Peak inspiratory pressure (PIP):

Defined as maximum desired pressure during each ventilation cycle.

Main determinant of tidal volume when using pressure-controlled ventilators.

Set at minimum pressure required to achieve chest movement with adequate air entry on auscultation in order to reduce complications from barotrauma.

Positive end-expiratory pressure (PEEP):

Defined as baseline pressure during expiration.

Minimum 'physiological' PEEP is 2 cmH_2O.

Effects are similar to CPAP with improvement in ventilation and oxygenation.

Start at levels of 4–7 cmH_2O. $PaCO_2$ may rise with increasing PEEP.

Ventilator rate:

Major effect on minute volume and thus $PaCO_2$.

Maximum rate on conventional ventilators is usually 150 breaths/min. Initial setting may vary from 20-100 bpm depending on gestational age of infant and underlying disease. Usually altered by changing the expiratory time.

Ratio of inspiratory to expiratory time (I:E ratio):

Normally ratios of 1: 1 to 1: 3 are used.

Reversed ratios with a prolonged inspiratory
time (e.g. 3:1) result in improved
oxygenation but are rarely used because of
risk of air leak as a result of air trapping.

Mean airway pressure (MAP):

Changes in flow, PEEP, PIP, inspiratory time
and ventilation rate will alter MAP.

Correlates directly with oxygenation.

High MAP is associated with increased risk of
barotrauma and air leak.

Main ventilator determinants for PaO_2 are FiO_2 and MAP.
Main ventilator determinants for $PaCO_2$ are PIP and ventilator rate.

Ventilator settings suggested in Table 9.3 are an initial guide.
Settings should be altered to obtain synchrony of the infant's respiratory effort with the ventilator by reducing inspiratory time and increasing the rate. If this fails muscle relaxation may be used but is rarely needed for babies <1000 g. Remember increased ventilation may be needed following relaxation as the infant's own efforts may have been contributing significantly to gas exchange.

Table 9.3. Suggested initial ventilator settings

	Infant with normal lungs	RDS infant < 2000 g	RDS infant > 2000 g
FiO_2	As indicated by oximetry	As indicated by oximetry	As indicated by oximetry
PIP (cmH_2O)	14–18	18–25	20–30
PEEP (cmH_2O)	2–3	3–5	3–6
Rate (bpm)	15–25	60–100	40–60
Inspiratory time (T_i) (s)	0.4–0.5	0.3–0.5	0.4–0.6

Monitoring during mechanical ventilation

➤ Arterial blood gases should be checked within 20 min of

starting mechanical ventilation and ventilator settings
adjusted to obtain satisfactory blood gases. Aim to keep
$PaCO_2$ in range of 5–6 kPa (38–45 mmHg) so that pH
remains >7.25 and PaO_2 should be in the range 7–10 kPa
(53–75 mmHg).

➤ Blood gases should be repeated within 30 min of alterations
to ventilator settings.

➤ When ventilation is stable, check blood gases at a minimum
of 4-hourly intervals.

➤ Oxygenation should be monitored continuously using pulse
oximetry and/or transcutaneous PO_2 monitoring (see p. 128).

Ventilatory management of specific respiratory conditions

🔀 Respiratory distress syndrome (RDS)

The aim of ventilation is to expand the lungs early with the lowest pressures possible to reduce the risk of lung damage.

➤ Assess the severity of the lung disease as soon as possible as
early treatment is most effective. This may be done by determining the pressure needed manually to ventilate the lungs,
the amount of oxygen to maintain normal oxygen saturation
and the chest X-ray appearance.

➤ Early initiation of CPAP or early administration of surfactant
reduce the severity of the course of the illness.

➤ Small babies prefer fast ventilator rates which may be necessary to obtain synchrony.

➤ Observe closely for improvement in the infant's condition,
weaning ventilatory support as tolerated.

➤ Wean by first lowering PIP, keeping $PaCO_2$ and pH levels
near the normal range. Then lower rate, keeping inspiratory time constant at approximately 0.4–0.5 s to prevent
air trapping. Inspired oxygen concentration should be
adjusted to keep PaO_2 and oxygen saturation in the normal
range.

✚ Meconium aspiration

A serious condition with high morbidity and mortality. Plugs of meconium result in air trapping and reduced pulmonary gas exchange. Complicated by air leaks and persistent pulmonary hypertension.

➤ In view of air trapping and increased airway resistance ventilate with prolonged expiratory times.

➤ Ensure adequate humidification.

✚ Persistent pulmonary hypertension of the newborn

Increased pulmonary vascular resistance causes R→L shunting, resulting in severe hypoxaemia. Hyperventilation with resultant alkalosis is effective in producing pulmonary vasodilatation but severe hypocarbia should be avoided.

➤ Achieve hyperventilation with low pressure and high rate if possible.

➤ Avoid high PEEP which may increase pulmonary vascular resistance.

➤ Calculate oxygenation index (OI) as a guide to outcome and requirement for ECMO or inhaled nitric oxide (INO):

$$OI = \frac{(MAP)\ (FiO_2) \times 100}{PaO_2}$$

➤ Wean very cautiously to avoid 'flip-flopping'.

✚ Pulmonary interstitial emphysema (PIE)

A major complication of mechanical ventilation resulting from barotrauma.

➤ Ventilate with fast rate and low pressure if possible to reduce barotrauma.

➤ If increased PIP is necessary, reduce inspiratory time to 0.2 s.

➤ High-frequency oscillatory ventilation (HFOV) may be useful (see p. 111).

Complications of mechanical ventilation

Acute complications:

Tube problems:
  trauma to nose, palate, larynx and trachea
  infection
  displacement
  blockage
  kinking

Circuit tubing problems:
  gas leaks
  water obstruction or inhalation
  kinking

Humidifier:
  overheating
  gas leaks
  infections, e.g. pseudomonas

Gas supply:
  failure
  wrong air/oxygen mix

Ventilator:
  failure
  raised pressure — pneumothorax, interstitial
  emphysema

Chronic complications

Airway:
  trauma with deformities of nose
  subglottic stenosis
  tracheal ulceration
  palatal groove

Lungs:
  bronchopulmonary dysplasia
  post-extubation collapse
  bronchial granuloma causing emphysema

Main causes of sudden deterioration on mechanical ventilation:

- Mechanical failure
- Tube blockage or displacement
- Pneumothorax
- Periventricular haemorrhage.

Check ventilator is working, disconnect and manually ventilate infant. If improvement occurs mechanical failure is likely. If no improvement, assess patency of tube and exclude pneumothorax.

If gradual deterioration, think of infection, patent ductus arteriosus or slowly progressive pulmonary interstitial emphysema.

Weaning from the ventilator

This is as important as ventilation therapy itself since the condition of the baby may be made worse by poor weaning. It is made easier by use of intermittent mandatory ventilation (IMV). This allows ventilation rate to be reduced and the infant to breathe between each mechanical ventilation. Patient-triggered ventilation (see p. 111) may be valuable in infants who are difficult to wean by minimizing the work of breathing.

Indications:

≺ Blood gases: $PaCO_2$ <6.5 kPa (50 mmHg)
                       pH >7.3
                       PaO_2 >7 kPa (53 mmHg)
≺ Ventilation: FiO_2 <0.5
                       PIP <25 cmH_2O.

Technique

➤ Prior to weaning ensure muscle relaxants have been discontinued, sedation reduced and maximum caloric intake obtained.

➤ When starting to wean, make small changes, reducing peak pressure first by 1–2 cmH_2O.

➤ Reduce inspired oxygen concentration by 3–5% at a time and ventilator rate by about 5 breaths/min. When lowering ventilation rate remember to adjust I:E ratio so that inspiratory time remains at about 0.4–0.5 s.

➤ Always check blood gases within 30–60 min of each ventilator change to ensure that $PaCO_2$ is not rising.

➤ Endotracheal CPAP can usually be employed when <40% oxygen is required and peak airway pressure is under 15 cmH_2O with low rate ventilation.

➤ Give respiratory stimulants such as aminophylline or caffeine during weaning to improve the chance of successful extubation.

Extubation

Extubation is usually attempted only after a successful period of some hours on endotracheal CPAP. An exception to this rule is the very immature infant who has been ventilated through a 2.5 mm tube, since breathing is difficult due to the high resistance in this narrow tube. Very immature infants may be successfully extubated when they can tolerate intermittent mandatory ventilation (IMV) of 10 breaths/min.

Technique

➤ Avoid feeding infant prior to extubation or empty stomach to prevent vomiting.

➤ Suction nasopharynx well.

➤ Remove tube on inflation to achieve adequate inflation and prevent post-extubation atelectasis.

➤ Place infant in well humidified O_2 hood, with FiO_2 concentration the same as that prior to extubation or if ≤1500 g, place on nasal-prong CPAP to lessen the likelihood of atelectasis.

➤ Half an hour after extubation, sample arterial blood gases.

➤ At 4 hours do a chest X-ray to look for collapse if FiO_2 has increased.

➤ Physiotherapy and gentle suctioning of the upper airways are helpful after extubation only if segmental collapse has occurred and it is tolerated by the infant.

New methods of mechanical ventilation

High frequency ventilation

Recent developments include very high frequency ventilation which is of three types:

1. High-frequency positive-pressure ventilation (60–200 breaths/min) uses conventional ventilators.
2. High-frequency jet ventilation (HFJV) (120–600 breaths/min) — ventilation with small pulses of gas under pressure at very rapid rates delivers very small tidal volumes.
3. High-frequency oscillatory ventilation (HFOV) (400–2400 breaths/min) — ventilation with small volumes of gas moving in and out of the airways resulting from piston- or diaphragm-generated action.

Indications:

≺ Severe pulmonary interstitial emphysema
≺ Intractable air leaks
≺ Intractable respiratory failure not responding to conventional ventilation
≺ Other indications may develop, such as use in very immature infants but trials are still ongoing.

Potential *advantages*:
   Reduction in MAP
   Reduction in air leaks and PIE
   Rapid improvement in ventilation with gradual improvement in oxygenation

Patient-triggered ventilation (PTV)

There are a number of ventilators triggered either by air flow or airway pressure changes. These have high sensitivity, short triggering delay and work without inadvertent PEEP even at fast ventilator rates. PTV is frequently unsuccessful in infants <28 weeks' gestation but for more mature babies may be a useful aid in weaning from the ventilator. They may also have a role in management of the larger baby who 'fights the ventilator'.

Other methods of treatment of respiratory failure

Inhaled nitric oxide (INO)

NO is synthesized in pulmonary endothelium and mediates vasodilatation over a very short period of time (half-life 3–6 s). When bound to haemoglobin, it is inactivated and, therefore, produces pulmonary vasodilatation without systemic effects. Used to treat babies with primary pulmonary hypertension in doses of 6–50 ppm. Nitrogen dioxide (NO_2) and methaemoglobinaemia need to be monitored and more controlled trials are needed to determine the optimal dosage of NO and the duration of therapy in babies with pulmonary hypertension from various causes. In term babies INO reduces the need for ECMO, but there are few trials in preterm babies.

Liquid ventilation

Perfluorocarbon is a vehicle for delivery of dissolved oxygen and removal of CO_2. Studies are ongoing, especially in the USA. May have a role in pulmonary hypoplasia.

ECMO

Extra-corporeal membrane oxygenation is used to treat respiratory failure in mature newborn infants who are unresponsive to other less invasive therapies. It is a form of cardiopulmonary bypass used in infants with severe meconium aspiration syndrome (MAS), pulmonary hypertension, congenital diaphragmatic hernia and RDS provided that the baby is >35 weeks' gestation (>about 2500 g). This high-tech intervention is only available in certain centres so most babies needing it must be transported.

Domiciliary oxygen therapy

Indicated for infants with chronic lung disease.

Equipment

Two supplies of oxygen are required:
1. home-based may be provided by an oxygen concentrator installed in the home or via large cylinders. In the long-term, an oxygen concentrator is often more convenient
2. mobile supply provided by small portable cylinders.
Low flow meter
Nasal cannulae
Monitoring – transcutaneous PaO_2 monitoring or pulse oximetry

Requires close follow-up and monitoring by staff in the community experienced in the use of domicillary oxygen.

Treatment of pneumothorax

Transillumination of the chest

This technique is used to make an immediate diagnosis of pneumothorax. If an infant receiving mechanical ventilation suddenly deteriorates, the chest may be transilluminated using a cold-light source (fibreoptic Minilight) in a semi-darkened room. There will be hyperlucency on the affected side. May not differentiate large from small pneumothorax so chest X-ray may be needed for confirmation.

 Very preterm babies may appear to transilluminate when using fibreoptic light when there is no pneumothorax.

Thoracocentesis

Needle aspiration of a pneumothorax

Immediate aspiration of a tension pneumothorax in a deteriorating infant (cyanosis, tachypnoea, circulatory failure, hypotension) is advisable even before radiographic confirmation. This may be performed with a 21 gauge scalp vein needle connected to a 3-way stop-cock and 20 ml syringe.

Technique

➤ Clean the skin with alcohol and povidone–iodine.

➤ Insert needle through the second intercostal space in the mid-clavicular line on the affected side.

➤ Air should be easily aspirated into the syringe, which can be emptied by turning off the 3-way tap.

➤ Repeat until no more air is obtained.

Chest drain insertion (Fig. 9.1)

There are two sites for insertion of the drain:

> *Anterior*: second or third intercostal space on or just lateral to the mid-clavicular line
>
> *Lateral*: fourth to sixth intercostal space, anterior axillary line

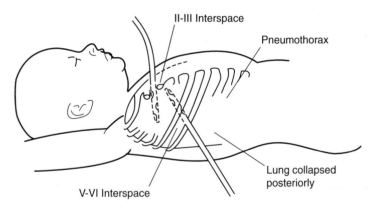

Figure 9.1. Sites for insertion of pleural drains in neonatal pneumothorax. Only one drain is usually necessary (see text).

Technique

➤ Prepare skin with full aseptic technique and infiltrate with 1% lignocaine as a local anaesthetic.

➤ Use 10–12FG pleural catheter (small babies may need 8FG).

➤ Make small incision in skin with scalpel. Blunt dissect through intercostal muscle and pleura with fine forceps.

➤ When approaching laterally rather than anteriorly, position baby on his side and aim the trocar towards the angle of Louis (sternum).

➤ Push and twist tube gently through incision into pleural space.

➤ Connect tube to under-water seal.

➤ Manipulate tube gently so that tip lies anteriorly in thoracic cavity (Fig. 9.1).

➤ Secure tube with suture and apply povidone–iodine cream to puncture site covered by gauze dressing.

➤ Tape tube securely to the chest wall using suitable tape.

➤ Chest radiography (AP and lateral films) to check tube position and resolution of pneumothorax.

➤ Consider applying continuous suction of 10–15 cmH$_2$O.

Removal of chest drain

Technique

The chest drain is removed when the respiratory problem has resolved.

➤ Tubing should be clamped when no bubbling has occurred for 24 hours.

➤ Remove tube 12–24 hours later if the infant's condition is unchanged.

➤ When the drain is removed, close the wound with a fine suture.

➤ Perform chest X-ray 2–4 hours after drain removal.

Arterial catheterization

Indications:

➤ Monitoring of blood gases in infants who require >40% O_2
➤ Continuous monitoring of blood pressure.

Sites used include umbilical, radial, posterior tibial and dorsalis pedis arteries.

Umbilical artery catheterization

Technique

➤ Use smaller (3.5FG or 4FG) catheters for infants <1200 g and larger catheters (5FG) for other infants.

➤ Insertion of an arterial catheter must be performed under full aseptic conditions.

➤ The anterior abdominal wall and cord stump should be gently cleansed with a dilute antiseptic solution (e.g. Savlon, povidone–iodine). Avoid alcoholic solutions, especially under radiant warmers as these can cause skin burns.

➤ Before cutting the umbilical cord, tie a piece of ribbon gauze around the base to control venous bleeding from the end (Fig 9.2b).

➤ Cut the cord at least 1 cm above the abdominal wall.

➤ Hold umbilical stump between finger and thumb or, if too short, use toothed forceps. Identify the arteries as small thick-walled and spiralling vessels in comparison to the larger thin-walled vein located superiorly. Dilate the mouth of one of the arteries using straight or curved iris (ophthalmological) forceps.

➤ Gently insert saline-filled catheter connected to a syringe with 3-way tap into the artery and pass into the aorta (Fig. 9.2b). There may be a flash of blood into the syringe when the artery is entered. Do not push too hard as tip of cannula may penetrate arterial wall.

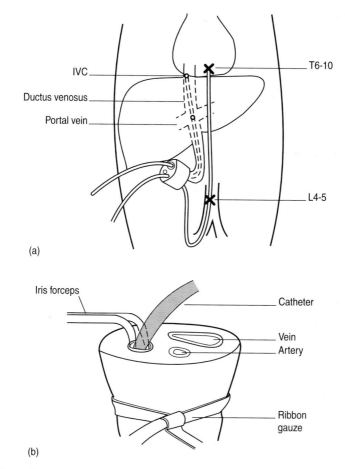

(a)

(b)

Figure 9.2. (a) Sites for umbilical catheter placement. X=arterial; O=venous. (b) Umbilical stump showing catheterization of the artery after dilation with iris forceps. Note the ribbon gauze tied around the base of the stump to prevent bleeding from the umbilical vein.

➤ Immediately after insertion, check legs and buttocks for pallor or blueness and palpate the femoral pulses.

➤ Stitch catheter to the cord stump and tape in 'goal-post' fashion (Fig. 9.3)

➤ Chest X-ray should be taken to confirm catheter position (Fig. 9.2a); ultrasound may also be used. If a catheter is in

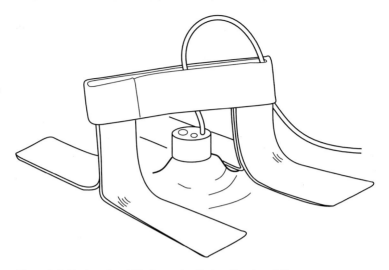

Figure 9.3. Taping of umbilical vessel catheters ('goal posts').

too far (above T5), then it should be withdrawn to below T6. If below T10 then it must either be withdrawn to the lower aorta (L4–L5) or totally replaced under aseptic conditions. Catheters that have been placed below L5 or those passing down the iliac artery should be replaced. *Under no circumstances should a non-sterile catheter be advanced into the umbilical artery.*

➤ After insertion, connect catheter and 3-way tap to an infusion pump delivering 5% dextrose at 0.5–1 ml/h to keep catheter open.

There are two commonly-used positions for catheter placement (Fig. 9.2a):
Lower aorta, below the renal arteries at L4–5
Upper aorta, above the diaphragm at T6–T10.

In general, use the high catheter position for infants <1500 g and the low position for bigger babies. High position allows longer functional use and does not increase risk of necrotizing enterocolitis.

Distance from shoulder to umbilicus is used to calculate the length of catheter that should be inserted to obtain correct placement in the aorta (Table 9.4).

Table 9.4. Umbilical artery catheter positions

Shoulder-umbilicus length (cm)	Umbilicus-lower aorta length (cm)	Umbilicus-upper aorta length (cm)
8	4	10
10	5–6	12
12	6–7	15
14	8	18
16	10	20
18	10–11	22

After Dunn (1966)

Removal

Arterial catheters are removed when regular monitoring is no longer required.

➤ Discontinue infusion for at least 1 hour before removal and close tap to arterial line.

➤ Tie purse string around umbilical stump and remove catheter slowly.

➤ Do *not* cover umbilicus after removal of catheter.

Complications

- Leg and gluteal blanching and cyanosis; if prolonged may lead to necrosis
- Major artery thrombosis: aorta, renal, mesenteric
- Emboli: clot or air
- Infection
- Haemorrhage

If leg or foot becomes pale and ischaemic, or blue, the arterial catheter must be removed immediately. After a while the other umbilical artery may be catheterized.

Radial artery catherization

The radial artery may be catheterized using a 22 gauge intravenous cannula connected to a T-connector. This allows frequent sampling with minimum disturbance to the baby and also measurement of pre-ductus oxygen tensions if the right radial artery is used.

Technique

> ➤ Check for patency of ulnar artery before catheterizing radial artery. Occlude both vessels, if on release of pressure on ulnar artery the hand becomes pink, ulnar flow is adequate (Allen test).

> ➤ Hold infant's hand supine in a neutral position. Palpate radial artery or outline vessel using a fibreoptic light.

> ➤ Cleanse skin and using 22 or 23 gauge intravenous cannula penetrate artery by directing cannula at an angle of approximately 30° to the skin just proximal to the wrist crease (Fig. 9.4).

> ➤ When flash back is obtained advance cannula, withdraw guide needle and connect to extension set.

Intermittent arterial sampling

Radial, posterior tibial or temporal arteries are the preferred sites for intermittent sampling. The temporal artery should *not* be used for permanent catheterization as cerebral embolization can occur. The brachial artery is an end-artery and as such

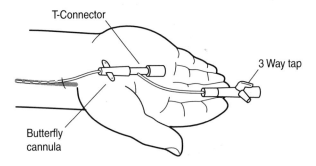

Figure 9.4. Catheterization of the radial artery.

percutaneous puncture is more hazardous. The median nerve may also be inadvertently damaged. Avoid femoral artery puncture as this can damage underlying hip joint.

Radial artery sampling

➤ Palpate radial artery at wrist. In the preterm infant, the vessel may be visible as a blue streak and can be outlined by transillumination.

➤ Before puncturing the radial artery, confirm presence of ulnar artery by palpation (see above). Use 23 or 25 gauge needle attached to 1 ml syringe which has been lightly coated with heparin (1000 units/ml).

➤ Insert needle at angle of 30° to skin surface just proximal to first wrist skin crease (Fig. 9.5). Aspirate a maximum 0.4 ml blood.

➤ Remove needle and cap sample.

➤ Occlude artery with firm pressure for 5 min to prevent haematoma formation.

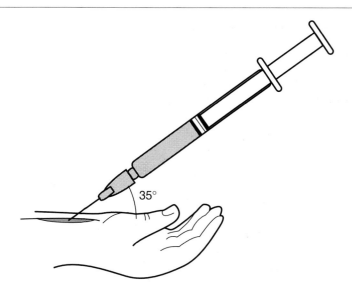

Figure 9.5. Site for intermittent radial artery sampling for blood gases.

Temporal artery sampling

Palpate branches of temporal artery and sample using 25 gauge needle.

Posterior tibial artery sampling

Locate artery midway between medial malleolus and back of Achilles tendon. Hold foot in neutral position. Sample as above.

Dorsalis pedis artery sampling

Hold foot partially plantar flexed. Locate artery between first and second metatarsal. Sample as above.

Venous catheterization

Venous sampling

Use any prominent superficial vein, e.g. antecubital, temporal or back of hand. If silastic line for parenteral nutrition is likely to be required, avoid using the temporal or antecubital veins (Fig. 9.6).

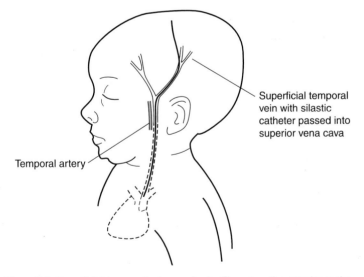

Superficial temporal vein with silastic catheter passed into superior vena cava

Temporal artery

Figure 9.6. Superficial temporal artery and vein. The artery lies anterior to the vein and may be used for intermittent arterial blood gas sampling. A silastic catheter is inserted into the vein and advanced to the superior vena cava.

Blood culture

Full aseptic technique should be used. Do not draw blood for culture from any indwelling catheter.

Use peripheral vein. Do *not* use femoral vein as it is impossible to clean the groin area effectively and the hip joint may be damaged.

Venous infusions

The technique is the same as that for adults. However, in view of the size of the patient, the following should be remembered.

1. Usual site — scalp, forearm, back of hand, foot.
2. Use i.v. cannula of appropriate size (18–26 gauge).
3. Be very gentle when advancing cannula as it is extremely easy to disrupt small veins.

Peripheral silastic catheters

Silastic catheters are often used for:

≺ Intravenous feeding of babies weighing <1000 g
≺ Prolonged parenteral nutrition
≺ Administration of drugs such as dopamine, tolazoline, hypertonic dextrose.

Preferred sites:
   Superficial temporal veins
   Antecubital vein
   Long saphenous vein

Technique

➤ Insert 19 gauge needle in the superficial temporal, antecubital or saphenous veins.
➤ Pass fine silastic catheter (0.635 mm outside diameter) through this needle and advance it to superior vena cava under strict aseptic conditions (Fig. 9.6).

➤ Slip needle back along the catheter and remove and connect catheter to an extension set.

➤ All catheter positions should be confirmed by radiography. If catheter is not radio-opaque, infuse radio-opaque dye prior to X-ray.

Umbilical venous catheterization

Umbilical venous catheterization is rarely used but may be indicated in the following circumstances:

≺ Resuscitation in the labour ward
≺ Exchange transfusion
≺ Blood gas sampling under conditions where arterial catheterization has failed
≺ Emergency volume expansion in collapsed infant.

Technique

Use full aseptic technique as for arterial cannulation.

➤ Locate umbilical vein — large, thin-walled vessel superior to umbilical arteries.

➤ Advance a saline-filled 5F catheter connected to a syringe into the vein for 5–10 cm to reach inferior vena cava. In practice only about 60% of venous catheters will pass through the ductus venosus to the vena cava, the others remaining in the liver or in the portal circulation.

➤ Place catheter tip at either of the two sites shown in Fig. 9.2, i.e. in the inferior vena cava or in the portal sinus (marked o).

Complications
● Infection
● Thrombosis of portal vein
● Pulmonary emboli
● Air embolus

Exchange transfusion

Indications:

◄ Blood group incompatibility, especially Rhesus
◄ Hyperbilirubinaemia from other causes
◄ Sepsis, sclerema or DIC (see p. 237)
◄ Drug intoxication due to diazepam, magnesium sulphate, mepivicaine.

Two techniques can be used.
    Isovolumetric technique
    Single vessel technique

The *isovolumetric technique* using an artery to withdraw blood and simultaneously infusing blood via a vein is the preferred method as it causes less circulatory disturbance. If possible use a peripheral artery and large peripheral vein, but if this is not possible the umbilical vessels may be used.

The *single vessel technique* using the umbilical vein to withdraw and infuse blood serially is now used less often because the risk of circulatory disturbance is greater.

Full aseptic technique should be used. The volume of blood exchanged should be 180 ml/kg (i.e. double blood volume) in order to achieve approx. 90% exchange of the baby's blood. Smaller volumes of blood may be exchanged when performed for conditions other than hyperbilirubinaemia.

Blood for neonatal exchange transfusion should be:
    Plasma-reduced red cells (Hct 0.55–0.60)
    ABO group of neonate
    Rhesus negative
    HIV, HBV, HCV and CMV negative
    HbS screen negative
    < 5 days old and preferably <72 hours
    Irradiated red cells if baby <1500 g.

Use equal amounts of blood warmed to body temperature in and out unless central venous pressure is initially high when a deficit of l0–20 ml may be allowed. In term babies, use 10 ml cycles taking 1–2 min per cycle and in preterm 5 ml taking 1 min per cycle.

Monitoring

➤ Continuous cardiorespiratory monitoring with ECG trace in all infants

➤ Regular measurement of blood pressure

➤ Continuous measurement of body temperature.

At the start of the exchange transfusion, store the first 10 ml of infant's blood for measurement of haemoglobin, bilirubin and red cell enzymes if indicated. At the end of the exchange transfusion, blood should be sent to the laboratory for haemoglobin, total and direct bilirubin, electrolytes, calcium, glucose and blood culture.

Complications

Metabolic acidosis
Hypothermia
Circulatory overload
Electrolyte disturbances: hyperkalaemia, hypernatraemia and
    hypocalcaemia
Acute dilatation of the stomach
Ischaemia of the intestine, perforation or necrotizing
    enterocolitis
Air embolism
Cardiac arrhythmias
Infection
Hypoglycaemia
Thrombocytopenia

Plasma exchange

Indicated for polycythaemia with packed cell volume >70% or >65% if symptoms present (see pp. 351–2). Use peripheral artery and vein if possible; if not, umbilical vein.

Same techniques as for exchange transfusion; volume needed

usually 20 ml/kg (p. 352). Use plasma or 5% salt-poor albumin as donor solution. Remove catheter(s) at end of exchange.

Heel stab

Capillary blood drawn from a heel stab may be used for routine samples if only a small volume of blood is needed.

Technique

➤ The medial part of the heel should be used for the stab (Fig. 9.7). Clean the skin with alcohol and then apply a thin layer of petroleum jelly before puncture to prevent the blood smearing over the skin.

➤ Use a disposable sterile lancet or stylet and insert to a maximum depth of 2 mm. Use of an automatic system has been shown to reduce pain.

➤ Allow blood to drip into collecting bottle.

If heel is warmed to 40°C for 3 min and free-flowing blood is obtained, measurements of pH, PCO_2, and PO_2 up to 7 kPa (53 mmHg) correlate with arterial samples (Table 8.3).

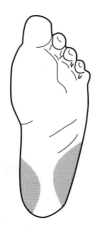

Figure 9.7. Site for heel stab (shaded area). The lancet should be used to pierce the medial aspect of the heel to a depth of 1–2 mm to obtain capillary blood.

Complications

Osteomyelitis of os calcis after deep incision
Tissue atrophy
Inclusion dermoids

Heart and respiration monitoring

Cardiorespiratory monitors pick up ECG trace from two chest leads and a lead on the right leg. The ECG is often displayed on screen and heart rate is shown both digitally and as a continuous trace. Respiration rate is also shown digitally and as a continuous trace. These traces can be stored in memory in small microprocessors for recall of trends. Alarm limits may be set with these monitors so that a heart rate limit of 100–200 beats/min is usual setting and apnoea alarm after 10 s.

Most of these monitors now include modules for pulse oximetry (see p. 129), transcutaneous PO_2 and PCO_2, invasive and non-invasive blood pressure, temperature and even EEG and are appropriate for babies requiring intensive care. Less sophisticated monitors of heart and respiration rate exist and are suitable for babies having high dependency or special care.

Simpler monitors are available to detect 'apnoea' or infant movement, using a compressible capsule attached to the abdominal wall or an air-filled mattress. These are unreliable as heart beat or seizures may cause sufficient compression of sensor to prevent alarm sounding when respiration has ceased. They may fail to detect obstructive apnoea, but are still requested by parents with previous SIDS or cot death. For discussion of home monitoring of babies with recurrent apnoea or siblings of SIDS, see p. 367.

Transcutaneous oxygen and carbon dioxide monitoring

A heated electrode measures oxygen tension across the skin. Use at 43°C if possible and for very immature babies at 42°C.

Should be calibrated fully prior to monitoring and at least 20 min allowed for stabilisation before taking readings.

Precautions:

Electrodes should be resited at least every 4 hours to prevent skin burns

May underestimate central PaO_2 in: hypotension; increased postnatal age; oedema, sclerema

> **!** Transcutaneous oxygen monitors may underestimate central PaO_2 in shocked babies.

Pulse oximetry

The pulse oximeter continuously monitors oxygen saturation with a sensor attached to the hand or foot. Oxygen saturation is then calculated by measuring oxyhaemoglobin as a proportion of total functional haemoglobin. As a ratio is measured rather than an absolute value, no external calibration is needed.

Advantages over transcutaneous monitors:

Ease of use: no calibration or warm up period

Fast response time

Easily portable

Simultaneous heart rate measurement

Less affected by peripheral oedema or poor perfusion

Causes no skin burns

Disadvantages:

Susceptible to patient movement

Frequent alarm calls

Accuracy and standards for babies not determined

Normal limits are not interchangeable between different makes of monitors

Altered slightly by jaundice and phototherapy

May cause pressure necrosis if applied too tightly

Now incorporated into cardiorespiratory monitors. Important to know which system is used to set upper and lower limits of oxygen tension. May have a place in domiciliary oxygen therapy for BPD (see p. 112).

Lumbar puncture (spinal tap)

Indications include:

≺ Suspected meningitis (sepsis work-up in ill infant)
≺ Unexplained apnoea
≺ Suspected subarachnoid haemorrhage
≺ Unexplained seizures
≺ Post-haemorrhagic hydrocephalus – therapeutic.

Technique

➤ Get an experienced nurse to hold the baby in the lateral decubitus or sitting position gently flexing the lower spine.

➤ Avoid neck flexion as this leads to upper airway obstruction.

➤ Prepare the site for puncture using full aseptic technique.

➤ Use a 22 G spinal needle with stylet to prevent a core of skin leading to a dermoid cyst in later life.

➤ Identify lumbar space L4–5 opposite iliac crest.

➤ Gently insert needle in direction of umbilicus until subarachnoid space is penetrated (slight give in needle, about 1 cm from skin in term infant, 0.5 – 0.75 cm in preterm).

➤ Remove stylet and allow CSF to drip out into 3 specimen containers.

➤ Remove the needle, and apply a small adhesive plaster.

Ventricular tap

 The decision to perform a ventricular tap should be taken by a senior doctor as complications such as porencephalic cysts can occur.

A ventricular tap may be needed to diagnose and treat ventriculitis. Antibiotics are sometimes given by this route (see p. 240).

Indications:

≺ Diagnosis of ventriculitis
≺ Non-communicating hydrocephalus — reduction of ICP
≺ Administration of intraventricular antibiotics.

Technique

➤ Full aseptic technique should be used after shaving the scalp.

➤ Gently insert a lumbar puncture needle with stylet at the lateral angle of the anterior fontanelle and angled towards the inner corner of the eye on the same side (Fig. 9.8).

➤ Once the skin has been pierced, remove the stylet and gently advance the needle until CSF wells up the needle (about 1–2 cm if the ventricles are dilated, or 3–4 cm in term babies with normal sized ventricles).

➤ Collect CSF from the ventricles by allowing it to drip into sterile bottles.

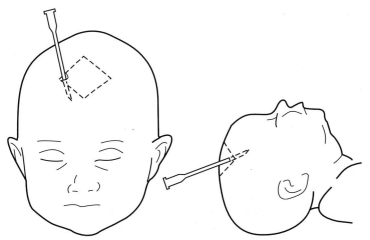

Figure 9.8. Line of insertion of lumbar puncture needle with stylet when performing ventricular tap.

➤ If the ventricle is not entered first time, withdraw the needle along line of insertion and try again at a slightly different angle. Use ultrasound scan for guidance.

 On no account should a syringe be attached to the needle to aspirate fluid as this may precipitate bleeding.

Subdural tap

This is rarely performed as ultrasound and CT scanning have largely replaced this technique for diagnosis of subdural haematoma and with improved obstetric care the need to decompress a large subdural haemorrhage is rare.

Technique

➤ Prepare site for tap using full aseptic technique.

➤ Insert a short wide-bore needle (Pitkin needle) or a 22 G spinal needle through the lateral angle of the anterior fontanelle, aiming laterally into the subdural space (about 0.5 cm).

➤ Once puncture of the dura is felt, withdraw the stylet and allow fluid to drain. If fluid is viscid, this may take several minutes.

Repeated taps may be needed as subdural effusions can re-accumulate.

Suprapubic aspiration

Indications for bladder tap:

≺ Inconclusive cultures of clean voided specimens (clean catch or bag)

≺ Suspicion of septicaemia in any ill infant prior to starting antibiotic therapy.

Contraindications are:

Abdominal distension with dilated loops of bowel
Bleeding disorder.

Technique

➤ Perform procedure at least 1 hour after the baby has passed urine to ensure a full bladder or identify full bladder using ultrasound.

➤ Prepare a wide area of skin over the lower abdomen using full aseptic technique.

➤ Use a number 21 G sterile disposable needle attached to a 10 ml syringe to puncture the skin 0.5–1.0 cm above the symphysis pubis in the midline.

➤ Gently advance needle towards the fundus of the bladder, angled upwards at 30° from the perpendicular.

➤ As the needle is slowly advanced, maintain gentle suction on the syringe until urine appears in it. It should not be necessary to introduce the needle further than 2.5 cm below the skin surface.

Pericardiocentesis

This is rarely needed and should be done by the most senior person available.

Indications:

◄ Pneumopericardium causing cardiac tamponade
◄ Drainage of pericardial effusion.

Technique

➤ Use a 21 G cannula connected to a 3-way tap and 10 ml syringe.

➤ Insert under the ribs to the left of the xiphisternum and advance up and to the left at 45° to the vertical and 45° from the midline.

➤ Keep gentle traction on the plunger of the syringe and at about 1 cm depth the pericardium should be entered and air or fluid withdrawn.

➤ Ultrasound guidance may be helpful if easily available.

➤ The cannula may be left in position and allowed to drain under water.

Paracentesis abdominis

Indications:

◄ Ascites — therapeutic if ventilation impaired or diagnostic
◄ Necrotizing enterocolitis following perforation.

Technique

➤ Prepare site using aseptic technique:

  right or left iliac fossa avoiding area lateral to rectus muscle where inferior epigastric artery lies and avoiding liver and spleen

  anterior midline approach 1–2 cm below the umbilicus. Ensure bladder is empty if using this site.

➤ Inject local anaesthetic and incise the skin, muscle and peritoneum with a scalpel before inserting cannula.

➤ Advance cannula carefully.

➤ Fluid can be withdrawn gently using a syringe or cannula left *in situ* for continuous drainage.

Cardioversion (see p. 294)

Cardiac massage (see p. 46)

Renal dialysis (see Ch. 19)

Nursing points

Baby

- Adequate local analgesia and sedation with morphine must be administered prior to any invasive procedure and consideration given to the need for further pain relief.
- Careful observation of the baby's condition and maintenance of temperature are important during and after all procedures. Specifically:
  - ➤ Monitor oxygenation, chest movements and colour of baby after intubation or ventilatory changes
  - ➤ Check circulation in appropriate limbs or areas of body following arterial cannulation
  - ➤ Ensure arterial and venous cannulation sites are kept visible and observe for haemorrhage or leakage
  - ➤ Monitor site of any invasive procedure, keep clean and handle gently
  - ➤ Half-hourly recordings of temperature and blood pressure during exchange transfusions.
- Continuous cardiorespiratory monitoring and strict fluid input/output chart to be kept during procedure.
- Lubricating eye drops, passive physiotherapy and careful positioning are important for babies given muscle relaxants for long periods. Ensure sedation is also given to these babies.
- Nursing the baby on a ventilator:
  - ➤ Ensure the endotracheal tube is firmly secured.
  - ➤ Note position of tube and check hourly for signs of displacement.
  - ➤ Keep tube patent by suctioning as needed: usually 3–6 hourly after first 24 hours using aseptic technique. Ventilator disconnections should be brief (<10 s).
  - ➤ After suctioning send aspirate twice weekly to laboratory for culture.
  - ➤ Ensure that warmed, humidified gases are being given to prevent heat loss and drying of airways.
  - ➤ Nurse baby semi-prone to avoid lung compression.
  - ➤ Avoid traction on tube by supporting tubing and connectors. This helps to prevent trauma to larynx and vagal stimulation which may cause bradycardia.
  - ➤ Change baby's position every 3 hours making sure that tubing does not kink by carefully re-positioning it.
  - ➤ Record oxygen concentration, ventilator pressures and rate, and humidity temperature every hour.
  - ➤ Increased surveillance is needed if muscle relaxants have been given: accidental disconnection or extubation can be very serious.

Paralysed babies need gentle passive exercises of limbs to prevent contractures.
➤ Avoid over-handling.
➤ Careful explanation of all care to parents.
● Nursing role in lumbar puncture:
➤ Basic pack with styletted spinal needle, local anaesthetic, lotions, collodion, universal containers and gowns, masks and gloves.
➤ Attach cardiorespiratory monitor and pulse oximeter if baby ill or unstable.
➤ Have oxygen, resuscitation masks, laryngoscope, endotracheal tubes, and suction ready for ill babies.
➤ Hold baby gently but firmly in left lateral position with right hand on occiput and left hand around the baby's thighs; avoid flexion of head. Upright sitting position is an alternative.
➤ Observe baby's colour and activity during procedure.
➤ Second nurse collects 12 drops or less of CSF in each of three sterile sample containers.
➤ Seal site with collodion and Band-Aid®.
➤ Baby should lie flat for at least 1 hour after procedure with minimal handling.

Family

● Explain the need for various procedures to parents.
● Results from any tests should be discussed with parents as soon as possible.
● If muscle relaxants are used explain the effects to the parents, as a motionless baby can cause great distress.

Equipment

● Grooves in the palate from the prolonged use of endotracheal and orogastric tubes can be prevented by fitting a dental plate.
● Check that resuscitation equipment, a pre-cut endotracheal tube, laryngoscope and introducer are readily available for all intubated babies.
● All ventilated babies should have a syringe, 3-way tap, cold light source and scalp vein needle readily available, in case of pneumothorax.
● When taking over the care of a baby, it is the responsibility of each nurse to check the alarms of all monitors are on and that their limits are set appropriately.
● Send the tip of all tubes and catheters removed from a baby for culture.

Staff

- Before beginning or assisting with a procedure, ensure there are adequate staff available to care for the remaining babies.

References and further reading

Anand KJS, Hickey PR (1987). Pain and its effects in the human neonate and fetus. *N Engl J Med* **317**: 1321.

Andreasson B, Lindroth M, Svenningsen NW, Johnson B (1988). Effects on respiration of CPAP immediately after extubation in the very preterm infant. *Pediatr Pulmonol* **4**: 213.

Angell C (1991). Equipment requirements for community based paediatric oxygen treatment. *Arch Dis Child* **66**: 755.

Black JA, Whitfield MF (1991). *Neonatal Emergencies*, 2nd edn. Oxford: Butterworth Heinemann.

Coldiron JS (1968). Estimation of nasotracheal tube length in neonates. *Pediatrics* **41**: 823.

Dear PRF (1987). Monitoring oxygen in the newborn: saturation or partial pressure. *Arch Dis Child* **62**: 879.

Dunn PM (1966). Localisation of the umbilical catheter by postmortem measurement. *Arch Dis Child* **41**: 879.

Elliott SJ (1991). Neonatal extracorporeal membrane oxygenation: how not to assess novel technologies. *Lancet* **337**: 476.

Finer N (1997). Inhaled nitric oxide in neonates. *Arch Dis Child* **77**: F81–4.

Fuhrman BP (1990). Perfluorocarbon liquid ventilation: the first human trial. *J Pediatr* **117**: 73.

Geggel RL (1993). Inhalational nitric oxide: a selective pulmonary vasodilator for treatment of persistent pulmonary hypertension of the newborn. *J Pediatr* **123**: 76.

Goldsmith JP, Karotkin EH (1996). *Assisted Ventilation of the Neonate*, 3rd edn. Philadelphia: WB Saunders.

Greenough A, Greenall F (1988). Observation of spontaneous respiratory interaction with artificial ventilation. *Arch Dis Child* **63**: 168.

Greenough A, Milner AD (1992). Respiratory support using patient triggered ventilation in the neonatal period. *Arch Dis Child* **67**: 69.

Halliday HL (1989). When to do a lumbar puncture in a neonate. *Arch Dis Child* **64**: 313.

Hudak BB, Allen MC, Hudak ML, Loughlin GM (1989). Home oxygen therapy for chronic lung disease in extremely low birth weight infants. *Am J Dis Child* **143**: 357.

Johnson RV, Donn SM (1988). Life span of intravenous cannulas in a neonatal intensive care unit. *Am J Dis Child* **142**: 968.

Kempley S, Bennett S, Loftus BG, Cooper D, Gamsu HR (1993). Randomized trial of umbilical arterial catheter position: clinical outcome. *Acta Paediatr* **82**: 173.

Levin DL, Morriss SC, Moore SS (1989). *A Practical Guide to Pediatric Intensive Care*, 2nd edn. St Louis: CV Mosby.

Marlow N (1998). High frequency ventilation and respiratory distress syndrome: do we have an answer? *Arch Dis Child* **78**: F1.

Ramsden CA, Reynolds EOR, Morley CT *et al* (1987). Ventilator settings for newborn infants. *Arch Dis Child* **62**: 529.

Silverman M (1992). Domiciliary oxygen therapy for children. Report of a Working Group of the Royal College of Physicians. *J R Coll Phys* **26**: 125.

Southall DP, Bignall S, Stebbins VA *et al* (1987). Pulse oximeter and transcutaneous arterial oxygen measurements in neonatal and paediatric intensive care. *Arch Dis Child* **62**: 882.

Tarnow-Mordi W (1988). How to ventilate premature babies. *Care Crit Ill* **4**: 26.

Tarnow-Mordi W, Wilkinson A (1986). Mechanical ventilation of the newborn. *Br Med J* **292**: 575.

UK Collaborative ECMO Trial Group (1996). UK collaborative randomised trial of neonatal extracorporeal membrane oxygenation. *Lancet* **348**: 75–82.

10 Respiratory Problems

In the newborn, respiration differs from the adult in being more rapid, more shallow and more irregular. This is due to lower pulmonary compliance and proportionately increased work of breathing. Despite the extra work of breathing, $PaCO_2$ and bicarbonate levels are lower than in adults. Chemical control of ventilation is discussed in Ch. 15.

 Respiratory problems are the commonest cause of serious neonatal illness and death. Accurate diagnosis and management are therefore imperative.

Respiratory distress usually presents as a combination of grunting, tachypnoea (respiratory rate >60 breaths/min), nasal flaring, sternal or subcostal retractions and cyanosis.

Causes of neonatal respiratory distress include:

- Respiratory distress syndrome (RDS)
- Transient tachypnoea of the newborn (TTN)
- Aspiration pneumonia (meconium, secretions or milk)
- Pulmonary air leaks: pneumothorax, interstitial emphysema, pneumomediastinum and pneumopericardium
- Pneumonia (congenital, especially group B streptococcal, and acquired)
- Congenital lobar emphysema
- Pulmonary hypoplasia
- Pulmonary haemorrhage
- Chronic lung disease: bronchopulmonary dysplasia, Wilson–Mikity syndrome
- Cardiac failure: congenital heart disease, PDA, supraventricular tachycardia, severe anaemia

- Persistent pulmonary hypertension (persistent fetal circulation)
- Metabolic acidosis (any aetiology, see p. 92)
- Cerebral irritation: asphyxia, haemorrhage, meningitis
- Congenital diaphragmatic hernia
- Airway obstruction: choanal atresia, Pierre Robin syndrome
- Tracheo-oesophageal fistula
- Drugs: methylxanthines, narcotic analgesia in labour, diazepam
- Over-heating or hypothermia
- Chest wall disorders: thoracic dystrophy, myasthenia gravis

In practice the first five conditions are the commonest and account for almost 90% of acute respiratory disorders. History, clinical findings and investigation of these common respiratory disorders of the newborn are shown in Table 10.1.

Approach to initial assessment of acute respiratory distress

A detailed knowledge of the antenatal and perinatal history is essential:

< Gestational age
< Maternal conditions that may affect the fetus: Rhesus incompatibility, diabetes, raised blood pressure, antepartum haemorrhage
< Evidence of intrauterine growth retardation (see p. 75)
< Factors related to infection: duration of rupture of the membranes; maternal pyrexia, discharge or uterine tenderness; results of vaginal culture; current antibiotic treatment
< Multiple pregnancy
< Treatment with antenatal corticosteroids
< Previous baby with RDS
< Labour: duration, complications, type of analgesia, mode of delivery
< Presence of fetal distress, need for resuscitation, cord pH.

Table 10.1. Differential diagnosis of respiratory distress

	RDS	PHT	GBS	TTN	MAS
Gestation	Usually preterm	Often term	Preterm or term	More often term	Usually post-term
Perinatal history	APH, IDM, rhesus, immature L/S ratio	Asphyxia, aspirin in pregnancy	Uterine inertia, asphyxia, PROM	IDM, C/S, asphyxia	Asphyxia, IUGR
Clinical features	Grunting prominent, gradual deterioration	Cyanosis prominent, sudden deterioration	Shock prominent, early apnoea, pulmonary haemorrhage	RR >60, mild distress	Meconium staining, over-inflated chest, progressive deterioration
Effect of oxygen	Improvement	Cyanosis unchanged	May improve	Improvement	May improve
Blood gases	Hypoxaemia, raised PCO_2, mixed acidosis	Marked hypoxaemia, low or normal PCO_2, metabolic acidosis, (R) radial/aorta difference	Hypoxaemia, metabolic or mixed acidosis	Mild hypoxaemia, low or normal PCO_2 mild metabolic acidosis	Hypoxaemia, metabolic acidosis
Chest X-ray	Under-inflation, reticulogranular mottling, air bronchogram	Over-inflation, clear lung-fields, cardiomegaly	Coarse infiltrates, collapse or mimic RDS	Over-inflation, streaking, ↑ pulm. vasc., pulm. oedema, slight cardiomegaly	Coarse infiltrates, overinflation ± pneumothorax
Treatment	CPAP helpful, IPPV surfactant replacement	CPAP unhelpful, IPPV, vasodilating drugs, ECMO	Penicilin, blood transfusion, ± mechanical ventilation	Oxygen, IPPV (rarely)	Airway suction at birth, may need IPPV, CPAP unhelpful
Outcome (mortality)	<25%	~20%	~40%	0%	~30%

RDS = respiratory distress syndrome; PHT = pulmonary hypertension (persistent fetal circulation); GBS = group B streptococcal pneumonia; TTN = transient tachypnoea of the newborn; MAS = meconium aspiration syndrome; APH = antepartum haemorrhage; IDM = infant of diabetic mother; PROM = premature rupture of membranes; C/S = caesarean section; IUGR = intrauterine growth retardation; L/S = lecithin/sphingomyelin; RR = respiratory rate; CPAP = continuous poitive airways pressure; IPPV = intermittent positive pressure ventilation ECMO = extracorporeal membrane oxygenation

Important points to note in the physical examination are:

≺ Estimated gestational age
≺ Level of activity
≺ Degree of cyanosis
≺ Severity of respiratory distress.

Cyanosis may be a late sign of hypoxaemia in the newborn. Fig. 10.1 shows the haemoglobin–oxygen dissociation curves for adult and fetal haemoglobin. With a shift to the left with fetal haemoglobin, cyanosis may not become apparent until PaO_2 is <5 kPa (38 mmHg). Also, if polycythaemia is present, the baby may appear cyanosed when PaO_2 is normal. Arterial blood gas tensions must be measured if infant needs >30% inspired oxygen.

Other factors causing a leftward shift in haemoglobin–oxygen dissociation curve (increased affinity of haemoglobin for oxygen) are:

● Reduced hydrogen ion concentration (increased pH)
● Reduced temperature
● Reduced $PaCO_2$
● Reduced 2,3-diphosphoglycerate concentration

Increases in all these factors shift the curve to the right (decreased affinity for oxygen).

Management of respiratory distress syndrome is discussed in detail; the general approach to other respiratory conditions is similar.

➕ Respiratory distress syndrome

Respiratory distress syndrome (RDS) or hyaline membrane disease is caused by surfactant deficiency and affects mainly the preterm infant. The incidence of RDS varies with gestational age (Table 10.2).

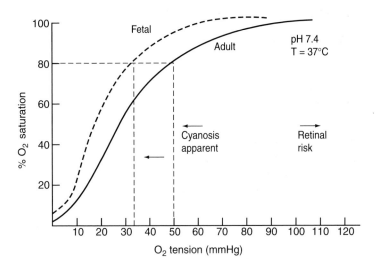

Figure 10.1. Haemoglobin–oxygen dissociation curves for fetal and adult haemoglobin. Cyanosis may appear late in hypoxaemia in the newborn. After Klaus and Fanaroff (1979).

The risk of RDS is increased by:

- Prematurity
- History of RDS in siblings
- Maternal diabetes or Rhesus isoimmunization
- Maternal hypertension without fetal growth retardation
- Male sex
- Second twin
- Birth asphyxia
- Antepartum haemorrhage.

The risk of RDS is reduced by:

- Prenatal steroids
- Prolonged rupture of membranes (2 days–1 week)
- Growth retardation from maternal hypertension or other causes
- Heroin or alcohol addiction

- Black infants
- Female sex.

 Prenatal steroid administration significantly reduces the incidence of RDS (by 50%).

Surfactant is produced by alveolar Type II cells and, by reducing alveolar surface tension, prevents alveolar collapse at end-expiration. The major components of surfactant are phosphatidylcholine (lecithin), phosphatidylglycerol (PG) and phosphatidylinositol (PI). Most of the phosphatidylcholine is in the form of dipalmitoylphosphatidylcholine (DPPC) which comprises 60% of surfactant. Several of the components of surfactant must be present for it to lower surface tension as DPPC alone is ineffective. Surfactant is produced from 22 to 24 weeks' gestation onwards.

Deficiency of surfactant leads to alveolar collapse, reduced lung volume, decreased lung compliance and ventilation/perfusion abnormalities. In RDS the lungs are stiff (low compliance) and high pressures are needed to expand them. In severe RDS, pulmonary hypertension with R→L shunting also occurs.

Hypoxaemia from ventilation/perfusion abnormalities leads to metabolic acidosis from cellular anaerobic glycolysis with lactic acid production. Respiratory acidosis is also present

Table 10.2. Incidence of RDS by gestational age

Gestation (weeks)	Babies with RDS (%)
26	90
28	80
30	70
32	55
34	25
36	12
38	3
40	<1–2

Prenatal steroids have reduced these incidence figures.

because of alveolar hypoventilation. The combination of acidosis and hypoxaemia reduces myocardial contractility, cardiac output and arterial blood pressure. Perfusion of kidneys, gastrointestinal tract and other non-vital organs is also reduced. Oedema and electrolyte disturbances occur.

There may be other co-existing problems of prematurity.

Radiologically, the areas of atelectasis appear as diffuse reticulogranular mottling and air in the major bronchi is contrasted against the white background as air bronchograms.

The natural progression of RDS consists of increasing oxygen requirements for 36–48 hours, then stabilization for 24 hours as the lungs begin to produce surfactant, followed by improvement after about 72 hours. By the end of 7 days, the baby with mild or moderate RDS should have completely recovered. Improvement is often heralded by a diuresis as a consequence of improved renal function. This natural progression is altered by early surfactant treatment (see p. 149).

Diagnosis

The diagnosis is based on the clinical picture of tachypnoea, grunting and nasal flaring and must be confirmed by chest X-ray. Severity of RDS may be graded as follows:

Grade I: Fine reticulogranular mottling, good lung expansion

Grade II: Mottling with moderate air bronchograms

Grade III: Diffuse mottling, heart borders just discernable, prominent air bronchograms

Grade IV: Bilateral confluent opacification of lungs ('white out')

 Note that the degree of atelectasis may be less prominent than expected if the baby is mechanically ventilated or treated with CPAP.

Very immature babies with RDS may present with apnoea rather than tachypnoea, or apparent asphyxia and assisted ventilation is frequently needed from birth. In these babies

surfactant replacement should be given as early as possible, either in the labour ward or after stabilization in the NICU.

Management

A successful outcome to this potentially fatal disease requires meticulous attention to detail. The management of RDS is complex and involves more than just support of ventilation. If, however, the underlying hypoxaemia and acidosis can be corrected, many of the other complications of RDS can be ameliorated.

Initial management

➤ Place infant in prewarmed incubator or under radiant warmer and attach pulse oximeter. Handling should be kept to a minimum.

➤ Give oxygen by headbox to keep saturation 92–95%.

➤ If >30% oxygen is required and infant is < 1.5 kg, start nasal CPAP, insert arterial catheter (see p. 116) and take a chest radiograph.

➤ If >1.5 kg, wait approximately 30 min to see if there is any improvement. If there is none and oxygen requirement >40%, insert arterial catheter and take radiograph.

➤ A chest radiograph is important to confirm clinical diagnosis (Table 10.1) and determine catheter position (see p. 117).

➤ Prophylactic or early surfactant should be strongly considered for all babies <30 weeks' gestation.

Initial investigations

≺ Glucose stix
≺ Blood gases and pH
≺ Haemoglobin, packed cell volume
≺ Blood pressure by arterial transducer or non-invasive means
≺ Blood culture, white cell count (IgM, CRP)
≺ Gastric aspirate; Gram stain and culture
≺ Chest X-ray.

Antibiotic therapy

Penicillin should be given to all babies with respiratory distress until cultures taken at birth prove negative.

Babies at *increased* risk of streptococcal pneumonia include:

≺ Vaginal swab grows streptococci
≺ Gastric aspirate shows polymorphs and Gram-positive organisms
≺ Any atypical features seen in infant (see p. 162).

Penicillin should be given to all babies with respiratory distress until infection has been excluded.

Monitoring

All infants on assisted ventilation should be continuously supervised by a trained nurse. Any clinical deterioration should be reported immediately.

The following measurements should be made initially:

≺ *Continuous*:
    heart rate
    respiratory rate
    transcutaneous PO_2 or oxygen saturation
    temperature (servo-control)
    blood pressure (transducer or non-invasive)
    inspired oxygen concentration (with analyser close to infant's face)

≺ *4-hourly (minimum)*:
    blood gases and pH
    glucose strip test

≺ *12–24 hourly*:
    urine output
    bilirubin if clinically jaundiced
    electrolytes (and calcium)
    haemoglobin or packed cell volume

Respiratory therapy

Continuous positive airway pressure (CPAP) should be commenced when PaO_2 is <8 kPa (60 mmHg) in 40% oxygen in babies >1500 g. Use endotracheal, mask or nasal-prong CPAP (see p. 102). Start with pressure of 6–8 cmH_2O and check frequent arterial blood gas samples until improvement occurs or respiratory failure develops. For babies of <1000 g, nasal-prong CPAP may be started soon after birth even if respiratory distress is minimal. This may prevent development of atelectasis.

Respiratory failure is present when any one of the following occurs on two consecutive blood gas analyses 20 min apart:

◁ PaO_2 <6 kPa (45 mmHg) in 60% oxygen on CPAP of 6–8 cmH_2O

◁ pH <7.20 (often associated with $PaCO_2$ over 10 kPa (75 mmHg))

◁ Intractable apnoea.

Mechanical ventilation is used under these circumstances or as initial management of very immature babies (either if nasal-prong CPAP fails or baby is apnoeic at birth and needs endotracheal intubation for resuscitation). Nasotracheal intubation may be preferable to orotracheal intubation as the tube is more firmly anchored and less liable to slip out or kink. Occasionally, damage to anterior nares or nasal septum can occur; this is less likely if the tube is not cut too short. The endotracheal tube is anchored by taping it securely to the face.

Initial ventilator settings and further management are described in Ch. 9.

Sudden deterioration when breathing spontaneously may be caused by:

- Pneumothorax
- Intraventricular haemorrhage
- Infection
- Airway problems, aspiration
- Apnoea.

Briefly inspect the airway and apply suction if secretions are present. Ventilate by hand with bag and mask; if the chest moves poorly, transilluminate for the presence of pneumothorax. If there is rapid improvement from bagging and transillumination is negative, observe closely. Check blood gases for respiratory failure. If transillumination is positive, treat for pneumothorax (see Ch. 9). If there is *little or delayed improvement*, consider:

- Infection
- Intraventricular haemorrhage
- Need for assisted ventilation.

If there is *rapid deterioration* on assisted ventilation: Disconnect from ventilator and bag by hand. If the baby improves there may be a ventilator problem, e.g. disconnection or improper ventilation settings.

If there is *no improvement* consider:

- Tube blocked or displaced
- Pneumothorax, interstitial emphysema
- Infection
- Intraventricular haemorrhage.

A more *gradual deterioration* may be due to infection, development of a patent ductus arteriosus or slowly progressive pulmonary interstitial emphysema.

Investigate by suctioning the airway, transillumination of the chest, chest radiography, cerebral ultrasound scan or echocardiogram as indicated. Ventilator settings may need to be increased for a short time.

Surfactant replacement

Surfactant replacement therapy has been shown to reduce mortality and complications such as pneumothorax and pulmonary interstitial emphysema in babies with severe RDS and also when used prophylactically in babies <30 weeks' gestation.

Two main types of surfactant have been used in clinical trials (natural, derived from animal lungs; and synthetic or protein-free) and many are now available for general clinical use (Table 10.3).

Table 10.3. Surfactant preparations in clinical practice

	Composition	Dose of phospholipids (mg/kg)	Volume (ml/kg)	Number of doses (suggested max.)
Synthetic				
ALEC™	DPPC:PG 7:3 (w/w)	100	1.2 ml*	4
Exosurf™	DPPC 13.5 mg Cetyl alcohol 1.5 mg Tyloxapol 1.0 mg	67.5	5	2
Natural				
Survanta™	Bovine lung mince plus DPPC, tripalmitin, palmitic acid, phospholipids 84% SP-B, SP-C 1%	100	4	4
Alveofact™	Bovine lung lavage Phospholipids 45 mg/ml SP-B, SP-C 1%	50	1.2	4
Curosurf™	Porcine lung mince Phospholipids 99% SP-B, SP-C 1%	100–200	1.25–2.5	3
Infasurf™	Calf lung surfactant lavage Phospholipids 95% SP-B, SP-C 1%	90–100	3	3

* Total dose.

The surfactant associated proteins in natural surfactants (SP-B, SP-C) ensure a more rapid onset of action. Inspired oxygen concentrations and ventilator pressures can usually be lowered within minutes of instillation of one of these preparations. In general, natural surfactants are given rapidly, e.g. Curosurf™ as a single or divided double bolus into the lower trachea or after turning the baby from side to side. It is recommended that Survanta™ be given in 4 divided boluses into each lung segment because of the larger volumes needed (4 ml/kg versus about 1.25 ml/kg for Curosurf™ and Alveofact™). Exosurf™ is usually given more slowly over 5–20 mins using an adaptor attached to the proximal end of the endotracheal tube, as tube blockage, reflux of surfactant or transient hypoxaemia may occur during more rapid instillation. These are uncommon complications after rapid bolus treatment with the natural surfactant preparations. Alec is used prophylactically as a rapid bolus dose of 1.2 ml, with subsequent doses given for continuing respiratory distress.

> **!** Babies should be monitored closely following surfactant administration.

More even distribution of natural surfactant is best obtained by a short period of manual ventilation after instillation. Once the baby is reconnected to the ventilator, inspired oxygen concentrations can be rapidly lowered with the aid of a pulse oximeter or transcutaneous oxygen tension monitor. If high ventilator rates (>60 breaths/min) are being used, it is usually possible to lower peak pressure soon afterwards. Movement of the chest wall remains the best guide to pressure requirements. Overdistension of the lung should be minimized by avoiding high flow rates and using low inspiratory times (0.3–0.4 s). With natural surfactants, levels of PEEP can usually be lowered (3 cmH$_2$O), but for synthetic surfactants higher PEEP levels are probably advisable (5 cmH$_2$O).

Blood pressure should also be carefully monitored after surfactant replacement and any hypotension corrected by infusion of colloid. Hypotension may be due to PDA which can be detected by Doppler echocardiography and managed with intravenous indomethacin (see p. 288). PDA may occur earlier on in the course of the disease after surfactant replacement, following a reduction in pulmonary vascular resistance. Pulmonary haemorrhage has been described in association with surfactant treatment of very immature babies; this is probably due to haemorrhagic pulmonary oedema secondary to a large L→R shunt across the PDA.

The type of surfactant preparation used and the timing of its use may be critical for optimal outcome. It is clear that natural surfactants work more rapidly than synthetic ones, and a recent meta-analysis has shown that mortality and pulmonary air leaks are reduced with natural surfactants, but the differences are not great. Several studies now suggest that the earlier in the course of RDS that surfactant is given the better the outcome. This is especially true for immature babies (<30 weeks' gestation). If endotracheal intubation is needed for resuscitation of these babies, they should probably be given surfactant soon afterwards unless they are particularly vigorous. For this form of prophylaxis or very early treatment, either a natural or synthetic preparation should probably be used in a dose of at least 60–100 mg phospholipid/kg. For later 'rescue' treatment of ill babies when a rapid response is desirable, a natural surfactant preparation may be more suitable. Because babies with established RDS are likely to have inhibitors of surfactant (proteins from the plasma) in the alveoli, a larger dose of phospholipid may be needed (100–200 mg/kg).

Not all babies respond optimally to surfactant. Some reasons for a poor response are:

- Wrong diagnosis:
    congenital pneumonia
    pulmonary hypoplasia
    ARDS
    pulmonary hypertension
    congenital heart disease
- Insufficient dose: if inhibitors present, may need 100–200 mg phospholipid/kg
- Maldistribution: given into one lung or even into stomach
- Pre-existing asphyxia and acidosis: correct first
- Overdistension of the lungs: reduce ventilator settings
- Development of PDA
- Development of pulmonary haemorrhage: exclude PDA
- Relapse: need for repeat doses.

Sedation

A morphine infusion (or other narcotic) should be considered for all babies having mechanical ventilation, especially those who breathe asynchronously with ('fight') the ventilator. A reasonable dose is 5–10 µg/kg/min.

In infants who fight the ventilator, faster rates (70–100 breaths/min) are often effective. If this fails, muscle relaxation may be used; vecuronium (0.05 mg/kg/h by infusion after a loading dose of 0.1 mg/kg) or atracurium have short half-lives, degrade independently of liver or renal function and have fewer side effects than some of the older muscle relaxants such as pancuronium. Prolonged infusion can however lead to accumulation in immature babies. Careful tube care is vital and accidental or prolonged disconnection should be avoided.

Muscle relaxants may lessen the risks of pneumothorax and chronic lung disease.

Other drugs have a very limited place in management except in the infant with very severe RDS and R–L shunting, secondary to pulmonary hypertension. This is an analogous situation to that found in persistent pulmonary hypertension (see p. 171).

Acid–base balance

Disturbances in acid–base balance should be corrected carefully (see p. 92).

Metabolic acidosis: the cause, e.g. hypovolaemia or sepsis, should be established and treated. If unexplained metabolic acidosis is present (pH <7.25 and base deficit >8 mmol/l), bicarbonate should be infused slowly. Use sodium bicarbonate 8.4% diluted 4:1 with 5 or 10% dextrose in a dose of 1 mmol/kg. Note that 1 ml of 8.4% bicarbonate contains 1 mmol.

 Repeated or excessive use of bicarbonate in RDS is both ineffective and dangerous, especially in the very immature infant.

THAM (tris-hydroxymethyl-amino-methane; Tromethamine USP) is an alternative to sodium bicarbonate but may not be readily available.

Respiratory acidosis: should be treated by assisted ventilation.

Hypovolaemia and hypotension

If the packed cell volume is <45%, this should be corrected with transfusion of whole blood or packed cells (see Ch. 21). Low blood pressure (mean arterial blood pressure in mmHg <gestational age) should be corrected with an infusion of 10–20 ml/kg of colloid (blood, plasma or 5% salt-free albumin). Inotropes (dopamine or dobutamine, starting at 5–10 μg/kg/min) should be considered where there is insufficient response to colloid.

Fluids, electrolytes and nutrition

Preterm infants with RDS often tolerate oral feeding poorly and this may lead to:

Increased oxygen consumption and lowered oxygen tensions
Abdominal distension and regurgitation
Necrotizing enterocolitis

Most babies <33 weeks' gestation require intravenous fluids, at least initially.

Fluid intake in severe RDS should be reduced because of decreased urinary output from decreased renal perfusion and increased capillary permeability. Account must be taken of increased insensible water losses under radiant heaters or phototherapy.

Start with 5 or 10% dextrose at 60–80 ml/kg/day. If infusion is required for >24 hours, electrolyte supplementation and amino acids will be required (see Ch. 11). Monitor sodium and potassium balance carefully for first 2–3 days in very immature babies.

Upon recovery, feeding can be started orally. Orogastric or transpyloric feeding are used (see Ch. 11), and small amounts of either expressed breast milk or formula can usually be started by the second day. It is not necessary to remove umbilical artery catheters before feeding.

Recovery

Weaning from the ventilator is described on p. 109. Gentle chest physiotherapy may be used after endotracheal extubation if there is segmental collapse, unless the infant does not tolerate handling. Nasal-prong CPAP may also facilitate extubation and prevent alveolar collapse (Ch. 9).

Later complications

Patent ductus arteriosus (p. 286)
Chronic lung disease (p. 167)
Retinopathy of prematurity (p. 87)
Neurological and developmental problems, intraventricular haemorrhage and periventricular leucomalacia (see Ch. 16 and 24)

✚ Transient tachypnoea of the newborn (TTN)

This is a relatively common respiratory disorder of both preterm and term infants. The cause may be delayed resorption of lung fluid and predisposing factors are:

- Perinatal asphyxia
- Caesarean section
- Maternal diabetes (or potential diabetes)
- Excessive maternal analgesia
- Oxytocin and excess hypotonic fluids in labour
- Neonatal polycythaemia.

Each of these conditions is associated with increased production of lung fluid or delay in its removal via trachea, pulmonary lymphatics or veins. Transient left ventricular failure may also be involved in pathogenesis.

Clinically, the disorder mimics mild RDS with tachypnoea predominant (up to 120 breaths/min) and minimal grunting or indrawing ('classical' TTN).

Radiographs show increased pulmonary vascular markings, mild cardiomegaly, hyperinflation of the lungs and fluid in costophrenic angles and horizontal fissure, resembling those of pulmonary oedema.

In some infants with radiographic findings of TTN there may

be very marked hyperinflation and pulmonary hypertension with R→L shunting (severe or 'malignant' type). These infants are usually very ill and resemble those with persistent pulmonary hypertension (see p. 171). Tricuspid regurgitation may be present with a loud pansystolic murmur. Echocardiography is helpful in distinguishing these two types of TTN (see Table 10.1).

Classical TTN is a short-lived illness with <40% oxygen needed to maintain normal arterial blood gases. Tachypnoea generally abates by 2–3 days. In infants who are distressed or have respiratory rates over 80 breaths/min, withhold oral feeds and provide fluids and calories intravenously. Exclude infection as streptococcal pneumonia can present like TTN. An alternative diagnosis should be considered when the illness is slow to resolve, e.g. congenital heart disease, particularly total anomalous pulmonary venous drainage or anomalous left coronary artery.

✚ Aspiration pneumonia

There are two distinct entities:
1. Meconium aspiration occurs predominantly in the post-term infant
2. Aspiration of milk or upper airways secretions, which is more common in the preterm infant

✚ *Meconium aspiration syndrome (MAS)*

Meconium staining of amniotic fluid occurs in about 10% of labours at term. It is more common in post-term and SGA babies and is often associated with intrauterine hypoxia. Its occurrence in preterm infants may indicate intrauterine infection (e.g. listeria or Gram-negative bacilli).

Management at delivery

➤ Perform pharyngeal suction before the onset of breathing.
➤ Aspirate any meconium found below the cords using a suction cathether.

➤ Reserve intubation of the trachea for depressed infants born after thick meconium staining of the liquor. Avoid lung lavage as this liquefies the meconium and helps drive it distally. If the baby is vigorous at birth, intubation is not necessary.

Such measures significantly improve outcome but not all MAS is preventable as it can occur *in utero* either before or during labour.

Massive meconium aspiration may lead to a very severe illness by three mechanisms:

1. Plugging of the small airways with hyperinflation as a result of a ball-valve mechanism. Atelectasis with ventilation/perfusion imbalance and profound hypoxia may occur
2. Meconium pneumonitis from chemical irritation, which may be delayed
3. Asphyxia causing pulmonary hypertension

Secondary infection may also occur since meconium is able to support a variety of bacterial growth *in vitro*. The eventual outcome may be determined by associated asphyxia which may also affect cerebral, myocardial and renal function.

Subsequent management

Any infant with significant meconium below the cords should be admitted to the neonatal unit irrespective of clinical condition immediately after resuscitation. Chest radiography should be performed (Table 10.1). Deterioration of these infants may occur slowly as the meconium tracks distally in the respiratory tract. Pneumothorax occurs in about 15% of infants.

In the neonatal unit initial management comprises:

➤ Observation

➤ Humidified oxygen to maintain SaO_2 >95%

➤ Gentle chest physiotherapy may be indicated if the chest radiograph is abnormal but handling should be kept to a minimum

➤ Antibiotics should be given in cases of massive meconium

aspiration. Surfactant treatment may have a role but, there is no role for corticosteroids in the early management of MAS

➤ If there has been severe asphyxia or there is acute hyper-inflation of the lungs, pulmonary hypertension may occur (see p. 171).

Even with aggressive management, the mortality rate in massive meconium aspiration is up to 30%. Chronic lung disease may occur in some infants who survive intensive mechanical ventilation.

✚ *Late-onset aspiration*

This usually occurs in a small preterm infant who becomes apnoeic during or soon after a feed. Milk can usually be seen in the hypopharynx or below the cords and should be aspirated from the airway with a suction catheter. The infant should then be bagged with 40% oxygen until spontaneous breathing recurs. Chest radiograph usually shows collapse or consolidation, especially of the right upper lobe. Antibiotic therapy is usually started after a sepsis work-up (see Ch. 14) because of the risk of super-imposed or underlying infection. The infant should be carefully monitored for a few days following this episode.

Recurrent attacks of apnoea with or without aspiration may be caused by gastro-oesophageal reflux. Barium swallow or oesophageal pH monitoring are indicated. Up to 70% of babies intubated for mechanical ventilation have recurrent bouts of aspiration. Thickening of the feed or transpyloric feeding may reduce this complication.

✚ Pneumothorax

Asymptomatic pneumothorax probably occurs in about 1 % of all newborns and does not need treatment.

Symptomatic pneumothorax usually occurs as a complication of:

- RDS or its treatment
- Meconium aspiration

- Over-zealous resuscitation
- Pulmonary hypoplasia, e.g. Potter's syndrome or diaphrgmatic hernia
- Post-thoracotomy
- TTN, aspiration pneumonia or other causes of low lung compliance
- Staphylococcal pneumonia with pneumatocoele (rare).

During mechanical ventilation, a syringe with 3-way tap and butterfly needle (19 or 21 gauge) should be readily available to drain chest in an emergency (see p. 113).

The incidence of pneumothorax in infants with RDS treated with assisted ventilation varies from 15 to 30%. In 10% the pneumothorax will be bilateral. Since the introduction of surfactant treatment pneumothorax has become less common and probably occurs in <10% of mechanically ventilated newborns.

Alveolar rupture allows air to track along the broncho-vascular space to the mediastinum and thence into the pleural space. The usual consequence is a tension pneumothorax and the pneumomediastinum is not always radiologically apparent.

> A syringe, 3-way tap and butterfly needle should be readily available whenever a baby is being ventilated.

Diagnosis

Tension pneumothorax may present as:

◁ Sudden deterioration
◁ Shift of the mediastinum (apex beat) away from the affected side
◁ Reduced breath sounds on the affected side
◁ Asymmetry of chest wall movement ('proud' hemithorax)
◁ Hypotension and poor perfusion in association with tachycardia or bradycardia.

Transillumination of the chest with a fibreoptic light often shows hyperlucency of the affected side (see p. 113). Anteroposterior

(AP) and cross-table lateral chest radiographs should be taken since collapsed lung may be pushed back against the posterior chest wall and the AP film may underestimate the extent of the pneumothorax. In RDS the lungs are less compliant so that major shift of the mediastinum may not occur and a small pneumothorax on X-ray may cause marked clinical deterioration.

Management

In very immature babies, treatment should not be delayed by waiting for a chest radiograph. Air should be aspirated with a butterfly needle initially, followed by the insertion of a pleural drain connected to an under-water seal (see Ch. 9). Adequate sedation and local analgesia should be used in all but the most critical situations.

Always check the position of pleural drain by radiography. If there is a poor response to drainage, the intercostal tube may be wrongly positioned. The commonest problem is where the tip of the drain is placed posteriorly below the air; this can be diagnosed with a lateral chest X-ray and the drain adjusted.

Other air leak conditions

Once an air leak has occurred in the newborn, air may spread from the mediastinum to reach the peritoneal cavity (pneumo-peritoneum) or the pericardial cavity (pneumopericardium), or into the neck, causing subcutaneous emphysema (uncommon in the newborn). Occasionally air will rupture into a pulmonary blood vessel causing generalized arterial air (pneumatosis arterialis) with sudden death. These forms of air leak are uncommon and their incidence has been further reduced by use of surfactant. They are still seen occasionally in very immature infants who need high ventilator pressures or those with pulmonary hypoplasia.

✚ *Pneumopericardium*

Pneumopericardium is usually a very serious condition with cardiac tamponade which often requires drainage. It presents with reduced cardiac output and decreased heart sounds; diagnosis should be confirmed radiologically. Pericardial drainage is a very skilled procedure and a senior doctor should be involved in management (see p. 133).

✚ *Pulmonary interstitial emphysema*

Pulmonary interstitial emphysema (PIE) may occur in infants with severe RDS needing mechanical ventilation. It may present with a profound deterioration in clinical condition and lead to pneumothorax with sudden deterioration. The diagnosis is confirmed by chest X-ray. Chronic lung disease is a long-term complication of survivors.

The condition is difficult to treat. High rate, low pressure ventilation may help and there may be a place for high frequency oscillation ventilation. Short periods of manual ventilation at high rates (120 breaths/min) may be effective in reducing the amount of PIE. It has been suggested that pleural drains be inserted cautiously to create pneumothoraces and improve pulmonary compliance but this is controversial.

Occasionally, the interstitial emphysema is confined to one lung, which may herniate over to the unaffected side. In this situation, selective intubation of the unaffected side may allow therapeutic collapse of the emphysematous lung for a period of 24–48 hours. Selective intubation of the right lung is easy to perform, but intubation of the left main bronchus is more difficult, particularly as the disposition of the main bronchi may be altered by mediastinal shift.

✚ Pneumonia

This may be congenital or acquired.

✚ *Congenital pneumonia*

The clinical and radiological picture of congenital pneumonia may be similar to RDS.

Predisposing factors in congenital pneumonia are:

- Prolonged rupture of the membranes
- Maternal illness with fever or foul-smelling liquor
- Maternal colonization with group B streptococci
- Birth asphyxia and aspiration of infected material.

Infection may be ascending, transplacental or follow aspiration during passage down the birth canal (see Ch. 14). The organisms most commonly isolated are β-haemolytic streptococci, coliforms, *Listeria monocytogenes*, bacteroides and occasionally staphylococcus or pseudomonas.

✚ Group B β-haemolytic streptococcal pneumonia

Early-onset group B β-haemolytic streptococcal (GBS) pneumonia is becoming an increasingly important cause of neonatal illness in the UK. From 10 to 30% of pregnant women carry this organism in the genital tract or rectum. Infants born to colonized women usually become colonized but only 1% of them develop serious illness. Serious sepsis occurs in about 3 per 1000 births with a mortality rate of 30–50%. GBS pneumonia may be very difficult to distinguish from RDS. One or more of the following findings may help with diagnosis:

- ≺ Early onset of apnoea
- ≺ Shock/hypotension
- ≺ Metabolic acidosis
- ≺ Pulmonary infiltrates on radiographs
- ≺ Blood-stained tracheal aspirate
- ≺ Neutropenia
- ≺ Streptococci seen on Gram stain of gastric aspirate
- ≺ Positive blood and gastric aspirate culture for streptococci.

Because of the ever-present risk of infection, all infants with respiratory distress should be treated initially with penicillin in high dose (see p. 147). If cultures prove negative, the antibiotic may be stopped after 2–3 days. If the diagnosis is confirmed, then a combination of high-dose penicillin and aminoglycoside (gentamicin or netilmicin) is effective since these antibiotics have a synergistic action against streptococci.

Hypotension is common in congenital sepsis and should be treated with colloid infusion (10–15 ml/kg), or inotropes. Transfusions with fresh blood are also helpful by providing opsonins to improve the newborn's white cell function. If there is neutropenia, granulocyte or buffy coat transfusions may help, although there is a theoretical risk of graft versus host disease. There may be a role for granulocyte colony stimulating factor, although this remains under study. Mechanical ventilation may be required (see Ch. 9).

 Hypotension is common in congenital sepsis and should be treated aggressively.

The overall mortality for this condition remains high (30–50%) despite early and apparently adequate treatment. The reasons for this may be:

- Intrauterine onset of infection
- Delay in diagnosis (confusion with RDS)
- Immature infants are often affected
- Affected infants may have immunological deficiencies.

The incidence of infection may be reduced by giving ampicillin (2–4 g i.v.) or penicillin intrapartum to women in preterm labour who are colonized with GBS. Antibiotics should also be given intrapartum to women with signs of chorioamnionitis (see p. 23).

➕ Listeriosis

Early-onset listeriosis has a similar clinical picture and high mortality; it has become more common in the UK partly as a result of imports of soft cheese made from unpasteurized milks. *Listeria monocytogenes* grows well at low temperatures so that these cheeses and pâtés should not be kept in the refrigerator. Maternal 'flu-like' illness is the usual antecedent and infection of the fetus is probably transplacental, although it is known that the newborn may become infected after aspirating contaminated amniotic fluid during birth. Meconium staining in premature labour is very uncommon and if present should raise the suspicion of congenital bacterial infection.

At birth the infant may have a maculopapular or petechial rash and hepatosplenomegaly. Leucopenia and thrombocytopenia are common and Gram-positive coccobacilli may be seen on smear of gastric aspirate.

Treatment with ampicillin and gentamicin is effective but a poor outcome can occur despite early treatment because of severe pulmonary involvement and coexisting meningitis. There is a 50% neonatal mortality and about 50% of survivors have significant disability.

Anaerobic organisms

Anaerobic organisms may also cause congenital pneumonia; *Bacteroides fragilis* has been isolated from some infants born after prolonged rupture of the membranes. There is usually foul-smelling amniotic fluid and the infants are also malodorous. Although the mother may have a fever and rigors, the infant usually has a relatively benign course, with mild pneumonia, jaundice, hypocalcaemia and lethargy. Ampicillin and gentamicin in combination have been used to treat this condition, although the organism is resistant *in vitro*. Clindamycin, metronidazole or chloramphenicol are occasionally required.

✚ *Acquired pneumonia*

This is common particularly in babies who are ventilated, the endotracheal tube acting as a direct route for bacteria to enter the lungs. There may have been obvious or 'silent' aspiration of feeds. Any organism may be involved but nosocomially-acquired bacteria, such as coagulase-positive and -negative staphylococci and Gram-negative bacilli (particularly coliforms), are common, and occasionally yeasts may be seen.

In *Staphylococcus aureus* pneumonia, the infant is often very ill and assisted ventilation is needed. Sclerema may be present. The chest X-ray initially may show non-specific changes and later lobar consolidation with pneumatoceles. Complications include pneumothorax and emphysema.

Treatment of acquired pneumonia involves suitable antibiotics, supplemental oxygen, assisted ventilation as indicated, and sometimes physiotherapy. A commonly encountered situation is where *Staph. epidermidis* is isolated from endotracheal secretions. This organism is often an 'innocent bystander', but should be treated when there has been any clinical deterioration or worsening of the chest X-ray.

✚ Pulmonary hypoplasia

This is now more frequently diagnosed.

It may be caused by:

- Oligohydramnios (renal agenesis, urinary tract obstruction, prolonged rupture of membranes)
- Lung compression (diaphragmatic hernia, lung cysts, pleural effusions, erythroblastosis, chondrodystrophies)
- Absent fetal breathing movements (anencephaly, neuromuscular disorders).

For a description of Potter's syndrome see p. 321.

Pulmonary hypoplasia may present as asphyxia at birth. The lungs are very stiff and difficult to inflate, and there is usually a poor response to resuscitation. Pneumothoraces and respiratory failure often develop. The chest X-ray shows small lungs with a bell-shaped thorax. Sometimes mechanical ventilation with high pressures is successful in 'opening up' the lungs but surfactant replacement is largely unsuccessful, as is ECMO. If pulmonary hypertension coexists, inhaled nitric oxide may be helpful. Liquid ventilation is being studied as a promising new treatment.

There is a high mortality and at autopsy the lung to body weight ratio is low, usually <0.01, but this ratio may be increased by mechanical ventilation. Absolute confirmation of the diagnosis requires more sophisticated autopsy analysis such as radial alveolar counts.

✚ Pulmonary haemorrhage

The incidence of this condition is decreasing and is now most commonly seen in streptococcal pneumonia or immature babies treated with surfactant. About 5% of infants weighing <1500 g treated with surfactant for RDS develop pulmonary haemorrhage.

Predisposing factors include:

- GBS pneumonia
- Surfactant treatment
- SGA infant
- Perinatal asphyxia
- Hypothermia and acidosis
- Coagulation disorder
- Severe erythroblastosis
- Hypoglycaemia
- Cardiac failure, especially left ventricular
- Oxygen toxicity.

The condition often presents with slight haemorrhage from an endotracheal tube in a baby receiving IPPV for some other reason. More often than not this is due to trauma from endotracheal suctioning. Occasionally, massive pulmonary haemorrhage occurs in an initially stable baby. In this situation, there is sudden collapse with frank, frothy blood in the mouth, nose and airway. There is increased opacification of the chest radiograph.

Management

Underlying sepsis, acidosis and hypothermia should be treated together with support of respiration and correction of coagulation disorder. Vitamin K and fresh blood transfusions should be given. It is possible to reduce the pulmonary bleeding by increasing the peak and end-expiratory pressures to cause tamponade to bleeding pulmonary capillaries. It may be necessary to use high pressures (peak up to 30–35 cmH$_2$O and PEEP 8–10 cmH$_2$O) to treat pulmonary haemorrhage successfully. If

PDA is confirmed, frusemide and indomethacin should be given.

The endotracheal tube may become blocked by fresh or clotted blood, but endotracheal suctioning should not be performed unless occlusion is suspected, as over-zealous suctioning may precipitate further bleeding.

✚ Chronic lung disease (CLD)

Bronchopulmonary dysplasia (BPD) was first described in the late 1960s. It was originally defined as chronic oxygen dependency at 28 days of life in a baby who had been ventilated, usually for RDS; however, this definition is no longer appropriate as more immature babies are now cared for. Changes of CLD may be apparent radiologically as early as 1 week. It is also apparent that many small babies who do not have an acute respiratory condition, but who require mechanical ventilation for apnoea, may develop chronic lung disease. There is still no generally agreed modern definition of CLD, but useful definitions are a need for supplemental oxygen at a corrected age of either 36 weeks' gestation or term.

The disorder appears to be becoming more common as increasing numbers of immature babies survive. Surfactant treatment has not reduced the risk of CLD and may have increased the absolute numbers of affected babies. The incidence varies but approximately 25–30% of babies following IPPV and 5–10% of all babies <1500 g develop CLD.

Predisposing factors are:

- Pulmonary immaturity
- Need for oxygen concentrations >60% for 5 days or more
- Positive pressure ventilation
- Endotracheal intubation
- Infection
- Pulmonary interstitial emphysema
- Patent ductus arteriosus and high fluid intake.

There is a continued debate about whether barotrauma (or volutrauma) or oxygen toxicity is responsible for CLD. Both high ventilator pressures and oxygen free radicals are probably important aetiological factors and the process involves inflammatory changes in the airways.

Clinically, affected babies have continued oxygen dependency, indrawing, wheezing, cyanotic spells and right-heart failure. Prolonged ventilator and oxygen dependency is a frequent presentation in the VLBW infant. Recurrent respiratory infections are common later in infancy.

Radiologically, four stages have been described but in severe cases there is pulmonary streaking, patchy over-inflation and emphysematous cysts:

Stage 1: indistinguishable from RDS (first week)

Stage 2: generalized opacity and pulmonary plethora (second week)

Stage 3: cystic changes with stranding (third week)

Stage 4: hyperinflation, widespread stranding, cardiomegaly (after fourth week)

Very immature babies may present with a need for supplemental oxygen from 10 days, with chest radiographs showing generalized haziness, equivalent to stage 2. These babies usually do not progress to develop cysts.

CLD usually improves spontaneously as new alveoli may be generated for at least the first 7 years of life. There is a normal increase in alveolar number from 30 million at birth to 300 million at 7 years.

Management

Vitamin E in large doses (100 mg/day) has been used to prevent BPD but its benefit is not proven (see also p. 350).

Treatment is largely symptomatic:

➤ Oxygen should be administered to keep arterial oxygen tension above 7 kPa (53 mmHg). Levels lower than this are associated with pulmonary vasoconstriction and right heart failure. Oxygen may be given to the baby at low flow rates using nasal cannulae, allowing increased mobility. It is important to increase the concentration of supplemental oxygen at times of short-term increased need, e.g. feeding and handling, and especially during blood sampling. Painful procedures should preferably be avoided or adequate analgesia provided. Note also that other procedures such as immunization and treatment for retinopathy of prematurity may cause a short-term deterioration in the clinical condition.

➤ Good nutrition is essential for adequate lung growth and repair. High protein and energy formula feeds in addition to vitamin supplements are needed (p. 183).

➤ Diuretics and fluid restriction may be indicated in the presence of PDA, excessive weight gain or cor pulmonale.

➤ Respiratory infections should be suspected whenever there is any clinical deterioration and treated appropriately.

Corticosteroids, particularly dexamethasone, have been used with some success in weaning ventilator-dependent babies, but use in spontaneously breathing infants is controversial. Treatment regimens vary considerably from centre to centre, e.g. 0.5 mg/kg/day in two divided doses for 3 days, reducing the daily dose by 50% every 3 days for a total of 12 days. It is important to reduce the dose to the lowest effective amount.

Steroids cause hyperglycaemia, hypertension, loss of weight and cardiac hypertrophy and may increase the risk of sepsis, bowel perforation and gastric haemorrhage.

> Corticosteroids should be used in the lowest effective dose to minimize side effects.

Other treatment strategies involve the use of dexamethasone early in the course of RDS (e.g. first 3 days) to prevent CLD. This facilitates weaning from the ventilator and may reduce the risk of CLD. Topical steroid use, e.g. budesonide by inhalation using a spacing device, may be effective with fewer side effects: clinical trials are currently being undertaken.

Outcome

Many babies have mild to moderate CLD and can be weaned from oxygen prior to discharge. Those with severe CLD may need domiciliary oxygen therapy for weeks or months after going home. Domiciliary oxygen treatment allows earlier discharge from hospital and may reduce the risks of developmental delay, and costs. Oxygen may be given by nasal catheter or spectacles at very low flow rates. Pulse oximeters should be used to assess oxygen needs (SaO_2 90–95%).

Careful discharge planning is essential, and should involve those who will continue to care for the baby in the community (family, general practitioner, liaison neonatal nurse, health visitor, respiratory technician, social worker, etc.). Parents should be educated about, and comfortable using, any specialized equipment. They should be taught how to perform cardiopulmonary resuscitation, and given advice regarding parental smoking and avoidance of infection.

Most infants recover gradually, but some continue to have symptoms throughout infancy with frequent respiratory infections and hospital admissions, particularly during the winter months when respiratory syncitial virus epidemics are common. There is a higher than average risk of wheezing in these babies, although not all go on to develop asthma.

✚ Wilson–Mikity syndrome

This is an uncommon chronic pulmonary condition of the preterm infant that resembles bronchopulmonary dysplasia. Usually, however, there is no preceding severe RDS or need for IPPV and at about 7–10 days of age a gradually progressive form of respiratory distress develops.

There is indrawing of the chest, rising respiratory rate and slowly increasing oxygen need to about 30%. The PCO_2 rises but there is a metabolic compensation and raised bicarbonate. Chest radiography shows streaky infiltrates, increasing densities with cystic changes and later over-inflation.

This chronic condition tends to improve after 4–8 weeks.

Aetiology is uncertain though there are many theories:

- Fluid retention from either excessive administration or chronic patent ductus arteriosus
- Mineral and vitamin deficiency (rickets)
- Recurrent aspiration
- Chronic deficiency of surfactant causing alveolar instability (chronic pulmonary insufficiency of prematurity (CPIP))
- Instability of the chest wall in the very immature infant
- Alveolar fluid leak and chronic inflammation.

Treatment is aimed at maintaining normal blood gases with added oxygen and CPAP to stabilize the alveoli if necessary. Fluid restriction and diuretics may be helpful but adequate intake of protein, energy, trace elements and vitamins should be ensured.

In most cases the disorder is self-limiting but some infants progress to terminal respiratory failure with worsening emphysema.

✚ Persistent pulmonary hypertension (PPHN) (see also Ch. 17)

In persistent pulmonary hypertension (or persistent fetal circulation) there is vasoconstriction of the pulmonary arteriolar bed with R→L shunting of blood across the ductus arteriosus and foramen ovale. This is abnormal after the first few hours of life.

Pulmonary hypertension in the newborn is poorly understood but may be primary or secondary type. In the *primary type* the pulmonary capillaries and arterioles are thickened. This has been associated with constriction of the ductus arteriosus *in utero* from maternal ingestion of aspirin or indomethacin. Chronic intrauterine hypoxia has the same effect (e.g. in placental insufficiency or maternal hypoxia), but many cases are idiopathic.

The causes of secondary pulmonary hypertension include:

- Severe birth asphyxia: hypoxaemia, acidosis
- Severe lung disease, e.g. RDS, meconium aspiration or TTN
- Some forms of bacterial pneumonia, e.g. listeriosis, group B streptococcus
- Congenital diaphragmatic hernia
- Pneumothorax
- Polycythaemia, hypoglycaemia

Diagnosis

The diagnosis of pulmonary hypertension is often difficult to make. The infant presents with respiratory distress and cyanosis, the liver may be enlarged and hypoxaemia is usually profound, suggesting cyanotic heart disease. Myocardial dysfunction is often associated with PPHN secondary to hypoxia, acidosis or hypoglycaemia.

Differential arterial blood gas sampling or oxygen saturation monitoring may reveal R→L shunting across the ductus arteriosus. The PaO_2 of blood from the lower aorta (post-ductus) will be lower than that of the right radial artery (pre-ductus). Similarly, SaO_2 measured from the legs or left hand will be less than that measured from the right hand.

The chest X-ray in primary pulmonary hypertension shows clear lung fields with hyperinflation and cardiomegaly. In secondary pulmonary hypertension, the chest X-ray has the appearance of the underlying condition. Echocardiography provides a useful non-invasive method of assessing pulmonary pressure and excluding underlying structural congenital heart disease.

Management

> ! Babies with PPHN are very labile and are likely to deteriorate even with minimal handling.

The underlying condition should be treated first.

Mechanical ventilation is usually necessary. Blood gases and pH should be kept within the normal range; arterial $PaCO_2$ should not fall below 3 kPa (23 mmHg) as this may lead to cerebral vasoconstriction and reduced cerebral blood flow. The baby should be adequately sedated as any stress can lead to deterioration. Muscle relaxants may be necessary. Hypoglycaemia and polycythaemia should be corrected by dextrose infusion and partial plasma exchange, respectively.

Pulmonary vasodilating drugs are used when PaO_2 is below 5 kPa (38 mmHg), despite maximum ventilation with 100% oxygen:

Tolazoline. May be used in a dose of 1–2 mg/kg as an intravenous bolus and, if effective, then as an infusion of 1–2 mg/kg/h if there is a satisfactory response. The drug should be infused in isotonic saline or 5% dextrose through a scalp vein. Side effects are hypotension (corrected by volume expansion or inotropes) and gastric bleeding. The response to tolazoline is measured by blood gas analysis 10 min after the bolus dose or continuously by pulse oximetry, and by echocardiography. A cutaneous flush is usually seen in responding infants. Deterioration in oxygenation may occur after administration of tolazoline if the blood pressure prior to treatment was low or low–normal.

Prostacyclin. May be a more effective pulmonary vasodilator drug but also causes systemic effects. The dose is 10 ng/kg/min.

Inhaled nitric oxide. Shows promise as a selective pulmonary vasodilating drug (see Ch. 9) but specialized equipment is required and further trials are needed before it enters routine use.

Babies who do not respond to any of these measures may respond to high frequency oscillatory ventilation, but some require extra corporeal membrane oxygenation (ECMO). The latter should be performed in a regional centre experienced in its use.

Typical criteria for referral for ECMO include:

◄ Gestation >34 weeks
◄ Birthweight >2.0 kg

≺ No bleeding disorder
≺ Failure to respond to maximal medical treatment
≺ Oxygenation index (OI) >25–40
  (OI = MAP x FiO$_2$ x 100/ PaO$_2$, where MAP is the mean airway pressure in cmH$_2$O and PaO$_2$ is the postductal oxygen tension in mmHg)

Infants with pulmonary hypertension may suddenly improve with, for example, PaO$_2$ increasing from 5 to 20 kPa (40 to 150 mmHg). Caution is required in reducing oxygen concentration or ventilation because these infants may 'flip-flop'; this is a sudden fall in PaO$_2$ upon reduction of ventilation or oxygen concentration and is thought to be due to increased reactivity of pulmonary circulation to oxygen and hydrogen ion concentrations.

Once initial improvement is seen, conventional ventilator settings (rate, pressure or both) and oxygen concentration should be cautiously lowered using the 'rule of twos', e.g. oxygen concentration lowered by 2%, peak pressure by a maximum of 2 cmH$_2$O, and ventilator rate by 2/min.

➕ Upper airway obstruction

This may cause problems soon after birth (see p. 40).

➕ *Choanal atresia*

This is an uncommon condition but causes a major emergency since babies are obligate nose breathers early in life. The presentation is of respiratory distress at birth relieved only by crying. In this situation an attempt should be made to pass a catheter through the nasal passages to confirm the diagnosis. Once confirmed a small oropharyngeal airway should be inserted until surgery is performed.

➕ *Pierre Robin syndrome*

This consists of a triad of micrognathia, cleft palate and glossoptosis and may cause acute airway obstruction as the tongue falls back. Insert a small oropharyngeal airway to push the tongue forward if there is respiratory embarrassment. Intubation can be difficult and babies with major airway obstruction may require tracheostomy. Surgery at a later date should be performed by an experienced maxillofacial surgeon.

✚ Congenital laryngeal stridor

This is usually due to laryngomalacia but occasionally to laryngeal webs or cysts. Laryngoscopy/bronchoscopy should be performed to make the diagnosis. Spontaneous improvement usually occurs in laryngomalacia, although symptoms are made worse by upper respiratory infections. Very occasionally tracheostomy is needed.

✚ Subglottic stenosis

This may be congenital or acquired. The latter is due to prolonged endotracheal intubation, especially if the tube is too big, but <1 % of ventilated babies need tracheostomy. Minor surgery to split the cricoid cartilage has been advocated as an alternative to tracheostomy. Affected infants may need repeated tracheal dilatation or laser treatment and laryngotracheal reconstruction is sometimes needed at about 2 years of age.

Nursing points

Baby

- Hypothermia causes increased oxygen consumption, therefore careful attention to temperature control is important.
- Endotracheal tubes (ET) cause discomfort. Gentle, infrequent handling will benefit the baby.
- Suctioning is a traumatic, invasive procedure which should be performed as required, not routinely. It may precipitate apnoea.
- Anticipate and prepare for specific problems in certain babies, e.g.:
  babies given *muscle relaxants* need extra care during handling and suctioning to avoid dislodging the ET

  big babies with *meconium aspiration syndrome* may appear decep-
    tively well before deteriorating
  babies with *early-onset streptococcal pneumonia* may appear well at
    birth, then develop tachypnoea before collapsing
  ventilated babies, particularly those with pulmonary interstitial
    emphysema, bronchopulmonary dysplasia and those requiring high
    peak inspiratory pressures, are at risk of developing pneumo-
    thoraces. A syringe, 3-way tap, cold light source and scalp vein
    needle (19 or 21 gauge) should be readily available in case of
    emergency
  continuous blood pressure monitoring should be used for babies being
    given *vasodilating drugs,* such as tolazoline, as these may cause
    hypotension.

Family

- Parents tend to watch monitors closely — careful explanation of their
  function is necessary.
- Encourage families to become involved in the care of their baby as
  they feel able.

Equipment

- Continuous monitoring reduces the necessity for handling the baby.
- Resuscitation equipment, an ET, laryngoscope and introducer should
  be kept ready next to all ventilated babies.
- The nurse taking over the care of a ventilated baby is responsible for
  checking the resuscitation equipment, monitors, ventilator and alarm
  settings at the beginning of the shift.
- Oral feeding tubes should be used for babies with respiratory problems rather than nasal tubes, to maintain a patent nasal airway.
- Transcutaneous oxygen monitor probes need to be resited at least 4
  hourly. They heat the skin causing local vasodilatation and can cause
  severe burns if left in one place for a prolonged period.

Staff

- A pre-discharge meeting involving the parents, hospital and community staff may be of benefit, particularly for babies with prolonged or
  ongoing respiratory problems.
- Some babies may require oxygen therapy at home. Liaison with community staff is vital to ensure the home circumstances are adequate
  and the necessary support is available.

References and further reading

Bohin S, Field DJ (1994). The epidemiology of neonatal respiratory disease. *Early Hum Dev* **37**: 73.

Corcoran JD, Patterson CC, Thomas PA, Halliday HL (1993). Reduction in the risk of bronchopulmonary dysplasia from 1980–1990: results of a multivariate logistic regression analysis. *Eur J Pediatr* **152**: 677.

Crowley P (1995). Antenatal corticosteroid therapy: A meta-analysis of the randomised trials, 1972 to 1994. *Am J Obstet Gynecol* **173**: 322.

Cunningham AS, Lawson EE, Martin RJ, Pildes RS (1990). Tracheal suction and meconium: a proposed standard of care. *J Pediatr* **116**: 153.

Emond D, Lachance C, Gagnon J, Bard H (1993). Arterial partial pressure of oxygen required to achieve 90% saturation of hemoglobin in very low birthweight newborns. *Pediatrics* **91**: 602.

Goldsmith JP, Karotkin EH (1996). *Assisted Ventilation of the Neonate*, 3rd edn. Philadelphia: WB Saunders.

Greenough A (1995). Meconium aspiration syndrome — prevention and treatment. *Early Hum Devel* **41**: 183.

Greenough A, Milner AD, Roberton NRC (eds) (1996). *Neonatal Respiratory Disorders*. London: Arnold.

Halliday HL (1998). Pulmonary disorders and apnoea. In: *Forfar and Arneil's Textbook of Paeditrics*. Campbell AGM, McIntosh, N, eds. 5th edn. Edinburgh: Churchill Livingstone, pp. 175–198.

Halliday HL (1992). Other acute lung disorders. In: *Effective Care of the Newborn Infant* eds, Sinclair JC, Bracken MB, Oxford: Oxford University Press pp. 359–384.

Halliday HL (1996). Natural vs synthetic surfactants in neonatal respiratory distress syndrome. *Drugs* **51**: 226.

HiFO Study Group (1993). Randomised study of high frequency oscillatory ventilation in infants *J Pediatr* **122**: 609.

Jobe AH (1993). Pulmonary surfactant therapy. *N Engl J Med* **328**: 861.

Klein MD, Whittlesey GG (1994). Extracorporeal membrane oxygenation. *Pediatr Clin N Am* **41**: 365.

Morrissey MSC, Bailey CM (1990). Diagnosis and management of subglottic stenosis after neonatal ventilation. *Arch Dis Child* **65**: 1103.

Ng PC (1993). The effectiveness and side effects of dexamethasone in preterm infants with bronchopulmonary dysplasia. *Arch Dis Child* **68**: 330.

Soll RF, McQueen MC (1992). Respiratory distress syndrome. In: *Effective Care of the Newborn Infant* eds, Sinclair JC, Bracken MB. Oxford: Oxford University Press, pp. 325.

Taeusch WH, Ballard RA, Avery ME (eds) (1991). *Schaffer and Avery's Diseases of the Newborn*, 6th edn. Philadelphia: WB Saunders.

Thibeault DW, Beatty EC, Hall RT *et al* (1985). Neonatal pulmonary hypoplasia with premature rupture of fetal membranes and oligo-hydramnios. *J Pediatr* **107**: 273.

11 Fluids and Nutrition

At birth, transplacental feeding stops and the baby must receive nutrition by the enteral or parenteral route.

Fluid requirements

Fluid requirements increase during the first week of life (Table 11.1). Intake should always be balanced against losses — renal and insensible. Remember that insensible losses can be extremely high for very immature babies and that these are further increased by the use of radiant warmers and phototherapy.

Table 11.1. Fluid and energy requirements

| | Volume (ml/kg/day) | | Energy | |
Day	Incubator	Radiant warmer	kcal/kg/day	kJ/kg/day
1	50–80	80–100	40–50	162–209
2	80–100	100–120	50–70	209–293
3	100–120	120–140	70–90	293–376
4	120–150	140–160	90–110	376–460
5	150	160–180	110–120*	460–502

*Energy needs are made up as follows:

resting expenditure	50 (209)	specific dynamic action	8 (33)
intermittent activity	15 (63)	faecal loss	12 (50)
occasional stress	10 (42)	growth allowance	25 (104)

Intravenous fluids are usually required in the following circumstances:

≺ Very low birth weight babies
≺ Severe respiratory distress, e.g. RDS, pneumonia
≺ Gastrointestinal problems, e.g. atresia, NEC

➢ Hypoglycaemia
➢ Other serious diseases, e.g. septicaemia, hypoxic ischaemic encephalopathy.

10% dextrose in water is the basic solution used. After 24 hours, electrolytes should be added depending on blood biochemistry.

Changes in water and sodium balance after birth occur when:

Loss of interstitial fluid causes early postnatal water loss (about 7% of body weight)
A physiological net negative water and sodium balance occurs

The aim is to minimize early sodium intake until this physiological postnatal diuresis/natriuresis occurs. After this postnatal adaption is over, sodium balance must be positive to allow growth. Renal salt wasting is common in very preterm infants resulting in sodium needs usually of 4–5 mmol/kg/day, but can be higher. Some babies may need 8–12 mmol/kg/day due to immature tubular resorption.

Clinical assessment of fluid and sodium balance is provided by:

≺ Vital signs
≺ Weight
≺ Fluid intake
≺ Urine output
≺ Serum and urine sodium concentration
≺ Serum and urine osmolality
≺ Urine specific gravity.

Excess fluid intake can occur, and has been incriminated in the pathogenesis of PDA, BPD, ROP and NEC in VLBW infants.

Babies may develop fluid retention because of:

• Excessive fluid intake or bicarbonate boluses
• Inappropriate ADH secretion
• Unrecognized hypovolaemia.

Approximate daily requirements of electrolytes are listed in Table 11.2. It is important to remember that electrolytes and water can be obtained from other sources — catheter flushes, sodium bicarbonate therapy, non-nutritional infusions (e.g. heparin, morphine, dopamine) and antibiotics (many penicillins contain relatively large amounts of sodium).

Table 11.2. Daily requirement of minerals

Mineral	Requirement (mmol/kg)
Sodium	2–4
Chloride	2–4
Potassium*	1–3
Calcium	0.5–1.0
Magnesium	0.25
Phosphorus	2–3

* Caution if reduced urine output.

Many antibiotics contain relatively large amounts of sodium and may result in excessive sodium load in immature babies.

Energy requirements

Energy requirements are shown in Table 11.1. After the first few days of life, the infant needs about 120 kcal/kg/day to support growth (15 g/kg/day).

The choice of feed for the preterm infant depends on severity of illness and degree of prematurity. Maternal breast milk or preterm formulas are given by the enteral route and parenteral feeding is used if enteral feeding is not possible. Nutritional care should be individualized for each baby, taking into account:

Degree of prematurity
Degree of prenatal undernutrition
Postnatal age

Concurrent disease
Enteral feed tolerance
Risk of NEC.

Enteral feeding

Human milk

Maternal breast milk is the best food for the newborn infant. Banked human milk is rarely used due to the potential risk of HIV transmission. It also has inadequate levels of protein, energy, calcium and phosphorus for the preterm infant. The initial concentrations of these nutrients are higher in the milk of mothers who have delivered preterm babies, but fall as lactation progresses.

The *advantages* of human milk are:
Defence against infection by supplying plasma
    immunoglobins and specific secretory IgA
Defence against necrotizing enterocolitis
Neurodevelopmental advantage for vulnerable premature
    infants
Better gastrointestinal tolerance than with formulas
Improvement of mother–baby bonding.

Microbiological examination of expressed breast milk (EBM) is not necessary if given to a mother's own infant. EBM must be refrigerated adequately and fed to the infant within 2–3 days of being expressed unless frozen.

The variable composition of preterm breast milk and the huge nutrient needs of preterm infants can be overcome by the use of human milk fortifiers in appropriate amounts. These improve growth rates by ensuring energy, protein and mineral intakes are optimized whilst retaining the benefits of breast milk.

The following questions should be considered when prescribing drug therapy to lactating mothers:
Is the drug therapy really necessary?
Can a safer drug be used?
Should levels of the drug be monitored in the infant?

Minimize drug exposure by asking the mother to take the drugs just after breast-feeding or before the infant is due to have a lengthy sleep.

Formula feeds

Formula milks have been designed to resemble breast rather than cow's milk. Low birth weight formulas have higher energy, protein, sodium, calcium, phosphorus, trace element and vitamin levels to meet the increased needs of preterm babies. The constituents of various milks are shown in Table 11.3. Preterm formula should be given until the baby weighs 1800 g and thereafter term formula should be considered.

Table 11.3. Constituents of milks

	Protein* (g/ 100 ml)	Fat (g/ 100 ml)	Energy kcal/ 100 ml	Energy kJ/100 ml	Ca	P	Na†	K	Fe
							mg/100 ml		
Fresh breast milk	1.2–1.5	4.0	65–75	272–313	35	15	15	60	0.08
Cow's milk	3.3	3.8	65	272	110	90	35	150	0.05
Typical term formula	1.5	3.6	67	281	60	35	18	85	0.04
Typical preterm formula	2.0	3.5	70	298	70	40	25	70	0.5

*Nitrogen content of milk produced by mothers of 28–30 weeks' gestation babies is 30% higher than at term.
† Preterm breast milk may contain more sodium than that from term mothers.

It is recommended that preterm formulas be enhanced with LCP (long chain polyunsaturated fatty acids) at levels typically found in breast milk. LCPs are lipids which are important in metabolism and as precursors of phospholipid biomembranes, particularly in the brain and retinal photoreceptors. Many manu-facturers have begun to add LCPs to both term and preterm formulas.

Other milk formulas may occasionally be fed to newborn babies. Soya protein formulae should be reserved for babies who are clearly allergic to cow's milk protein and should not be used for prolonged periods in preterm babies. Elemental formu-las (e.g. Pregestamil™) are occasionally indicated when gut function is poor following NEC or infection or there are signs of malabsorption. The role of follow-on formulae for preterm infants after hospital discharge is not clear.

Minerals and vitamins

Iron

Preterm infants have low iron stores at birth. Depletion of these stores is exacerbated by frequent blood sampling and decreased erythropoiesis. Early anaemia should be corrected by blood transfusion. The recommended iron intake for preterm babies is 2 mg/kg/day after 6–8 weeks of age. Early anaemia should be corrected by blood transfusion as iron administration in early life may increase the risk of infection. Iron supplements should be discontinued when full mixed feeding is established. The role of erythropoieten in the management of anaemia of prematurity has not been adequately established.

Vitamins

Most formulas have adequate amounts of vitamins. It is stan-dard practice to give multivitamin drops to preterm babies to ensure adequate intake of vitamin D of at least 400 interna-tional units/day, e.g. Abidec (0.6 ml) or Children's Vitamin Drops (10 drops) per day for preterm infants until aged 6 months.

Calcium and phosphorus

Preterm babies are prone to reduced bone mineralization in early life, which in severe cases may result in metabolic bone disease or osteopenia of prematurity (rickets, fractures). The main cause is inadequate substrate (calcium, phosphate) intake. Breast milk is inadequate in meeting calcium and phosphate needs and it is often impossible to meet these by TPN. Although preterm formulas do supply adequate calcium and phosphate for preterm babies, absorption may be poor.

Recommendations:

➤ All preterm babies should receive supplementary vitamin D using a multivitamin preparation as above.

➤ EBM should be supplemented with phosphorus using fortifiers.

➤ If osteopenia develops, supplement with calcium and phosphate.

Route of feeding

Babies <34 weeks' gestational age cannot co-ordinate sucking and swallowing, have delayed gastric emptying and therefore usually require tube feeding in early life.

Orogastric is preferred to *nasogastric* feeding as less obstruction is caused to the airway. *Orojejunal* feeding has not been shown to have the expected advantages of improved feed tolerance and decreased aspiration; it is used for infants with delayed gastric emptying or severe gastro-oesophageal reflux.

Correct placement of a gastric tube should be checked by aspirating fluid and checking acidity of the aspirate with litmus paper. Feeds may be given as intermittent boluses, usually by gravity feeding or continuously by syringe pump. If continuous orogastric feed is used, place the syringe pump below the baby with the nozzle pointing upwards to allow separated fat to be given to the baby.

Method of placing a jejunal tube:

➤ Stiffen silastic tube by placing it briefly in refrigerator.

➤ Measure tube from lips to stomach, add 8 cm and mark with tape.

➤ Place baby on right side and pass tube through mouth into stomach; aspirate for acid reaction.

➤ Leave for 30 min, then pass tube 2 cm every 30 min until mark has been reached.

➤ Tape firmly in position.

➤ Aspirate to check for alkaline reaction.

➤ Start feeds when in position (can be checked on next radiograph).

➤ Feed continuously, never by bolus.

Initiation of feeding

The fetus swallows fluid during intrauterine life, and this may prepare the gut for enteral feeding. Small amounts of enteral feeds trigger gut hormone surges in preterm infants; these are trophic for the gut. Early enteral feeding has been shown:

> To decrease cholestasis and metabolic bone disease
>
> To improve maturation of intestinal function
>
> *Not* to increase incidence of NEC
>
> It is recommended that minimal enteral feeding is given to all preterm babies, except those at greatest risk of NEC.

The following feeding schedule is recommended:

➤ Sick VLBW infants — start continuous feeds at 0.5 ml/h and increase slowly provided there is no evidence of ileus.

➤ Larger preterm infants — feed by bolus every 1–2 hours. Most infants weighing >1500 g tolerate 3 hourly intermittent feeds.

Observe all infants for feeding intolerance: distension, vomiting, large gastric residuals. Attainment of full enteral feeding may take weeks in the sickest babies. When attained, feed at 160—180 ml/kg/day. Higher intakes are allowed for breast fed babies, SGA babies and those needing catch-up growth. Allow demand feeding when bottle or breast feeding is fully established.

Parenteral nutrition

Parenteral nutrition (PN) may be total (TPN) or more usually partial when used to supplement enteral feeding.

Neonatal PN is indicated when gastrointestinal function is compromised by malformation, disease or immaturity. The aim, however should be to attain full enteral nutrition as soon as possible.

Protein

Parenteral amino acids must be adequate in quality and quantity to support nitrogen retention and growth in premature infants. In the past, amino acid solutions have been associated with hyperammonaemia, hyperphenylalaninaemia and metabolic acidosis. The latest solutions (Primene™, Vaminolact™) contain the conditionally essential amino acids as well as true essential amino acids, have low phenylalanine concentrations and are carbohydrate and electrolyte free. 3 g/kg/day of amino acids will support growth at intrauterine rates if adequate energy intake is given.

Recommended schedule for amino acid delivery:

➤ Use the latest generation of amino acid solutions

➤ Commence at 1 g/kg/day on day 2 of life

➤ Increase by 0.5 g/kg/day to a maximum of 3.5 g/kg/day

➤ Reduce intake if unexplained metabolic acidosis or high blood urea.

Carbohydrate

Preterm infants have significantly greater relative glucose needs than term infants, primarily due to brain: body mass ratio.

Hypoglycaemia (blood glucose <2.6 mmol/l) is due to low glycogen stores, low glucose production or excess insulin secretion. It is not always associated with abnormal neurological signs.

Hyperglycaemia occurs frequently in ELBW infants, causing osmotic diuresis, dehydration, weight loss and may predispose to

IVH. There is no fixed definition; blood glucose ≥ 11 mmol/l is commonly associated with persistent glycosuria (>50 mmol/l). Causes include endogenous hepatic gluconeogenesis during glucose infusion with decreased peripheral glucose utilization, insulin resistance and slow response to glucoregulatory hormones. It may be treated with parenteral glucose restriction or insulin infusion.

Recommended schedule for carbohydrate delivery:

➤ Commence glucose at 4–5.5 mg/kg/min (60–80 ml/kg/day of 10% dextrose) on day 1

➤ Gradually increase during first week of life

➤ If hyperglycaemic on appropriate glucose intake, give continuous insulin infusion until normoglycaemia (4–8 mmol/l) returns

➤ Parenteral fluids equivalent to a maximum of 12.5% and 15% dextrose are given by peripheral and central venous line, respectively.

Insulin infusion is prepared as 10 units/kg soluble insulin in 10 ml of 20% albumin and 40 ml of 10% dextrose given at 0.5 ml/kg/h (0.1 units/kg/h) and titrated to keep glucose at 4–8 mmol/l. If glucose <4 mmol/l, stop insulin. If insulin needs are >1 ml/h, double the concentration of insulin infusion.

Lipid

Lipid emulsion provides an iso-osmotic energy-rich parenteral solution plus essential fatty acids. As little as 0.5 g/kg/day soybean oil emulsion, such as Intralipid™, will prevent essential fatty acid deficiency. Many complications have been linked to lipid emulsion usage in preterm infants, but more recent studies suggest that lipid emulsion is safe for neonatal TPN, provided the following strict dosage guidelines are followed:

➤ Use 20% rather than 10% lipid emulsion

➤ Commence lipid at 0.5 g/kg/day

➤ Increase by 0.5 g/kg/day to a maximum of 3.0 g/kg/day

➤ Infuse lipid for 20 h/day

➤ Check lipid levels twice a week and adjust accordingly

➤ Lower lipid to 1.0 g/kg/day if sepsis, rising bilirubin, or deteriorating condition.

Intralipid™, which contains 50% linoleic acid and 100% long-chain triglycerides is the most commonly used lipid emulsion. Mixed lipid emulsions (50% MCT, 50% LCT) have been used in research studies and appear promising. MCT are predominantly lipids of 8 and 10 carbon atoms and do not require carnitine for metabolism. Since pure MCT emulsion does not supply essential fatty acids, mixed MCT/LCT solutions are recommended.

Other additives

PN should also contain electrolytes, minerals, trace elements and vitamins.

Sodium — see enteral feeding

Potassium — hyperkalaemia is common in ELBW infants, due to immature distal tubular function, and intake should be restricted

Calcium and phosphorus — impossible to supply adequate amounts by the parenteral route

Zinc, copper, manganese, iodine and fluoride — supplied in trace element solutions such as Ped-El™

Selenium — not contained in current solutions; an important antioxidant that should be supplied to preterm infants (25.5 nmol/kg/day)

Water-soluble vitamins are not stored in the body so they must be provided daily. They should be administered separately from fat-soluble vitamins

Fat soluble vitamins, especially vitamin A, are low in body stores of preterm infants. They can be provided as Vitlipid™, which is added to a 20% lipid emulsion

Administration

Continuous venous access is crucial for the delivery of PN and can be infused via:

Peripheral vein
Central vein
Umbilical vein

Peripheral PN is used for babies who are expected to move on to full enteral feeds quickly, provided dextrose concentration is <12.5%. *Central* PN is used for babies who will need it for a prolonged period. Central venous catheters provide reliable and prolonged venous access, with a low risk of infection and major complications, and allow use of hyperosmolar solutions (see p. 123).

> **!** Use of peripheral venous lines for PN may result in inadvertent undernutrition because of 'down time' when re-erecting lines.

Monitoring and delivery

PN use in the newborn requires:
Intensive medical and nursing care
Close collaboration with an experienced pharmacy
   department
Frequent biochemical monitoring using microtechniques

The following should be measured *daily or more frequently:*

➤ Serum urea, electrolytes and calcium

➤ Full blood picture and platelet count

➤ Acid–base balance

➤ Glucose strip testing of blood and urine

➤ Urine specific gravity and analysis

➤ Body weight and fluid balance.

The following should be measured *weekly:*

➤ Body length by stadiometer

➤ Head circumference by non-stretchable tape measure

➤ Serum lipid levels and liver, renal and bone profile.

The following should be measured *when appropriate:*

➤ Abdominal girth

➤ Faecal occult blood

➤ Blood cultures

➤ Trace element levels

➤ Specialized body composition analysis.

PN should be prepared under strict aseptic conditions in the pharmacy with a laminar flow hood and terminal filtration prior to delivery.

It is important that each unit has a regimen for PN use in the newborn. PN should be prescribed daily using the most recent weight and individually for each baby. Allow for carbohydrate-free solutions (amino acids, vitamins, trace elements) when prescribing PN and decrease volume proportionally as enteral feeds increase. Consider suboptimal nutritional intake due to non-nutritional parenteral fluids (heparin, analgesia, sedation, respiratory stimulant). Avoid interruption of TPN for administration of colloid or drugs.

Complications

Appropriate PN prescription and frequent monitoring should prevent or detect the following problems:

Bacteraemia (*Staphylococcus epidermidis*) or fungaemia

Extravasation of nutrient infusate and skin sloughing

Central venous catheter dislodgement or thrombosis

Cholestatic jaundice — use minimal enteral nutrition

Inadvertent undernutrition

Nursing points

Baby

- Great care must be taken of infusion sites to reduce the frequency with which intravenous lines need to be resited, and to note and stop extravasation of infusions quickly.
- Care must be taken with tube feeding to ensure the tube is not dislodged, leading to aspiration.
- The baby's weight and occipitofrontal head circumference should be monitored regularly and plotted on the appropriate percentile chart.
- Blood glucose strip test estimations are required regularly for babies receiving intravenous nutrition. Hyperglycaemia may be an early sign of sepsis.

Family

- Parents should be told of the benefits of breast feeding and the mother encouraged to express milk, even if it is only for a short while.
- Every breast feeding mother should be taught how to hand express breast milk, about physiology of lactation, use of mechanical breast pumps, how frequently to express and how to store breast milk.
- Parents should be shown how to tube feed their baby and encouraged to visit for as many feeds as possible. The importance of checking the position of the tube before a feed must be emphasized to prevent aspiration.
- Help and advice may be needed with early feeds, whether the baby is breast or bottle feeding.
- The choice of baby milk formulae available should be discussed with the parents.

Equipment

- If continuous feeds of breast milk are given, the infusion pump should be placed below the level of the baby, with nozzle uppermost, to avoid loss of supernatant fat.
- Electric breast pumps should be available, in a quiet room on the neonatal unit for mothers to use when visiting.
- Parenteral nutrition packs should be connected up using an aseptic technique.
- If a central line is used for parenteral nutrition, another intravenous line is required for drug administration.
- Dental plates should be fitted to those babies requiring prolonged orogastric or oral endotracheal tubes, to prevent palatal grooves.

Staff

- All new staff should receive training about breast feeding to ensure consistency and adequate support is given to parents.
- Every neonatal unit should have a feeding policy manual for staff to refer to.

References and further reading

Barker DJP (1992). Fetal growth and adult disease. *Br J Obstet Gynaecol* **99**: 275.

Draper G, McNinch A (1994). Vitamin K for neonates: the controversy. *Br Med J* **308**: 867.

Ferguson AE, Tappin DM, Girdwood DWA, Kennedy R, Cockburn F (1994). Breast feeding in Scotland. *Br Med J* **308**: 824.

Gross SJ, Slagle TA (1993). Feeding the low birthweight infant. *Clin Perinatol* **20**: 193.

Heird WC (1992). Parenteral feeding. In: *Effective Care of the Newborn Infant* (eds, Sinclair JC, Bracken MB). Oxford: Oxford University Press, pp. 141–60.

Kashyap S, Schulze KF, Forsythe M, Dell RB, Ramakrishnan R, Heird WC (1990). Growth nutrient retention, and metabolic response of low birthweight infants fed supplemented and unsupplemented preterm human milk. *Am J Clin Nutr* **52**: 254.

Lucas A, Morley R, Cole TJ, Lister G, Lesson-Payne C (1992). Breast milk and subsequent intelligence quotient in children born preterm. *Lancet* **339**: 261.

Steer PA, Lucas A, Sinclair JC (1992). Feeding the low birthweight infant. In: *Effective Care of the Newborn Infant* (eds, Sinclair JC, Bracken MB) Oxford: Oxford University Press, pp. 93–140.

12 Glucose, Calcium and Electrolyte Disturbances

Glucose, calcium and electrolyte values for the first few days of life may vary. Low glucose, calcium and sodium levels may cause apnoea and seizures.

Glucose metabolism

Glucose is the major energy source of the fetus, crossing the placenta from maternal serum by facilitated diffusion. The newborn's blood glucose level at birth is the same as umbilical venous blood or about 70% of maternal blood levels. After birth, blood glucose level falls as glucose produced from the breakdown of glycogen in the liver and from gluconeogenesis is insufficient to maintain blood glucose at fetal levels (see Fig. 3.1). When feeding is started, blood glucose slowly recovers at 2–4 hours of age.

✚ Hypoglycaemia

Traditionally defined as a blood glucose <1.5 mmol/l (25 mg/dl) in the first 24 hours of life and <2 mmol/l (35 mg/dl) thereafter. However, evidence from follow-up studies of preterm babies suggests that hypoglycaemia should be redefined as a blood glucose level < 2.6 mmol/l (45 mg/dl).

 Early detection and treatment is essential as symptomatic hypoglycaemia may cause cerebral damage.

Causes of hypoglycaemia:

- Depleted glycogen stores:
  - intrauterine growth retardation
  - prematurity
  - delayed feeding
  - chronic asphyxia
  - hypothermia
- Fetal hyperinsulinaemia:
  - infant of diabetic mother (IDM)
  - severe Rhesus isoimmunization
  - Beckwith's syndrome
  - nesidioblastosis
- Other:
  - adrenal insufficiency
  - exchange transfusion
  - sepsis
  - congenital heart disease
  - galactosaemia
  - maternal drugs
  - glycogen storage disease
  - congenital hypopituitarism

Symptoms are non-specific:

- ≺ Tremor ('jittery')
- ≺ Apnoea
- ≺ Refusal to feed
- ≺ Seizures
- ≺ Cyanosis
- ≺ Hypothermia
- ≺ Heart failure.

 Symptoms of hypoglycaemia are non-specific and diagnosis may be missed unless a high index of suspicion is maintained.

Blood glucose measured in whole blood in the laboratory or using a bench top blood glucose electrode in the neonatal unit should be used for diagnosis. Erroneously low glucose values may be obtained from capillary samples and from samples allowed to stand in room air prior to analysis.

Reagent strips for glucose measurement either alone or with a reflectance colorimeter are neither accurate nor precise and should only be used for screening or measuring trends. Any abnormal or borderline values should be checked by a laboratory method.

Management

Management includes:

- Identification of infants at risk and monitoring blood glucose.
- Prevention of hypoglycaemia by early enteral feeding (within 1 hour of birth) and avoiding environmental stresses such as cold.
- Prompt treatment of established hypoglycaemia.

Monitoring

Fetal hyperinsulinaemia (e.g. IDM) results in hypoglycaemia as early as 30 min after birth (see Fig 3.1). Check blood glucose at birth and 30 min later. If stable, repeat 3–4 hourly until 24 hours of age.

Babies with depleted glycogen stores (e.g. SGA) will present with hypoglycaemia at about 2–4 hours of age and this will last for 48 hours or longer. Check blood glucose 3-hourly for 48 hours until feeding has been well established and glucose levels have stabilized.

Treatment (see Fig. 12.1).

If the baby is asymptomatic give an enteral feed if tolerated, and repeat test for glucose level. If this is still <2.6 mmol/l, give intravenous 10% dextrose as below.

Intravenous dextrose

Should be given for immediate correction of symptomatic hypoglycaemia. Give an intravenous bolus of 10% dextrose 200 mg/kg (2 ml 10% dextrose in water/kg) after determining venous glucose level for confirmation of diagnosis. Follow with a continuous infusion of 10% dextrose at 6–8 mg/kg/min (3–5 ml/kg/h) to avoid rebound hypoglycaemia (see Appendix X).

Some babies may need 15–20% dextrose administered via a central venous line to meet their requirements. When the baby is normoglycaemic and tolerating oral feeds, reduce dextrose slowly to avoid rebound hypoglycaemia.

Glucagon

0.1 mg/kg intramuscularly or subcutaneously may be given acutely if intravenous access is difficult. Beware of rebound hypoglycaemia. Usually ineffective in babies with depleted glycogen stores, e.g. SGA.

 Glucagon is useful if intravenous access is difficult but may cause rebound hypoglycaemia.

Other treatments should *only* be used after further investigation. Check blood insulin, cortisol, glucose and growth hormone during a hypoglycaemic episode.

Hydrocortisone

If the baby needs >12 mg/kg/min of dextrose to maintain blood glucose, hydrocortisone 5 mg/kg 12 hourly may be given intravenously or orally. Once normoglycaemic, withdraw intravenous fluids first and when the baby has been stable for several days discontinue hydrocortisone.

Diazoxide

May occasionally be needed for hyperinsulinaemic infants, e.g. nesidioblastosis. Give diazoxide 10–25 mg/kg/day divided into 3 doses orally. Side effects include hypotension, sodium retention and hirsutism.

Persistent hypoglycaemia is discussed in Ch. 20.

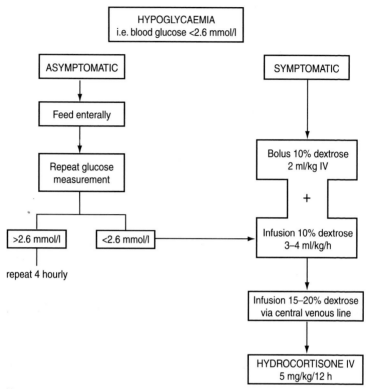

Notes:
1. Blood glucose measurement by strip method may be inaccurate. Confirm hypoglycaemia by laboratory analysis.
2. Babies with symptomatic hypoglycaemia who fail to respond to above management, should be referred to a paediatric endocrinologist.

Figure 12.1. Management of the infant with hypoglycaemia

✚ Hyperglycaemia

Defined as a blood glucose >8 mmol/l (150 mg/dl).

Common problem in preterm babies, particularly if receiving total parenteral nutrition. If blood glucose >11 mmol/l (180 mg/dl), may cause osmotic diuresis and electrolyte disturbances. There may be an increased risk of cerebral haemorrhage if serum osmolality rises >300 mOsm/l.

Causes of hyperglycaemia:

- Prematurity
- Parenteral nutrition
- Stress: sepsis, asphyxia, intracranial haemorrhage
- Drugs: steroids, theophylline
- Neonatal diabetes mellitus — rare.

 Hyperglycaemia may be an early sign of sepsis.

Management

➤ If blood glucose is >11 mmol/l, reduce strength of dextrose infusion then reduce rate of infusion if blood glucose remains high. An insulin infusion should be considered if hyperglycaemia persists.

➤ Infuse 0.1 unit/kg/h of soluble insulin intravenously and titrate the dose to keep glucose at 4–8 mmol/l .

➤ Measure blood glucose every 15 min at the start of insulin infusion and maintain glucose infusion to avoid abrupt changes in blood glucose.

Calcium and magnesium metabolism

Calcium, phosphorus and magnesium levels are higher in the fetus than the mother. There is active transport of these minerals against a gradient *in utero*, enabling the fetus to grow. After birth, serum calcium and magnesium levels fall until 48 hours of age, stabilize and then rise. In the newborn there is a deficient parathyroid response to hypocalcaemia because persistent fetal hypercalcaemia leads to parathyroid suppression. Also, increased serum phosphate as a result of reduced renal excretion exacerbates the hypocalcaemia. Spontaneous increase in parathormone occurs after 3 days.

There is a complex interrelationship between serum magnesium and serum calcium, both being controlled by parathormone. Hypomagnesaemia is usually accompanied by hypocalcaemia and both may be corrected by the administration of magnesium sulphate.

✚ Hypocalcaemia

Defined as total serum calcium <1.8 mmol/l (7 mg/dl) or ionized calcium <0.7 mmol/l (3 mg/dl).

Early hypocalcaemia (within days 1–3) is a result of perinatal events causing an exaggeration in the expected postpartum fall of calcium

Causes of early hypocalcaemia:

- Prematurity
- RDS
- Asphyxia
- Infants of diabetic mothers (IDM)
- Sepsis
- Exchange transfusion.

Late hypocalcaemia (within days 5–7) is usually the result of a congenital defect.

Causes of late hypocalcaemia:

- Maternal hyperparathyroidism
- Hypoparathyroidism (e.g. Di George syndrome)
- Maternal and fetal hypovitaminosis D
- Renal failure
- Hypomagnesaemia
- Feeding of unmodified high phosphate milk (now rare).

Symptoms include irritability, seizures or lethargy and apnoea. Hypocalcaemia of itself would appear to be benign even if seizures are present; underlying cause may determine the long-term outcome.

Management

Give calcium supplements orally if asymptomatic and if tolerating feeds. Oral preparations of calcium are hypertonic and therefore intravenous 10% calcium gluconate is the preparation of choice for oral use. Give 2.0 mmol/kg/day divided 4–6 hourly into feeds.

Take care with calcium infusions:

> **!** *Extravasation* can lead to severe necrosis of the skin. Solutions with >8 mmol/l00 ml calcium should not be infused by pump

> **!** Do *not* mix with bicarbonate or fluids containing phosphate as precipitation will occur

> **!** Do *not* give intra-arterially or via umbilical venous catheters placed near the heart or within the liver

> **!** *Always* give intravenous boluses of calcium slowly with ECG monitoring

If seizures are present, hypocalcaemia should be corrected by slow intravenous infusion of 10% calcium gluconate, 0.2–0.5 ml/kg, diluted 1: 4 with 5% dextrose. As bradycardia and arrhythmias can occur during infusion, give slowly over approx. 15 min with ECG monitoring. Follow by continuous intravenous calcium supplementation of 2.0 mmol/kg/day. If baby is tolerating feeds, oral supplementation with calcium is preferred, as above.

> **!** Hypocalcaemia will not be corrected by giving calcium if serum magnesium is low: correct hypomagnesaemia if present.

✚ Hypercalcaemia

Defined as a total serum calcium >2.75 mmol/l (11 mg/dl) or ionized calcium >1.4 mmol/l (5.6 mg/dl).

Causes of hypercalcaemia include:

- Excessive administration of calcium

- Drugs, e.g. thiazide diuretics
- Hypophosphataemia — common in VLBW babies on PN or breast milk
- Neonatal hyperparathyroidism.

Usually asymptomatic but can cause reduced intestinal motility.

Management

Treat the underlying cause and give adequate fluid replacement.

Frusemide 1 mg/kg/dose 2–4 hourly is effective in the short term by enhancing renal excretion of calcium.

✚ Hypomagnesaemia

Defined as a serum magnesium level <0.6 mmol/l (1.5 mg/dl). Usually transient. Symptoms are similar to hypocalcaemia.

Treatment only necessary if symptomatic. Give 0.2 ml/kg of 50% magnesium sulphate by deep intramuscular injection to prevent skin necrosis. One dose is usually sufficient.

Electrolyte disturbances

✚ Hyponatraemia

Defined as a serum sodium <130 mmol/l (mEq/l).

Early hyponatraemia in VLBW infants is generally due to inappropriate ADH secretion and late hyponatraemia due to inadequate sodium intake.

Causes of hyponatraemia are:

- Inappropriate ADH secretion:
    asphyxia
    meningitis
    pneumonia
    mechanical ventilation
- Inappropriate i.v. fluids:
    low sodium intake

excessive fat emulsion
hyperglycaemia
- Increased loss of sodium:
    diarrhoea, vomiting
    renal tubular acidosis
- Drugs:
    diuretics
    indomethacin
    mannitol
- Other:
    renal failure
    cardiac failure
    adrenal insufficiency
    maternal hyponatraemia

Severe hyponatraemia (<120 mmol/l) is associated with apnoea or seizures. Other symptoms include apathy, hypotonia, hypotension and paralytic ileus.

Management

➤ Anticipation of increased sodium losses and adequate replacement (see below) in preterm babies.

➤ Fluid restriction — commonly the only treatment necessary if inappropriate ADH secretion is present.

➤ Sodium replacement — appropriate if there is inadequate intake or loss of sodium. Replace slowly intravenously over 48 hours after calculating sodium deficit:

Sodium deficit = (135 – plasma sodium) × 0.6 × body weight (kg)

Remember to add deficit to maintenance requirements of sodium when administering infusion.

If the baby has serious symptoms, hypertonic saline, 4 ml/kg of 2.7% or 3% solution, may be given by infusion slowly over 1 hour.

Oral replacement is satisfactory for chronic losses in asymptomatic infants.

➕ Hypernatraemia

Defined as a serum sodium >145 mmol/l (mEq/l).

Causes are:

- Dehydration: radiant warmers, immature infants
- Vomiting and diarrhoea
- Mismanaged intravenous fluids
- Excessive use of sodium bicarbonate
- Osmotic diuresis: hyperglycaemia
- Congenital hyperaldosteronism.

Preterm infants become rapidly dehydrated if fluid is withheld or abnormal losses occur. The very preterm infant has very high insensible water losses which increase with radiant warmers or phototherapy. Hypernatraemia occurs frequently in the first 24–48 hours in babies of <28 weeks' gestation. This can be rapidly followed by hyponatraemia resulting from inadequate sodium intake and excessive urinary losses.

> **!** Hypernatraemia is often asymptomatic but there is an increased risk of cerebral haemorrhage due to increased serum osmolality.

Management

Reduction of serum sodium should be achieved gradually over 48 h using dextrose or normal saline in dextrose (1:5). Give 20 ml/kg plasma or albumin prior to dextrose if infant is volume depleted.

➕ Hyperkalaemia

Defined as a serum potassium > 7.0 mmol/l (mEq/l).

Causes:

- Haemolysis: sample via heel stab

- Impaired renal excretion:
    renal failure
    adrenal insufficiency
- Acidosis, shock, hypoxia
- Increased intake:
    intravenous fluids
    blood transfusion
    penicillin.

Most commonly results from haemolysis after heel stab sampling. If potassium is high repeat test from a venous or arterial sample.

Symptoms include lethergy, hypotonia, ileus, arrythmias, cardiac arrest.

ECG changes of hyperkalaemia:

≺ Tall peaked T waves
≺ ST depression
≺ Wide QRS complexes
≺ Prolonged P–R interval.

Management

➤ Stop all potassium administration

➤ Calcium gluconate produces a transient reduction in cell membrane threshold altering the ECG changes. Give 0.5–1.0 ml/kg over 15 min intravenously.

➤ Give sodium bicarbonate 1–2 mmol/kg i.v. — enhances exchange of potassium into the cells. Transient effect only.

➤ Give resonium A (sodium polystyrene sulphonate, an ion exchange resin) 1g/kg/day orally or rectally.

➤ If ECG changes persist give salbutamol 6μg/kg bolus intravenously.

➤ Glucose and insulin are also effective. Give 1 g/kg glucose (10 ml/kg 10% dextrose) mixed with 0.25–0.5 units soluble insulin intravenously. Give over 1 hour. Effect only transient.

➤ Peritoneal dialysis may occasionally be needed.

> Treatment of hyperkalaemia must be prompt and associated with ECG monitoring.

✚ Hypokalaemia

Defined as a serum potassium <3.0 mmol/l (mEq/l).

Causes:

- Inadequate intake
- Diuretic treatment
- Alkalosis
- Vomiting and diarrhoea
- Hyperadrenalism.

Symptoms include lethargy and muscle weakness.

Management

Treatment is with potassium replacement therapy provided renal function is normal (see p. 181). Avoid infusing solutions with >5 mmol/100 ml of potassium.

✚ Hypo- and Hyper-chloraemia

Causes of hypochloraemia

- Metabolic alkalosis:
    bicarbonate therapy
    hypokalaemia
- Respiratory alkalosis:
    mechanical hyperventilation
- Inadequate intake
- Diuretic therapy
- Vomiting and diarrhoea
- Chloridorrhoea (excessive loss in stool is rare).

Causes of hyperchloraemia

- Excessive intake
- Metabolic acidosis:
    shock
    hypoxia
    diarrhoea
    renal failure
- Respiratory acidosis:
    RDS
    pneumonia.

Management

In hypochloraemia, increasing intake is effective and in hyperchloraemia correction of the underlying cause is essential.

Nursing points

Baby

- Regular glucose strip test estimations and urinalysis for glycosuria are important for babies having parenteral nutrition. Hyperglycaemia may indicate early sepsis. Medical staff should be informed of blood glucose <2.6 mmol/l or >8–10 mmol/l.
- Care is needed with repeated heel stabs which may cause osteomyelitis of the os calcis. Blood glucose strip testing may be performed whenever blood is obtained for other investigations, such as blood gas analysis or serum bilirubin estimation.
- Anticipate those babies particularly at risk from these conditions and monitor blood glucose strips and urinalysis, including specific gravity, regularly. These babies include the very preterm and those with:
    ◄ Radiant heaters in use
    ◄ Vomiting and diarrhoea
    ◄ Bowel problems, e.g. obstruction, necrotizing enterocolitis
    ◄ Sepsis
    ◄ Renal problems — may be secondary to asphyxia or periventricular haemorrhage
    ◄ Diuretic or indomethacin treatment.

- Monitor closely for signs of hypocalcaemia, hypoglycaemia or hyponatraemia. These may include seizures, the signs of which may be subtle: lethargy, apnoea, irritability, hypotonia.

Family

- Careful explanation to parents of metabolic problems is needed.

Equipment

- Extravasation of infusions containing calcium can cause severe skin necrosis. Sites of such infusions should always be visible, checked at least half-hourly and stopped immediately if there are signs of redness or leakage. Umbilical vessels should not be used for these infusions.
- Infusions containing calcium should not be given through the same cannula as parenteral nutrition or solutions containing bicarbonate, as precipitates may form.

Staff

- All staff should be taught the correct technique for performing a heel stab.

References and further reading

Cornblath M, Schwartz R (1976). *Disorders of Carbohydrate Metabolism in Infancy*, 2nd edn. Philadelphia: WB Saunders.

Cowett RM (1985). Pathophysiology, diagnosis and management of glucose homeostasis in the neonate. *Curr Prob Pediatr* **15**: 11.

Hirata T, Brady JP (1977). *Newborn Intensive Care: Chemical Aspects*. Springfield, IL: Charles C Thomas.

Koh HHG, Aynsley-Green A, Tarbit M, Eyre JA (1988). Neural dysfunction during hypoglycaemia. *Arch Dis Child* **63**: 1353.

Koh HHG, Eyre JA, Aynsley-Green A (1988). Neonatal hypoglycaemia — the controversy regarding definition. *Arch Dis Child* **63**: 1386.

Lin HC, Maguire C, Oh W, Cowett R (1989). Accuracy and reliability of glucose reflectance meters in the high risk neonate. *J Pediatr* **115**: 998.

Lucas A, Morley R, Cole TJ (1988). Adverse neurodevelopmental outcome of moderate neonatal hypoglycaemia. *Br Med J* **97**: 1304.

Louik C, Mitchell AA., Epstein MF, Shapiro S (1985). Risk factors for neonatal hyperglycaemia associated with 10% dextrose infusion. *Am J Dis Child* **139**: 783.

Lyon AJ, McIntosh N, Wheeler K, Brooke OG (1984). Hypercalcaemia in extremely low birthweight infants. *Arch Dis Child* **59**: 1141.

Pryds O, Christensen NJ, Friis-Hansen B (1990). Increased cerebral blood flow and plasma epinephrine in hypoglycemic, preterm neonates. *Pediatrics* **85**: 172.

Reid MMcC, Reilly BJ, Murdock AI, Swyer PR (1971). Cardiomegaly in association with neonatal hypoglycaemia. *Acta Paediatr Scand* **60**: 295.

Tsang RC, Donovan EF, Steichen JJ (1976). Calcium physiology and pathology in the neonate. *Pediatr Clin North Am* **23**: 611.

Williams AF (1997). Hypocalcaemia of the newborn: a review. *Bull World Health Organ* **75**: 261–90.

13 Jaundice

Bilirubin metabolism

Red cell destruction releases globin, iron and unconjugated bilirubin (indirect reacting). This bilirubin exists in two forms: albumin-bound and free. Free bilirubin can cause kernicterus (see p. 220). In liver cells, bilirubin is conjugated by glucuronyl transferase, becomes water-soluble and direct reacting. Bilirubin is excreted in bile into the duodenum where stercobilinogen is formed which may be reabsorbed and excreted in urine as urobilinogen (Fig. 13.1).

In newborns, conjugated bilirubin may become unconjugated by action of β-glucuronidase in the gut and may be reabsorbed to undergo reconjugation in the liver — the *enterohepatic circulation of bilirubin*.

Factors involved in physiological jaundice are:

- Reduced red cell survival (40–60 days)
- Polycythaemia, bruising, cephalhaematoma
- Reduced Y and Z protein (ligandins)
- Inadequate calories, dehydration
- Reduced glucuronyl transferase activity
- Enterohepatic circulation
- Shunt bilirubin (20%) from haem pigments
- Alteration of hepatic blood flow at birth.

Reduced red cell survival and shunt bilirubin mean that bilirubin production in the newborn is at least twice that of the adult per kg of body weight.

Jaundice in the newborn is frequently benign and may resolve with no treatment. Well term infants who develop jaundice at

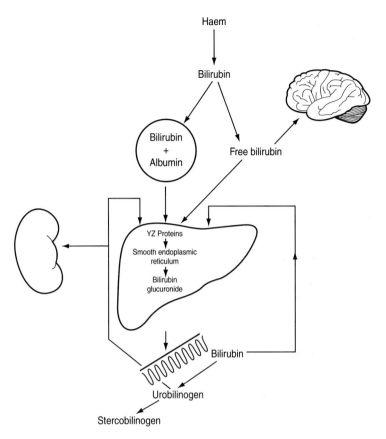

Figure 13.1. **Bilrubin metabolism**

>48 hours of age rarely need further investigation. Those babies at greatest risk and who require close observation and bilirubin monitoring are:

≺ Infants whose jaundice begins within 24 hours of birth
≺ Infants with blood group incompatibility
≺ Preterm infants
≺ Ill infants
≺ Infants with prolonged jaundice (>14 days).

Causes of neonatal jaundice are described in Table 13.1.

Table 13.1. **Causes of neonatal jaundice**

• Physiological jaundice	Aetiology: see above. Onset after 24 hours, reaches peak at 4–5 days but lasts longer in preterms. Peak levels usually <200μmol/l but exaggerated in dehydration, poor energy intake and breast-fed infants
• Isoimmune haemolytic disease	Rhesus (anti D), ABO or rarer antibodies: anti-c, anti-E, Duffy, Kell. Jaundice onset within 24 hours and Coombs' test positive.
	Maternal O/infant A worse than maternal O/infant B
• Other haemolytic disease	Glucose-6-phosphate dehydrogenase deficiency (aspirin, sulphas), pyruvate kinase deficiency, congenital spherocytosis or elliptocytosis, thalassaemia. May occur in infants of Mediterranean, African or Chinese origin
• Infection	Septicaemia, urinary infection, TORCH infections, viral hepatitis, syphilis
• Haemolysis from	Haematoma, excessive bruising, polycythaemia
• Galactosaemia	Urine Clinitest™ positive but Clinistix™ negative
• Hypothyroidism	Prolonged jaundice and absent femoral epiphyses (see Table 13.5)
• Drugs	Phenothiazines, novobiocin, vitamin K
• Cystic fibrosis	
• Biliary atresia or hepatitis	Prolonged jaundice with raised direct bilirubin
• Breast milk	Low fluid intake may accentuate 'physiological jaundice'. Also prolonged jaundice from abnormal progesterone metabolite in breast milk which competes with bilirubin for conjugation with glucuronyl transferase. Kernicterus unlikely even though bilirubin levels as high as 400 μmol/l may occur
• Rare inherited enzyme deficiencies	Inborn errors of metabolism: send urine for amino acid and sugar chromatograms
• Pyloric stenosis	

Infants jaundiced during first 24 hours of life

Likely to be due to blood group incompatibility but infection may also be the cause.

 All babies who develop jaundice during the first 24 hours of life or who have significant jaundice within 48 hours need investigation.

Investigate babies with early jaundice as follows:

➤ Haemoglobin, WCC, blood film

➤ Blood groups: mother and infant for incompatibility

➤ Coombs' test

➤ Urine for reducing substances.

If these investigations are negative or the baby is unwell, look for infection (bacterial or viral, see p. 225), and consider other rarer causes such as glucose-6-phosphate dehydrogenase deficiency.

Blood group incompatibility

Rhesus isoimmunization

15% of women are Rhesus negative (D antigen). Other Rhesus antigens can cause haemolysis (c, E). With the introduction of anti-D in 1969, the number of affected babies has fallen dramatically (number of exchange transfusions has dropped to <10% of the peak reached in 1970).

Antenatal management

Babies at risk are identified by routine screening of Rhesus–negative pregnant women for Rhesus antibody. Amniocentesis was traditionally used to estimate severity by measuring bilirubin concentration and optical density difference. In severe cases cordocentesis is used during the second trimester to measure cord haemoglobin and then transfuse the fetus directly to prevent hydrops. May reduce need for early delivery.

Postnatal management

After birth cord blood samples should be sent to assess severity:

➤ Haemoglobin

➤ Bilirubin

➤ Coombs' test

Treatment with phototherapy or exchange transfusion is used as indicated in Table 13.4 and p. 216–218.

> ❗ Continued low-grade haemolysis may continue for up to 3 months after birth, therefore babies should be followed up for detection of late anaemia.

ABO incompatibility

About 10% of group O women have IgG anti-A and anti-B haemolysins which cross the placenta (normally anti-A and anti-B are IgM antibodies and do not cross the placenta). First babies may be affected (unlike Rhesus) and the severity does not usually increase in subsequent pregnancies. ABO incompatibility is 3–4 times more common than Rhesus isoimmunization but rarely causes severe problems. Presentation is usually within the first 24 hours with highest bilirubin levels on third and fourth days. Coombs' test is may be only weakly positive and late anaemia is rarely a problem.

Preterm infants

Jaundice commoner because of hepatic immaturity and shorter red cell survival. Slower intestinal transport times with delayed passage of meconium may also be important. Meconium contains 1 mg bilirubin/g. Preterm infants at greater risk of kernicterus because of reduced bilirubin binding. In addition, hypoxia and hypoglycaemia cause increased free fatty acid levels which may displace bilirubin from albumin and acidosis decreases bilirubin binding and facilitates entry of free bilirubin into cerebral cells. Drugs that displace bilirubin from its albumin-binding sites (Table 13.2) should be used with caution in the preterm infant. Two drugs which may be weak displacers (e.g. aminophylline and methicillin) may be synergistic if given together.

Table 13.2. Drugs that displace bilirubin from albumin

Sulphonamides	Indomethacin
Salicylates	Oxacillin, azlocillin, carbenicillin, ticarcillin, methicillin
Sodium benzoate (parenteral diazepam)	Gentamicin, ceftriaxone, moxalactam
Frusemide, ethacrynic acid	Digoxin, aminophylline

Free fatty acids and haematin also displace bilirubin from albumin. This means that exchange transfusion must be performed at lower total bilirubin levels (Table 13.3, Fig. 13.2) but, preterm infants tolerate exchange transfusion less well than term infants.

Table 13.3. Suggested maximum safe bilirubin levels

Baby's weight	Safe level (μmol/l)
<1000 g	150–200
<1500 g	200–250
<2000 g	250–300
<2500 g	300–350

Ill infants

Infants who are clinically unwell and who are jaundiced must be fully investigated. Infection should be excluded by full sepsis

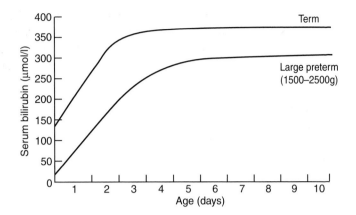

Figure 13.2. Maximum safe bilirubin levels for well term and preterm infants.

work-up. Acidosis should also be excluded or corrected. Blood film, blood groups of mother and infant and Coombs' test should also be done. If these initial investigations are negative, investigate for metabolic disorders and seek advice.

Management of early jaundice

The primary aim of management is to keep serum bilirubin below neurotoxic levels. Maximum safe levels of bilirubin are not known but suggested levels for different birth weights are given in Table 13.3 and Fig. 13.2.

There are at least 3 methods of reducing high bilirubin levels:
1. Phototherapy
2. Exchange transfusion
3. Drugs: phenobarbitone, oral agar

Phototherapy

Reduces bilirubin levels, but may also be used prophylactically in very immature infants with, for example, marked bruising. Works by converting bilirubin into water-soluble compounds which can then be excreted in the bile without conjugation.

Delivery of phototherapy is traditionally by overhead fluorescent lights. White lights are most commonly used but blue or green lights may be more effective. Blue light may result in uncomfortable side effects in staff such as dizziness and nausea.

Potential risks for the baby include:
- Retinal damage
- Increased insensible water loss
- Thermal instability
- Masking of sepsis
- Loose stools
- Rashes
- Bronzing if direct bilirubin raised

Another method for phototherapy uses a fibreoptic light system that delivers light to a pad or blanket. This method has several advantages over traditional methods — as the phototherapy pad is cool thermal instability and increased insensible water loss are not a problem; masking the eyes is probably not necessary and the baby may be held and fed during the process.

Bilirubin levels for initiating phototherapy are shown in Table 13.4. In a well term baby without incompatibility many would now suggest that treatment is not necessary until bilirubin is at the higher end of the range (350 μmol/l).

Table 13.4. Bilirubin levels for initiating phototherapy and exchange transfusion

	Bilirubin levels (μmol/l)	
	Phototherapy at	Exchange at
Normal term infant (no incompatibility)	280–350	360–450
Normal term infant but incompatibility	200–250	360
Well preterm infant >1500 g	200–250	280–360
Well preterm infant <1500 g	150–200	200–250
Sick preterm infant >1500 g	100–150	200–250
Sick preterm infant <1500 g	Any level	150–200

The following precautions should be taken during standard phototherapy:

➤ Cover the eyes without pressure (pad and bandage)

➤ Watch fluid balance carefully (increase fluid intake)

➤ Watch for temperature instability (check temperature 4-hourly)

➤ Watch for 'masked' sepsis (examine infant every 6 hours)

➤ Do not use if direct bilirubin is high (bronzing)

 Visual assessment of jaundice is not valid once phototherapy has commenced — check serum levels.

Exchange transfusion

This technique is described in Ch. 9, p. 125.

Indications:

≺ Obviously ill infant:
  anaemia, hydrops
≺ Cord blood findings:
  Haemoglobin <11 g/dl in Rhesus disease (bilirubin >120 μmol/l, Coombs' test positive)
≺ Prevention of kernicterus: Just under neurotoxic levels
  — see Fig. 13.2 and Table 13.3
≺ Other:
  DIC
  sclerema,
  polycythaemia
  some drug overdoses

Exchange transfusion soon after birth is usually performed to correct anaemia; later exchange transfusions are performed when bilirubin levels approach neurotoxic range and other methods have failed. Exchange transfusion should lower bilirubin levels by over 60%. About 2 hours after the procedure there will be a rebound rise in bilirubin level as tissue bilirubin equilibrates with plasma level. Hypoglycaemia may occur during or after exchange transfusion because Rhesus babies have hyperinsulinaemia (hypertrophy of islet cells, perhaps due to glutathione released from haemolysed red cells) and acid citrate dextrose (ACD) blood provides a glucose load which stimulates insulin release.

Drugs

Phenobarbitone

Ineffective unless used prenatally. Works by inducing glucuronyl transferase.

Oral agar

Plain agar has been shown to bind bilirubin in the gut and thus decreases enterohepatic circulation of bilirubin. Oral agar (500 mg in 10 ml distilled water 6 hourly before feeds) is said to be as effective as phototherapy in reducing bilirubin levels in term infants with physiological jaundice. The effect of phototherapy can be enhanced by combining its use with oral agar. Oral agar is not widely used in the UK or USA.

Emergency management of severe erythroblastosis (hydrops fetalis)

➤ Most will be delivered by elective caesarean section. Experienced personnel must be present.

➤ Resuscitate (see Ch. 4). May need intubation to stabilize. May need aspiration of pleural and peritoneal effusions. If intraperitoneal fetal transfusion has been performed within the previous 7 days, unabsorbed blood may splint the diaphragm and should be removed by paracentesis (p. 134).

➤ Catheterize umbilical vein. Check haemoglobin, bilirubin, Coombs' test. (NB Coomb's test may be negative if recent IUFT.) If central venous pressure >10 cmH$_2$O, remove 10 ml blood/kg; if normal or low, stabilize and transfer to neonatal unit.

➤ Mechanical ventilation if evidence of RDS, severe heart failure or pulmonary hypoplasia, all of which are associated with hydrops.

➤ Early exchange transfusion with semi-packed cells to increase a low haemoglobin; no deficit unless CVP high. Blood should be donor fresh if possible but certainly <48 hours old, cross-matched and CMV, HBV and HIV negative.

➤ May occasionally need digoxin and diuretics (p. 285), or peritoneal dialysis (p. 316).

➤ Clotting screen 1 hour after completion of exchange transfusion.

Kernicterus

Term used to describe yellow staining of the basal ganglia and nuclear areas of the brain in newborn babies dying with severe jaundice. Rarely seen in well term babies unless bilirubin levels are very high but yellow staining of the brain has been seen in preterm babies at low serum bilirubin levels.

Factors predisposing to kernicterus are:

- Immaturity
- Low serum albumin
- Hypoxia, acidosis, sepsis or hypoglycaemia.

Initially infant has non-specific signs such as poor suck, lethargy and hypotonia. Within hours the condition progresses to fever and hypertonia of extensor muscle groups leading to opisthotonos and retrocollis (trunk and neck arching). There may also be convulsions and downward rolling of the eyes or 'setting-sun' sign. Preterm babies may not exhibit the typical signs but may develop apnoea with increased tone.

Management

If kernicterus is suspected, immediate exchange transfusion should be given after infusion of albumin 1 g/kg.

The presence of signs of kernicterus is not an indication to abandon treatment as permanent neurological damage may be lessened or even prevented by prompt action. Failure to treat may result in the full-blown syndrome of choreoathetosis, spastic diplegia, high-tone hearing loss, mental retardation and failure of upward gaze.

Infants with prolonged jaundice

Defined as clinically apparent jaundice 10 days after birth in a term infant and 2 weeks after birth in a preterm infant. Breast feeding is the commonest cause in the term infant (at least 2% of breast-fed babies) and non-specific 'hepatitis' (or cholestasis) in the VLBW infant (Table 13.5). If due to breast feeding, there is an association with haemorrhagic disease of the newborn; therefore, ensure the infant has been given an appropriate dose of Vitamin K. Rarely should breast feeding be stopped and kernicterus has not been reported in the absence of coexistent haemolytic disease. Ensure adequate fluid intake and reassure mother. Occasionally phototherapy is needed.

Raised direct bilirubin (cholestasis) in the VLBW infant recovering from intensive care is common (1–2%). Probably due to a combination of problems: intravenous feeding, chronic infection and possibly ascending cholangitis. Often coexists with osteopenia of prematurity and chronic lung disease (p. 167).

The following investigations should be performed:

➤ Total and direct bilirubin

➤ Full blood count and film

➤ Urine culture

➤ Thyroid function tests

➤ Clinitest™/Clinistix™ on urine and chromatogram.

 All babies jaundiced after 14 days should have direct bilirubin measured

Table 13.5. **Causes of prolonged jaundice**

● Sepsis	Especially in ill infant, urinary infection or septicaemia
● Breast milk	Breast milk jaundice
● Hypothyroidism	Screen T4 and TSH. Other clinical signs often absent*
● Galactosaemia	Usually vomiting and sepsis picture. Test urine and send urinary chromatogram
● Inspissated bile syndrome	Follows severe haemolytic disease especially if exchange transfusion needed. Raised direct bilirubin; usually responds to conservative management. Liver biopsy may show giant cell hepatitis
● Cystic fibrosis	Uncommon presentation of this disorder
● Immaturity	Especially if bruised and fed with intravenous amino acids
● Obstructive jaundice	Hepatitis: infections, errors of metabolism, galactosaemia, drugs; biliary atresia, cholestasis, inspissated bile syndrome, parenteral nutrition, α_1-antitrypsin deficiency; choledochal cyst
● Delayed passage of stool	Increased enterohepatic circulation. Intestinal obstruction or extreme immaturity
● Pyloric stenosis	Occasional early presentation
● Syndromes	Gilbert's (impaired hepatocyte uptake and reduced intracellular binding proteins), Crigler–Najjar (impaired conjugation), Dubin–Johnson, Rotor (impaired transport mechanisms)

*Neonatal signs of hypothyroidism: prolonged pregnancy, high birth weight, large fontanelle, hypothermia, peripheral cyanosis, lethargy, poor feeding, delayed passage of meconium, prolonged jaundice, oedema, respiratory distress. Treat with thyroxine (see p. 340).

If direct bilirubin is raised (>20% total bilirubin) there is some urgency in differentiating biliary atresia from neonatal hepatitis as laparotomy and corrective surgery are more successful if done before 6–8 weeks.

Investigations to differentiate biliary atresia from hepatitis:

➤ Liver enzymes and α-fetoprotein

➤ Ultrasound scan of biliary tree

➤ Radioisotope excretion scan (HIDA scan)

➤ Liver biopsy.

Conservative management of neonatal hepatitis usually leads to resolution: treat any underlying infection, ensure adequate oral nutrition, especially fat-soluble vitamins A, D, E and K, and consider treatment with metronidazole.

Nursing points

Baby

- Remove baby's eye mask before handling to allow eye contact and normal stimulation.
- Healthy babies who are fully breast-fed do not require dextrose or water supplements whilst under phototherapy. They should be allowed to feed on demand to replace any fluid deficit.
- Monitor temperature regularly.
- Ensure insensible fluid losses are accounted for in fluid intake whilst under phototherapy or radiant heaters.
- Half-hourly recordings of temperature and blood pressure, continuous cardiorespiratory monitoring and strict fluid input/output chart to be recorded during exchange transfusions.

Family

- Note maternal blood group and antibody status.
- Explain the physiology of jaundice in appropriate terminology to the family.
- Anticipate the need for use of phototherapy lights and explain their use to parents, including the need to cover the baby's eyes, nursing the baby naked and the likelihood of loose stools and rashes.

- Prepare parents for the possibility of the serum bilirubin estimation rising slightly when phototherapy is stopped.
- If breast milk jaundice is diagnosed, reassure the parents that there is no need to stop breast feeding and explain the condition fully.

Equipment

- Consider using a tinted perspex shield to shade the baby's face and eyes instead of a mask.
- The use of Biliblankets™ allows treatment to continue uninterrupted while the baby is being held and fed.
- Following an exchange transfusion the tip of the catheter should be sent for culture.

Staff

- Adequate staffing levels on postnatal or transitional care wards should ensure that babies are not admitted to NICU simply for phototherapy.

References and further reading

Dodd KL (1993). Neonatal jaundice — a lighter touch. *Arch Dis Child* **68**: 529.

Newman TB, Maisels MJ (1989). Bilirubin and brain damage: what do we do now? *Pediatrics* **83**: 1062.

Newman TB, Maisels MJ (1992). Evaluation and treatment of jaundice in the term newborn; a kinder gentler approach. *Pediatrics* **89**: 809.

Yao TC, Stevenson DK (1995). Advances in the diagnosis and treatment of neonatal hyperbilirubinaemia. *Clin Perinatol* **22**: 741–58.

14 Fetal and Neonatal Infection

For discussion of cross-infection measures see p. 83. Maternal infection is discussed in Ch. 3. Early fetal infections are often caused by viruses. Some of these can be remembered by the mnemonic TORCH (toxoplasmosis — a protozoa, rubella, cytomegalovirus and herpes simplex), but there are others including HIV, parvovirus B19 and the hepatitis viruses. These are uncommon by comparison to perinatal bacterial infection (Table 14.1).

Table 14.1. Incidence of perinatal infection

Organism	Mother/1000 pregnancies	Fetus/1000 pregnancies	Newborn/1000 live births
Toxoplasma	1.5–6.4	1.3–7.0	0.05–1.0
Rubella virus			
epidemic year	20–40	4–30	2–6
interepidemic	0.1–1.0	0.2–0.5	0.25
Cytomegalovirus	30–140	5–15	1–5
Herpes simplex virus	1–10	Rare	0.1–0.5
Treponema pallidum	0.2	0.1	0.2
All bacterial infections	—	—	3–5

TORCH infections

Infants with TORCH infection are frequently small for gestational age, may have a rash, hepatitis, chorioretinitis, CNS findings and failure to thrive (Table 14.2). Such babies may be screened by measuring cord blood IgM (normal <0.2 g/l). If a TORCH infection has occurred, cord IgM >0.25 g/l in about

60% of babies. A more specific search for elevated TORCH titres is generally not warranted unless there are very strong clinical indications, or screening IgM is elevated.

Pregnant caregivers should avoid contact with babies who have congenital viral infections.

✚ Toxoplasmosis

This is uncommon in UK, but more common in France and Spain (3–6/1000 births) where undercooked meat may be the source. Hand washing is important as infection may also be contracted from young cats and their faeces. Infection is confirmed by presence of toxoplasma-specific IgM in the infant's serum. Acquired toxoplasmosis is treated with sulphadiazine (50–100 mg/kg/day, 12 hourly), pyrimethamine (1 mg/kg/day, once daily) and folic acid. Spiramycin has been used in pregnancy in some countries (3 g daily from diagnosis to the end of the pregnancy), but there have been no controlled trials of its use and no definite proven benefit in countries with a low prevalence rate.

✚ Rubella

Epidemics of rubella formerly occurred about every 7 years. The infection rate has fallen with the introduction of mass immunization and congenital rubella is now rare in developed countries. Children are immunized at around 15 months with the MMR vaccine. Seronegative women are at risk and should be immunized, but should not become pregnant for 3 months after vaccination. First-trimester infections are the most serious, causing CNS and cardiovascular defects. After 14 weeks of pregnancy, the only adverse effect on fetus is deafness. Infants with congenital rubella should be isolated and should be considered contagious up to 1 year of age unless viral cultures are negative.

✚ Cytomegalovirus (CMV)

Probably the commonest fetal viral infection, although most babies are unaffected. Of women susceptible to CMV, the risk

Table 14.2. Clinical features of TORCH infections

	TO	R	C	H
Central nervous system				
Encephalitis	+	+	+	+
Microcephaly	+	+	+	+
Hydrocephaly	+	+	+	+
Intracranial calcification	+	+	+	+
Psychomotor retardation	+	+	+	+
Hearing loss	+	+	+	?
Eye				
Chorioretinitis	+	0	+	+
Pigmented retina	+	+	0	0
Keratoconjunctivitis	0	0	0	+
Cataracts	0	+	0	+
Glaucoma	+	+	0	0
Visual impairment	+	+	+	+
Reticuloendothelial system				
Hepatosplenomegaly	+	+	+	+
Liver calcification	+	?	+	+
Jaundice	+	+	+	+
Haemolytic anaemia	+	+	+	+
Petechiae	+	+	+	+
Lymphadenopathy	+	+	0	0
Heart				
Myocarditis	+	+	+	+
Congenital heart disease	+	+	+	+
Bone lesions	+	+	+	?
Skin				
Vesicular lesions	0	0	0	+
Pregnancy complications				
Abortions, stillbirths prematurity, IUGR	+	+	+	+

+ = occurs; 0 = does not occur, ? = uncertain.
After Kadar (1979).

of primary infection during pregnancy is approximately 1%. Primary CMV infections during pregnancy are usually asymptomatic, but the risk of fetal infection is about 50%. Only 5–10% of congenitally infected infants have clinically apparent disease, but of these the mortality rate is 30%, and 90% of survivors have significant sequelae. Infants may present at birth with hydrops, thrombocytopenia, microcephaly and neurological deficits.

> **!** Congenital CMV-related CNS defects may not present until later in childhood.

CNS defects may not present until later childhood; 6% have late-onset sensorineural deafness. Postnatal infection may be acquired from blood transfusion, leading to pneumonitis and jaundice, so CMV negative blood must be used.

There is no effective treatment for established disease. Ganciclovir has been used but is highly toxic.

⊞ *Herpes simplex virus (HSV)*

The incidence of neonatal HSV infection is low, although rates vary from country to country (up to 0.5/1000 births in USA, 0.2 /1000 in UK). There are two sources of infection: *genital*, acquired during passage down the birth canal, and *orocutaneous*, from active lesions on the mother or caregivers (the latter is uncommon). There is a 50% risk of transmitting infection to the neonate if vaginal delivery occurs in a woman with active primary genital herpes. If caesarean section is performed before labour or within 6 hours of membrane rupture, the risk is reduced to <10%. Seventy per cent of infected newborns are born to women without obvious active lesions. Re-activation of infection in the mother is less likely to lead to infection in the baby as levels of anti-HSV antibodies are higher and virus is shed for shorter periods of time than in a primary infection.

Infection may be local or systemic. *Local infection* produces a vesicular rash on the presenting part, occurring on its own or as part of a systemic illness. This may become disseminated in

80% of cases if treatment is not commenced. *Systemic infection* may localize particularly to the lung (presenting by 3–7 days) or CNS, leading to meningoencephalitis, focal seizures and cranial nerve palsies; or become disseminated with fever, vomiting, lethargy, jaundice, bleeding from DIC (25%) and collapse. Disseminated disease usually presents in the first 1–2 weeks and localized disease in second or third week. Diagnosis is by electron microscopy of vesicle scraping and culture of virus. Polymerase chain reaction (PCR) assay of HSV–DNA in cerebrospinal fluid can provide a rapid and non-invasive method for the diagnosis of HSV encephalitis.

The infected infant should be isolated. Intravenous adenosine arabinoside (vidarabine, 15–30 mg/kg/day in 12 hourly i.v. infusions for 10–14 days) plus acyclovir (30 mg/kg/day, 8 hourly, for 10–14 days) may help, but mortality and morbidity are high. Treatment of mothers or staff with cold sores is empirical. Affected persons should wear masks and not handle the baby for 24 hours and local treatment with acyclovir should be given for up to 3 days.

Other congenital viral infections

✚ *Hepatitis B virus (HBV)*

Many countries screen all pregnant women for HBsAg. There is a high carrier rate in mothers from South-East Asia, especially Chinese; these, and others at high risk (e.g. i.v. drug abusers) should be included in any targeted screening programme. There is a high risk of vertical transmission to baby at birth if e-antigen is present.

Prevention is by vaccinating infants at risk. Give 0.5 ml (10 μg) anti-HBV vaccine intramuscularly into anterolateral thigh at birth and repeat at 1 and 6 months. To give protection until the vaccine becomes effective, give 200 IU of anti-HBV globulin intramuscularly in a different muscle as soon as possible after birth. Breast feeding should be discouraged in developed countries but may be important for other reasons in less-developed countries.

Precautions to avoid self-innoculation include care with contaminated needles, wearing gloves and visor at delivery and careful handling of infected secretions. Health care workers who are at risk of contracting hepatitis B because of exposure to blood should also be vaccinated. It should be remembered that immunization takes up to 6 months to become active.

✚ *Hepatitis C virus (HCV)*

Mothers at risk of HCV infection are similar to those at risk from HBV or HIV. There is little information about transmission of infection to the baby; in one small study of babies born to anti-HCV positive mothers, 80% of babies were anti-HCV negative by 12 months of life, with approx. 20% of babies having detectable HCV-RNA by 4 months. Neonates are potentially at risk from blood transfusion and donated blood should be screened for HCV.

Chronic hepatitis C in childhood appears to be a mild disease, at least in its early stages.

✚ *Human immunodeficiency virus (HIV)*

HIV is an RNA-containing lentivirus. Approximately two-thirds of HIV-positive mothers give birth to seropositive babies and 15–20% of these retain anti-HIV antibodies beyond 18 months of life and are at risk of developing AIDS. 75% of childhood cases of HIV are acquired vertically at birth from mothers with HIV. Infection may be acquired from infected blood or breast milk but these routes are rare in developed countries. However, donors to human milk banks should be tested for HIV and their milk pasteurized, and donated blood should also be screened.

Exposure to HIV may be confirmed by antibody detection in peripheral blood using ELISA or Western blot analysis. HIV positive antibody testing in an infant aged <18 months indicates maternal infection but does not diagnose infection in the infant; a definitive diagnosis can only be made by virus culture or detection of viral DNA by polymerase chain reaction methods (PCR). If either test is positive, it should be repeated immediately to confirm infection. If PCR or viral culture continues to remain negative at 4 months of age, there is a >95% chance of being uninfected. Viral p24 antigen testing is less sensitive than culture or PCR.

The maternal records should be checked for documentation of other infections which might affect the baby, e.g. TORCH, sexually transmitted disease, hepatitis B and C and tuberculosis. Infection with HIV rarely causes symptoms before 1 month of life. HIV-related initial signs and symptoms include *Pneumocystis carinii* pneumonia, and persistent lymphadenopathy, hepatomegaly and splenomegaly which appear around 6 months of life, usually preceded by hyper-IgG, A, M. Persistent oral candidiasis is a frequent precursor of AIDS. Approximately 30% of infected children present with AIDS within 6 months.

 Babies of mothers at risk of contracting HIV should also be screened for sexually transmitted diseases and hepatitis B and C.

Treatment regimens may vary but should be given under the supervision of those experienced in their use. During labour and delivery, the mother should be given an intravenous infusion of zidovudine (ZDV, 2 mg/kg i.v. over 1 hour, followed by a continuous infusion of 1 mg/kg/h) until the cord is clamped. The baby should be commenced on ZDV syrup 2 mg/kg/dose, 6-hourly within 8–12 hours of birth, and continued for 6 weeks. ZDV is toxic and expensive and its use must be monitored closely, particularly for haematological toxicity.

Prophylaxis for *Pneumocystis carinii* infection should be started in all babies at 6 weeks, when ZDV treatment is stopped. Treat with co-trimoxazole, given as trimethoprim 5 mg/kg/day and sulphamethoxazole 25 mg/kg/day, orally in two divided doses, 3 times per week on consecutive days. Prophylaxis beyond 4–6 months should be given to infected infants or to those whose infection status is indeterminate.

✚ *Varicella virus (chickenpox, zoster)*

> **!** If maternal chickenpox occurs within 4–5 days before delivery and 2 days afterwards, severe infection of the newborn can occur.

In pregnancy, varicella infection can lead to a severe pneumonitis in the mother. For non-immune women exposed to varicella through intimate contact, zoster immune globulin (ZIG or VZIg) should be given to modify severity of disease in the mother and reduce the risk of fetal infection. Maternal isolation is necessary. Infection in the first trimester can cause cicatricial skin lesions along sites of major nerves in the limbs, and eye and brain lesions. The risk to the fetus is only about 2%. However, if maternal infection occurs within 4–5 days before delivery and 2 days afterwards, severe infection of the newborn can occur. Mortality is approx. 30% untreated. ZIG (VZIg), 0.05 ml/kg i.m. should be given to baby at birth who can then be nursed with mother. Severe neonatal varicella may still occur despite giving ZIG at birth. For these babies intravenous acyclovir (60 mg/kg/day) should be given 8-hourly. Postnatal exposure to varicella is less risky although very immature babies (<28 weeks' gestation) and those born to mothers with no immunity should be protected with ZIG.

The situation sometimes arises where an older sibling develops chickenpox whilst the mother is in hospital having a baby. If the mother has had chickenpox in the past, both mother and baby may safely go home. If she has not, or there is uncertainty, the baby should be given ZIG and allowed home. The mother should, if possible, avoid close contact with the older child until the lesions have all crusted over.

✚ *Respiratory syncitial virus (RSV)*

Although not a cause of congenital infection, RSV can be a problem in neonatal nurseries where it may cause outbreaks in the winter months. Symptoms may vary from none to lethargy, poor feeding, rhinitis and tachypnoea. A small proportion of babies may require mechanical ventilation. The influenza, parainfluenza and rhinoviruses may cause a similar picture. Infection is typically passed on from parents or older siblings, who may have few symptoms themselves.

The ex-preterm nursery graduate who has had chronic lung disease is particularly at risk after discharge from the unit. Infection can be rapidly diagnosed by immunofluorescent assay of RSV antigen in nasopharyngeal secretions. Treatment involves isolation, careful hand washing and supportive measures. Nebulized ribavirin has been advocated but its use is probably best restricted to those babies who are at greatest risk, i.e. those with severe underlying lung or cardiac problems. Prophylaxis with hyperimmune RSV globulin is a promising additional therapeutic option for high risk preterm babies.

Bacterial infections

Severe bacterial infection in the newborn is mainly a problem in preterm babies and those receiving intensive care. The newborn has reduced defenses against infection:

1. *Decreased humoral immunity*: only IgG crosses the placenta (IgM contains specific bactericidal antibodies to Gram-negative organisms)
2. *Decreased cellular immunity*: still debated but the preterm infant probably has impaired cell-mediated immunity
3. *Decreased white cell activity:* phagocytosis reduced due to deficient opsonizing antibody and impaired chemotaxis
4. *Deficient complement system*
5. *Secretory IgA* from colostrum and breast milk will not be provided for bottle-fed baby

Risk factors for congenital bacterial infection:

- Preterm infant, especially male sex
- Prolonged rupture of membranes >24 hours

- Maternal infection — fever, leucocytosis, tender uterus, foul discharge suggesting chorioamnionitis
  recent urinary tract infection
  colonization with group B streptococcus
  Shirodkar suture (cervical cerclage)
  poor socioeconomic status
- Antepartum haemorrhage, especially abruption
- Early respiratory distress (p. 161).

Consider performing a sepsis work-up and starting antibiotic cover if any of these risk factors are present.

The commonest bacterial pathogens are coliforms, group B β-haemolytic streptococci, staphylococci, pseudomonas, listeria and others, e.g. klebsiella, haemophilus, serratia, pneumococci, enterococci and anaerobes. Infection may be congenital or acquired (nosocomial).

The route of infection may be:
Transplacental (rare)
Ascending, usually in the presence of ruptured membranes
Aspiration during passage down the birth canal
Direct invasion after birth, e.g. via umbilical cord, skin, indwelling lines or other equipment

Presentation

Signs of sepsis in the newborn:

≺ Pallor or mottling, shock
≺ Lethargy
≺ Hypotonia, poor Moro reflex
≺ Temperature instability (may be masked by servo-controlled incubator)
≺ Poor feeding, vomiting
≺ Glucose intolerance (often hyperglycaemia)
≺ Bloody stools or diarrhoea
≺ Apnoea, tachypnoea, cyanosis
≺ Tachycardia, bradycardia
≺ Omphalitis, abdominal distension

≺ Splenomegaly, hepatomegaly, enlarged kidneys
≺ Irritability, seizures
≺ Jaundice
≺ Abnormal bleeding, petechiae
≺ Sclerema.

Note that these are non-specific and numerous. Specific signs often present quite late in the illness, so that in any baby who is preterm or is receiving care and whose clinical condition changes, infection should be sought.

 Signs of sepsis in the newborn are numerous and non-specific.

Congenital infection predominantly presents as respiratory distress or apnoea, because infected material is aspirated at the time of birth, causing bronchopneumonia. This may progress to septicaemia or meningitis. *Nosocomial infections* may also present as septicaemia, pneumonia or meningitis but in addition osteomyelitis, urinary tract infection, skin infections and conjunctivitis may occur.

Laboratory investigations in suspected sepsis

➤ Relevant cultures: blood, CSF, urine, skin, external ear, throat, rectum, cord, amniotic fluid, gastric aspirate, catheter tips

➤ Microscopy: CSF, urine and gastric aspirate (Gram stain)

➤ Full blood picture (see Table 14.3)

➤ Acute phase reactants: C-reactive protein (CRP), erythrocyte sedimentation rate (ESR), cytokines: interleukins, tumour necrosis factor

➤ Radiographs: chest if respiratory signs, abdomen if NEC suspected

➤ Others (if indicated): immunoglobulins, blood gases, calcium, electrolytes, coagulation studies

➤ Histopathology of placenta and cord

Table 14.3 shows abnormalities that may occur on the blood film in neonatal sepsis.

When two or more tests are abnormal the likelihood of infection being present is significantly increased (about 90% positive predictive value). However, changes in C-reactive protein (CRP), white cell count and other markers of infection may be delayed. Blood cultures rarely become positive before 12 hours of incubation. The best test is a high index of suspicion; antibiotics should not be withheld until results of cultures have returned as this may be too late.

Table 14.3. **Blood film in neonatal sepsis**

Extreme shift to the left (band: segmented neutrophil ratio >0.2, see Appendix V)
Leucocytosis (>20 000/mm³ and over 60% neutrophils)
Leucopenia (<5000/mm³)
Toxic granulation of neutrophils
Fragmentation of red cells
Reticulocytosis
Thrombocytopenia (<100 000/mm³)

Management

Antibiotic treatment is the mainstay (see p. 245). Any baby with suspected infection (see above) should have a sepsis work-up and be given antibiotics. If all cultures subsequently prove negative, antibiotics can be stopped in 2–3 days if the baby is well. Proven infections (positive cultures) should be treated for at least 5–7 days with appropriate antibiotics by the intravenous route.

A combination of antibiotics should be given, usually a penicillin and an aminoglycoside (see Appendix II). The choice of penicillin is determined by the likely organism, e.g. group B β-haemolytic streptococcus — benzylpenicillin; staphylococcus — flucloxacillin; listeriosis and enterococcus — ampicillin. The third-generation cephalosporins are often used in the treatment of neonatal infection (p. 246). Late-onset infections are most commonly caused by coagulase negative and, occasionally, coagulase positive staphylococci, and a combination of flucloxacillin and netilmicin, or vancomycin may be needed (see below).

In addition to antibiotics, infants with infections need supportive care with intravenous fluids and nutrition, electrolyte and acid–base balance correction. Hypotension should be managed by volume expansion or infusion of dopamine. Bleeding disorder may be improved by giving fresh plasma and vitamin K. Exchange transfusion with fresh blood provides opsonins and can be useful in septicaemia and sclerema . A single volume exchange transfusion (80 ml/kg) may be performed as described on p. 125.

Granulocyte or buffy coat transfusions may be of benefit, although there is a potential risk of graft-versus-host disease in very immature, immunocompromized babies. Intravenous immune globulin (IVIG) has been used both in the prophylaxis and treatment of neonatal infections. Preliminary results from trials are encouraging, although its use on a regular basis is not yet widespread. Recombinant human granulocyte colony stimulating factor (G-CSF) has been used in chemotherapy-associated neutropenia, in both adults and children. Recent reports suggest that it may also be useful in severe neonatal infection, where the myeloid precursor pool becomes depleted, although more research is needed. A typical dose would be 10 μg/kg by i.v. infusion over 30 min, once daily.

✚ Congenital pneumonia

This may mimic respiratory distress syndrome (see p. 161).

✚ Septicaemia/bacteraemia

The onset of septicaemia may be early or late. Early infection is usually secondary to congenital pneumonia, although radiographic changes in the latter may be non-specific or minimal. The umbilicus may also be the portal of entry. Organisms frequently involved are coliforms, Group B β-haemolytic streptococcus (GBS), listeria, and other Gram-negative bacilli such as klebsiella.

Early onset

Early-onset infection with GBS or listeria may cause a very severe illness with circulatory collapse and DIC, leading to rapid demise unless aggressive treatment is instituted. Around 10–30% of pregnant women carry GBS in the genital tract or rectum. Babies born to these mothers will be colonized with the organism but only 1% will develop serious illness. Despite treatment the mortality rate is still high, at around 30%.

Listeria monocytogenes infection may be acquired transplacentally, following a maternal 'flu-like' illness. There may be meconium staining in premature labour although this is not specific to listeriosis. At birth the baby may have a maculopapular rash, hepatosplenomegaly and DIC. There is a 50% mortality rate, with significant disability in up to 50% of survivors.

Pseudomonas may cause infections similar to those caused by *Escherichia coli* but the mortality is higher. It occasionally presents with a pink macular rash associated with a marked vasculitis and necrotic lesions. Infections with serratia often resemble pseudomonas and occur in very immature infants who have been treated with broad-spectrum antibiotics.

Anaerobic infections (see p. 164), e.g. bacteroides, should be suspected in the presence of maternal illness, prolonged rupture of membranes, a foul-smelling baby or scalp abscesses.

Late onset

Late-onset septicaemia is usually due to staphylococci (both coagulase-negative and -positive) and is often acquired from indwelling lines. Methicillin-resistant *Staph. aureus* (MRSA) has emerged in recent years and may cause outbreaks within neonatal units. These organisms are resistant to most anti-staphylococcal antibiotics but usually respond to vancomycin.

In septicaemia or bacteraemia, the baby may present with non-specific signs or apnoea and bradycardia, lethargy and worsening jaundice. There may be an associated respiratory illness or cerebral signs due to meningitis.

Investigate with cultures (see above) and start intravenous antibiotics. A suitable combination is benzylpenicillin and an aminoglycoside such as gentamicin or netilmicin. Penicillin should be given in high dose if GBS is suspected or isolated, and ampicillin may be substituted for benzylpenicillin if listeria is likely. Cephalosporins such as cefotaxime, ceftazidime or ceftriaxone may also be used, particularly for coliform infections, but are probably better reserved as second-line treatment unless meningitis or pseudomonas infection are strongly suspected. The duration of treatment in proven septicaemia should be 7–10 days. Doses of antibiotics are given in Appendix II. Aim to keep trough serum gentamicin level in therapeutic range 0.5–1.0 mg/l; trough levels > 4.0 mg/l are ototoxic. Peak levels should be 5–8 mg/l (Table 14.4).

✚ *Sclerema*

This is a woody hardening of the subcutaneous tissues associated with infection, but is now rare. The changes first appear in the buttocks and legs but spread to the back and chest. The exact cause of changes in subcutaneous fatty tissues is unknown, but both hypothermia and reduced peripheral circulation may be underlying factors. Staphylococcal or streptococcal infections may be found. Therapy includes correction of metabolic and other abnormalities (hypoxia, hypothermia, acidosis, hypoglycaemia and coagulation disorder). Antibiotics should always be started if not already being administered. Exchange transfusion with fresh blood may help, perhaps by providing opsonins and other serum factors that enhance the ability to fight underlying infection. Steroids should not be given. Sclerema is associated with a poor prognosis.

✚ *Meningitis*

Early-onset infection is often caused by coliforms. GBS and listeria may cause late onset meningitis. Symptoms are usually non-specific, e.g. vomiting and lethargy. Seizures, high-pitched cry and tense anterior fontanelle occur later. If in doubt perform a lumbar puncture.

> ⚷ A lumbar puncture should be performed whenever there is any possibility of meningitis.

Antibiotics (cefotaxime, or a penicillin and an aminoglycoside) should be started or their dosage increased (see Appendix II). If there is clinical deterioration, persistent fever and increasing ventricular size, intraventricular antibiotics may be given. CT or MRI of the brain should be considered in order to exclude a subdural effusion or abscess when there is a persistent pyrexia or delayed improvement.

Duration of parenteral therapy is usually 2–3 weeks. Lumbar puncture should be repeated after 3 days and possibly again after 2 weeks to help determine response and duration of treatment. For poor responders, cefotaxime or chloramphenicol may be helpful as both penetrate well into CSF. If chloramphenicol is used, serum should be assayed (see below). Despite intensive care and newer antibiotics, outcome remains disappointing with 30–50% mortality and a significant proportion of survivors (perhaps 30–50%) have subsequent disability.

Survivors of meningitis should have hearing screening performed.

✚ *Urinary tract infection (UTI)*

Urinary tract infection occurs in about 1–2% of newborns. It is commoner in boys. Presentation may be with poor feeding, vomiting and jaundice. Urine for culture can be obtained by suprapubic aspiration (see Ch. 9), clean catch or by uribag. Urine obtained by suprapubic aspiration is least likely to be contaminated. Culture of urine collected by clean catch or uribag method may be contaminated, so take several specimens for culture and transport rapidly to the laboratory. All cultures should reveal the same organism $> 10^5$/ml, with pus cells. Treat with parenteral antibiotics for 7–10 days, followed by oral prophylaxis with trimethoprim 2–5 mg/kg/day. Renal tract imaging should be performed to look for renal anomalies (10–20%) and vesico-ureteric reflux (see Ch. 19). 25–50% of babies will have a recurrence of UTI.

✚ *Osteomyelitis*

May present up to 6 weeks after a septicaemia or bacteraemia, commonly staphylococcal, but may be due to other organisms such as salmonella. Bones most commonly affected are the tibiae, other long bones, vertebrae and maxilla. The skull bones and os calcis may be sites of iatrogenic infection secondary to scalp electrodes and heel stabs, respectively. Presenting signs are usually non-specific but later localized redness, tenderness, oedema and loss of movement occur. The infected site should be aspirated for culture. Radiological changes of bone rarefaction and lysis, and periosteal elevation do not occur until 10–14 days after presentation. Treatment should begin with flucloxacillin or fusidic acid in high doses and an orthopaedic opinion sought. Osteomyelitis in the newborn may lead to deranged bone growth if the metaphysis or epiphyseal plate are damaged. The duration of antibiotic therapy is at least 6 weeks. Skeletal survey should be performed on all infants about 4–6 weeks after a proven staphylococcal septicaemia.

Superficial infections

✚ Pemphigus

Also called scalded skin syndrome. This is a generalized bullous eruption which is often rapidly fatal. Prompt treatment with fluids and intravenous antibiotics is imperative.

✚ Septic spots

These can be differentiated from erythema toxicum by smear for Gram stain: septic spots contain polymorphs and organisms, often staphylococci; erythema toxicum lesions contain eosinophils with no organisms.

✚ Omphalitis

This presents as an erythematous and indurated area around the cord stump which may have a serous or purulent exudate. There is a danger of local and systemic spread which can be rapid.

Superficial staphylococcal infections are potentially dangerous and isolation with strict hand washing is essential. Local therapy with alcohol swabs and antiseptics, e.g. hexachlorophane, is helpful but ill infants should also have systemic antibiotics. Mupirocin (pseudomonic acid) is a local antibacterial agent with powerful activity against MRSA. To reduce colonization it should be applied liberally to carrier sites (nares, umbilicus and perianal area).

✚ Conjunctivitis

Caused by chemical, bacterial or viral agents. Chlorhexidine used to swab the maternal perineum or silver nitrate to prevent ophthalmia neonatorum may cause a purulent-looking neonatal conjunctivitis. This will be present on first day and will be culture-negative.

Ophthalmia neonatorum is caused by *Neisseria gonorrhoeae* (gonococcus), a notifiable disease in the UK. Severe conjunctivitis presenting within 24–48 hours, especially if bilateral with oedema of the eyelids, may be gonococcal infection. Swabs from both infant and mother should be taken (smear shows Gram-negative, intracellular diplococci) and penicillin eye drops should be started. These are given half hourly for the first 8 hours and then 4 hourly for 7 days. Systemic penicillin should also be given until results of culture are available. Prompt and aggressive therapy is necessary to prevent corneal damage and blindness. The mother and her contacts will also need treatment and referral to a genitourinary medicine specialist.

Chlamydia trachomatis is sexually transmitted and may cause conjunctivitis, typically presenting towards the end of the first week of life. Earlier presentation may occur if there has been prolonged rupture of the membranes. About 25% of babies born to infected mothers become infected. Less than 15% are symptomatic and approximately 25% of these develop pneumonia. The respiratory component is often mild and radiological findings much worse than the clinical picture. Babies with chlamydia conjunctivitis should be treated with oral erythromycin (40 mg/kg/day) for 10–14 days, and topical erythromycin or tetracycline eye ointment.

Conjunctivitis is also caused by staphylococci, streptococci and coliforms. Chloramphenicol eye ointment is effective for most cases of bacterial conjunctivitis but treatment should be guided by results of eye swabs taken prior to treatment.

Fungal infections

Fungal infections in the newborn are most commonly caused by candida spp., although others such as malassezia spp. and cryptococcus can occur. Candida can present as mild superficial mucocutaneous infection or more serious systemic illness.

Superficial infection

Candida is frequently picked up from the mother at birth and takes about 7 days to grow on moist areas such as the mouth and perineum. Infection may be encouraged by the use of broad spectrum antibiotics and parenteral nutrition. Superficial infection of mouth with thrush may make the infant reluctant to feed and candidiasis of the perineum may cause a fiery-red scaly rash affecting the intertriginous areas. Nystatin suspension 100 000 units/ml given after feeds for 7 days and nystatin cream applied to perineal infection are usually effective.

Systemic candidiasis

This is largely confined to the preterm infant. Predisposing factors include impaired host defenses, parenteral nutrition and indwelling lines, prolonged use of broad-spectrum antibiotics and chronic illness. Use of dexamethasone for chronic lung disease does not seem to predispose to candidiasis.

Signs of infection are non-specific (lethargy, apnoea, poor colour, abdominal distension) but in severe cases joint effusions (particularly the knee) or renal failure may occur. Occasionally, the renal tracts may be obstructed by fungal balls. Candida meningitis may be difficult to diagnose, sometimes found only at autopsy.

Candida can be cultured from the blood, urine, faeces and CSF. The organism is difficult to grow so several samples should be sent for culture and a high suspicion maintained in the very immature baby who deteriorates but has negative bacterial cultures. The presence of budding yeasts in a suprapubic aspirate of urine is diagnostic.

Treatment is with anti-fungal agents in addition to general supportive measures. First line management usually consists of a combination of amphotericin B and flucytosine.

Amphotericin B

Given intravenously, gradually increasing stepwise from 0.25 to 1.0 mg/kg/day. An alternative regimen is 0.6 mg/kg/day throughout the treatment period. Side effects include fever, renal toxicity, bone marrow suppression and severe electrolyte disturbance. Recently, a liposomal preparation of amphotericin has become available. This appears to have fewer side effects and higher doses of up to 5 mg/kg/day can be tolerated. Amphotericin B has been given intraventricularly in a dose of 5 μg into each ventricle on alternate days when candida meningitis has been diagnosed.

Flucytosine

Excreted by the urinary tract and can be given orally or intravenously. It should not be used as a single agent. The dose is 100–150 mg/kg/day, in four divided doses. The major side effect is severe bone marrow suppression, so blood levels must be monitored along with regular blood counts. Other side effects include hepatic and renal impairment.

Fluconazole

Fluconazole and other fungistatic agents have been used and appear to have fewer side effects. Fluconazole has a long half-life, is well absorbed when given orally and can be given in a dose of 6 mg/kg/day, once every 2–3 days. It is being used more frequently as a first-line treatment but relapses following cessation of treatment have been recorded.

The mortality of systemic fungal infections ranges from 15 to 50%, but there is a trend towards better survival with prompt and aggressive treatment. CNS involvement is associated with a poor prognosis and neurological sequelae are common.

Antibiotics in the newborn

The absorption, distribution, metabolism and excretion of drugs are different in the neonatal period. Many physiological factors influence the pharmacokinetics of antibiotics in the newborn, e.g. biotransformation, extracellular fluid volume, protein binding and renal function. Also, enzyme systems may be deficient, e.g. glucuronyl transferase. Antibiotic dosage depends upon gestational and postnatal age as well as weight and renal maturity. Appendix II gives dosage recommendations for newborns based on birth weight and postnatal age. The duration of antibiotic therapy depends on the diagnosis and result of cultures.

Penicillins

In general, these are safe and effective for treatment of streptococcal, pneumococcal and staphylococcal infections. Adverse reactions to penicillins are rare in the newborn, though bolus injections have caused seizures from CNS toxicity.

Ampicillin has a broad spectrum of activity and can be used against pathogens such as enterococci, coliforms, proteus and *Listeria monocytogenes*. Benzylpenicillin (pencillin G) does not penetrate well into CSF and the dose should be doubled for treatment of meningitis. Procaine penicillin G is used to treat congenital syphilis. Cloxacillin and flucloxacillin are antistaphylococcal penicillins, resistant to β-lactamase produced by hospital staphylococci. Flucloxacillin is the antibiotic of choice for staphylococcal infections unless methicillin-resistant *Staphyloccus aureus* (MRSA), which should be treated with vancomycin (p. 247), or teicoplanin, although there are few trials of the latter in the newborn.

A penicillin and aminoglycoside combination is commonly used as initial treatment for suspected or confirmed bacterial infections in the newborn.

Aminoglycosides

These antibiotics act on microbial ribosomes to inhibit protein synthesis. There is a risk of renal or oto-toxicity unless correct doses are used (see Appendix II). The risk of ototoxicity is related to both peak and trough serum levels of antibiotic and to cumulative dose, as well as concurrent treatment with frusemide. Aminoglycosides are usually given intravenously but can be given intramuscularly if the infant has a large enough muscle mass and is not shocked. If the drug is given intravenously, a 20 min infusion results in serum concentrations comparable to those after intramuscular injection. Netilmicin closely resembles gentamicin in antimicrobial activity, pharmacology, clinical efficacy and toxicity. However, it is more effective *in vitro* against pseudomonas than gentamicin or amikacin and may be less likely to cause ototoxicity. It may be preferred for late onset *Staphylococcus epidermidis* infection (total daily dose 6 mg/kg/day), in combination with flucloxacillin.

When using aminoglycosides, serum levels should be measured, particularly in very preterm infants or those with renal impairment. Recommended blood levels of various antibiotics are shown in Table 14.4.

Table 14.4. **Recommended blood levels of antibiotics**

	Peak (mg/l)	Trough (mg/l)
Gentamicin	5–8	<2
Netilmicin	9–12	<2
Amikacin	20–30	<8
Vancomycin	25–40	<10
Chloramphenicol	10–25	<5
Amphotericin B	0.2–4	—
Flucytosine	50–80	—

Blood levels are usually monitored after three doses of drug. Blood sample for Peak taken 1 hour after i.v. injection (except flucytosine – 2 hours); for Trough just before injection.

Cephalosporins

The third-generation cephalosporins achieve significant concentration in CSF. They are effective *in vitro* against most Gram-positive and -negative bacteria, but antimicrobial activity is approximately one-tenth that of benzylpenicillin. They may be used in the treatment of ampicillin-resistant klebsiella–enterobacter infections in combination with aminoglycoside and for suspected meningitis. Cefotaxime penetrates CSF well and cef-tazidime has activity against psuedomonas.

The use of cephalosporins probably should be limited to the management of proven Gram-negative septicaemia/meningitis, and not as first-line therapy as there are reports of resistant strains emerging.

Chloramphenicol

There are few indications left for the use of chloramphenicol in the newborn. It may be given for infection caused by organisms resistant to aminoglycosides or to infants not responding to conventional antibiotics after a trial period. Adequate antibiotic levels in CSF are achieved after oral administration in appropriate doses and chloramphenicol may be used to treat neonatal meningitis. 'Grey baby syndrome' is a complication of chloramphenicol therapy due to increased serum concentration of free and conjugated drug leading to collapse. Excessive doses, immaturity of glucuronyl transferase and reduced renal function combine to cause this complication. Early signs are vomiting, poor sucking, respiratory distress, abdominal distension and diarrhoea. In appropriate doses, 'grey baby syndrome' is not seen (see Appendix II). Because of its long half-life, chloramphenicol is given at 24-hour intervals for the first week and 12 hourly in the second. Blood dyscrasias have not been reported in newborn. Serum levels should be measured (therapeutic range 10–25 mg/l; toxic levels >50 mg/l).

Vancomycin

This is effective against methicillin-resistant *Staph. aureus* (MRSA), nosocomial strains of *Staph. epidermidis* and *Clostridium difficile*. Total daily dose 20–30 mg/kg/day in divided doses, although this should be halved in very immature sick infants. Check serum levels after 48 hours and aim to keep peak levels in the range 25–40 mg/l and trough <10 mg/l.

Metronidazole

This is effective against anaerobes and is often used to treat necrotizing enterocolitis and congenital pneumonia in 'smelly' babies. The dose is 22.5 mg/kg/day, given 8 hourly by infusion over 20–30 mins.

Ciprofloxacin

This is a synthetic quinolone bactericidal antibiotic which works by inhibiting bacterial DNA-gyrase. Ciprofloxacin has a wide spectrum of activity including pseudomonas and serratia, but its use in the newborn may be limited because it inhibits the metabolism of theophylline in the liver and may also damage joint cartilage in growing animals.

Teicoplanin

This is a relatively new glycopeptide antibiotic with similar properties to vancomycin. It is active against a wide range of organisms, including staphylococci, most listeria, and Gram-positive anaerobes. CSF penetration is unpredictable. Few side effects have been reported but leucopenia, thrombocytopenia and altered liver function have been described. A suggested regimen is a loading dose of 16 mg/kg i.v. followed by 8 mg/kg/day i.v. once daily.

Immunization of preterm babies

Preterm babies can be given diphtheria, tetanus and pertussis (DTP) vaccine, Haemophilus influenza type b (Hib) vaccine, and oral polio vaccine (OPV) at 2, 3 and 4 months of life. No correction needs to be made for prematurity.

If the baby remains in hospital, only DTP/Hib should be given to avoid cross infection with live polio virus in the neonatal unit. OPV can be given on the day of discharge.

In babies who have been on high-dose corticosteroids, vaccination with live vaccines should be postponed for 2–3 months, or an inactivated vaccine given, e.g. inactivated polio vaccine 0.5 ml i.m. Some babies who have had chronic lung disease may become a little unwell after immunization with pyrexia, irritability and occasionally need supplemental oxygen for a short time.

The only definite *contraindications* to immunization with pertussis are ongoing degenerative CNS disease and previous hypersensitivity to vaccine. The general practitioner should be notified on discharge of what vaccinations have been given to the baby.

Babies who are at risk of tuberculosis through contact with affected family members (e.g. immigrants from the Indian subcontinent), should be given BCG vaccine. The dose is 0.1 ml by intradermal injection. Those giving the vaccine should be familiar with the injection technique. Babies at risk of exposure to HIV should be screened for TB by Mantoux testing but should not receive BCG.

For vaccination of infants at risk of hepatitis B, see p. 229.

Nursing points

Baby

- Early diagnosis of infection often relies on a high index of suspicion and recognition of non-specific signs.
- Toxic blood levels of aminoglycosides may cause hearing impairment. Regular estimation of blood levels is important.
- Purulent ophthalmia neonatorum and neonatal meningitis are notifiable conditions in the UK.

Family

- Note any history of maternal infections or contacts during pregnancy.
- The importance of hand washing must be emphasized to families and other visitors and taught by example by staff.
- Inactivated polio vaccine should be given to babies who have recently been on systemic steroid treatment, or whose family members or contacts would be at risk from exposure to live polio virus.

Equipment

- Servo-controlled incubators may mask temperature instability. Careful observations of such recordings are required.
- All equipment should be changed and cleaned regularly. Every NICU should have a policy manual giving more specific guidelines.
- Adequate spacing between cots and incubators is important.

Staff

- Each NICU should have an Infection Control Officer to advise on specific measures.

- All new staff should be taught the importance of strict hygiene and hand washing and shown the correct technique and appropriate solutions to use.
- Pregnant staff or those trying to conceive should not care for babies with certain infections, e.g. cytomegalovirus, chickenpox, rubella.

References and further reading

American Academy of Pediatrics. Committee on Pediatric AIDS (1997). Guidelines for the evaluation of the HIV-exposed infant. *Pediatrics* **99**: 909.

Berger M (1991). Use of intravenously administered immune globulin in newborn infants: prophylaxis, treatment, both, or neither? *J Pediatr* **118**: 557.

Dobson SRM, Baker CJ (1990). Enterococcal sepsis in neonates: features by age at onset and occurrence of focal infection. *Pediatrics* **85**: 165.

European Collaborative Study (1991). Children born to women with HIV-1 infection: natural history and risk of transmission. *Lancet* **337**: 252.

Goldfarb J (1993). Breastfeeding: AIDS and other infectious diseases. *Clin Perinatol* **20**: 225.

Greenough A (1994). The TORCH screen and intrauterine infections. *Arch Dis Child* **70**: F163.

Issacs D, Moxon ER (1991). *Neonatal Infections*. Oxford: Butterworth Heinemann.

Kadar N (1979). TORCH infections: a significant health hazard to pregnant women. *J Mat Child Health* **4**: 430.

Klein JO (1990). From harmless commensal to invasive pathogen: coagulase-negative staphylococci. *N Engl J Med* **323**: 339.

McIntosh D, Issacs D (1993). Varicella zoster virus infection pregnancy. *Arch Dis Child* **68**: 1.

Ng PC (1994). Systemic fungal infections in neonates. *Arch Dis Child* **71**: F130.

Northern Neonatal Network (1996). *Neonatal Formulary.* London: BMJ Publishing Group.

Peckham CS, Logan S (1993). Screening for toxoplasmosis during pregnancy. *Arch Dis Child* **68**: 3.

Remington JS, Klein JO (1994). *Infectious Disease of Fetus and Newborn Infant* 4th edn. Philadelphia: WB Saunders.

Scott LL, Hollier LM, Dias K (1997). Perinatal herpes virus infections. Herpes simplex, varicella and cytomegalovirus. *Infect Dis Clin North Am* **11**: 27.

Task Force on Pediatric AIDS (1992). Perinatal human immunodeficiency virus (HIV) testing. *Pediatrics* **9**: 791.

Troendle-Atkins J, Demmler GJ, Buffone GJ (1993). Rapid diagnosis of herpes simplex virus encephalitis by using the polymerase chain reaction. *J Pediatr* **123**: 376.

Whitelaw A (1990). Treatment of sepsis with IgG in very low birthweight infants. *Arch Dis Child* **65**: 347.

15 Apnoeic Attacks

Apnoea in newborn is defined as cessation of breathing for >15–20 s and may be associated with bradycardia (heart rate <100 beats/min) and/or cyanosis/desaturation (SaO$_2$ <80%). The commonest cause is apnoea of prematurity but this diagnosis can only be made after exclusion of other causes.

Causes of recurrent apnoea:

- Hypoxia, especially severe RDS, CLD
- Sepsis, especially group B streptococcal septicaemia and meningitis
- Airway obstruction: aspiration, blocked nares, neck flexion or extension, face mask
- CNS disorders such as cerebral oedema or haemorrhage, seizures, kernicterus
- Cardiovascular: hypotension, PDA
- Metabolic disturbances such as hypoglycaemia, acidosis, hypocalcaemia and hyponatraemia
- Anaemia
- Gastro-oesophageal reflux
- Temperature instability especially hyperthermia
- Excessive pharyngeal stimulation and secretions
- Excessive handling
- Drugs such as maternal narcotic and analgesic drugs
- Discomfort or pain
- Apnoea of prematurity.

Apnoeic attacks occur in at least 30% of newborn infants of <34 weeks' gestation. Onset of apnoea of prematurity may be delayed until the third day of life or later. Apnoea within the first 24 hours suggests infection or severe RDS as an underlying cause.

Periodic breathing is a regular sequence of respiratory pauses of 10–20 s interspersed with periods of hyperventilation of 4–15 s, and occurring at least 3 times/min. It is not associated with cyanosis or bradycardia.

Apnoea of prematurity

Apnoea and periodic breathing are very common in the preterm infant. The aetiology is not completely understood but immaturity of medullary respiratory centres or chemoreceptors may cause irregular stimulation of breathing. Inspiratory and expiratory centres in the brainstem control ventilation (Fig. 15.1). They are influenced by sensors (central and peripheral chemoreceptors) which monitor arterial blood to maintain normal arterial oxygen tensions and pH. Response of the preterm respiratory centres to hypercarbia and hypoxaemia is different from that of the mature infant. Normally these chemical changes cause stimulation of respiration with increase in rate and depth of breathing (increased minute ventilation) but in the preterm infant the opposite often occurs: hypercarbia causing no response and hypoxaemia depressing respiration to cause central apnoea.

Apnoea of prematurity often has its onset on the third day of life and is not associated with other disease processes. The more immature the infant, the greater the incidence of apnoea. May also be associated with hypoxia, REM sleep, catecholamine deficiency and respiratory muscle fatigue.

Airway obstruction may also be important in about 10% of preterm babies, and a further 50% have a mixed picture of central immaturity and obstruction. However, the distinctions between obstructive, central and mixed apnoea are becoming increasingly blurred as research suggests similarity in their underlying pathophysiology.

Periodic breathing and apnoea of prematurity usually disappear at approx. 36 weeks' gestation but may occasionally persist until several weeks past term.

> **!** Diagnosis of apnoea of prematurity should only be made after exclusion of other causes.

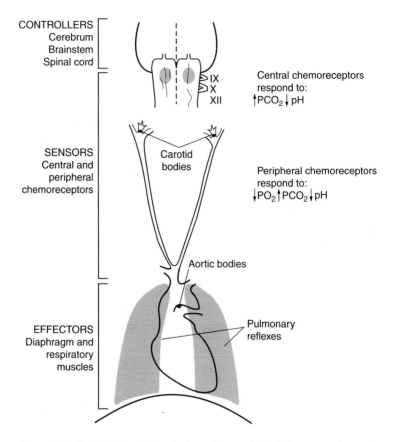

CONTROLLERS
Cerebrum
Brainstem
Spinal cord

Central chemoreceptors
respond to:
↑PCO_2 ↓pH

SENSORS
Central and
peripheral
chemoreceptors

Carotid
bodies

Peripheral chemoreceptors
respond to:
↓PO_2 ↑PCO_2 ↓pH

Aortic bodies

EFFECTORS
Diaphragm and
respiratory
muscles

Pulmonary
reflexes

Figure 15.1. Control of breathing: brain centres, peripheral chemoreceptors and effectors in man. Adapted from Brady and Gould (1984).

Investigation of apnoea (and bradycardia)

➤ Examine infant closely: look for signs of infection, airway obstruction, seizures or patent ductus arteriosus.

➤ Note incubator temperature and oxygen concentration.

➤ Laboratory investigations: full blood picture and platelets; blood culture; blood glucose, electrolytes, pH and calcium.

➤ Chest radiography.

➤ Examination of CSF if meningitis is suspected.

➤ US scan of brain.

Management of recurrent apnoea

Any underlying cause should first be corrected (see above). Apnoea of 15 s or more, especially with bradycardia, can be serious and needs action as outlined below:

➤ Search for underlying cause(s) and correct.

➤ General measures:
  continuous monitoring of heart rate, respiratory rate and oxygen saturation
  maintain temperature at lower end of neutral thermal environment (NTE)
  maintain normoxaemia by cautious increase in ambient O_2 concentration
  position infant prone, avoid airway obstruction

➤ Specific measures:
  stimulation: stroking, rocking, waterbeds
  continuous positive airway pressure (CPAP)
  mechanical ventilation
  drugs: caffeine, theophylline/aminophylline, doxapram

Repeated stimulation

Stroking, gentle rubbing or rocking prevents or shortens apnoeic attacks by increasing input to the respiratory centre. Rocking water beds reduce frequency of short apnoeic attacks but require an adequate and safe method of heating them.

Continuous positive airway pressure (CPAP)

Reduces frequency of apnoeic attacks by improving oxygenation and correcting alveolar collapse. May also reduce upper airway obstruction, stabilize the chest wall and stimulate receptors in nose, mouth and pharynx. Apply using nasopharyngeal tube or nasal prongs (see Ch. 9).

Drugs

Aminophylline, theophylline, caffeine and doxapram are used as respiratory centre stimulants.

Theophylline compounds

These are phosphodiesterase inhibitors and act by increasing the sensitivity of the respiratory centre to raised CO_2 tensions. Other effects are stimulation of the diaphragm, positive inotropic and chronotropic actions on the heart, mild diuresis (improved cardiac output) and increased heat production through utilization of brown fat. A loading dose of 6 mg/kg aminophylline (5 mg/kg theophylline) should be given slowly intravenously over at least 10 min followed by 1–3 mg/kg 8 hourly as maintenance. May also be given orally. After 24–48 hours of theophylline therapy, serum levels should be measured to keep them in therapeutic range (10–18 mg/ml). Side effects include tachycardia, hyperglycaemia and glycosuria, jitteriness, vomiting and haemorrhagic gastritis.

Caffeine

Has a wider margin of safety than theophylline and has been shown to be as effective in reducing apnoea. Loading dose is 10 mg/kg orally followed by 2.5 mg/kg once daily. Can be given intravenously but if extravasation occurs can cause severe skin necrosis so avoid this route if possible.

Doxapram

May be used when apnoea is resistant to treatment with caffeine or theophylline. Recommended dose is 1 mg/kg/h by infusion but doses as high as 2.5 mg/kg/h may be necessary in unresponsive infants. Side effects include jitteriness, abdominal distension, vomiting, hypertension. Avoid if infant has had seizures or is at risk of seizures.

Mechanical ventilation

Used for infants who are resistant to treatment with CPAP or drugs. Often needed for very immature babies, those with septicaemia and respiratory failure with acidosis. Low pressure, slow rate ventilation is often all that is necessary.

Long-term outcome

Prognosis depends on the cause of the apnoeic spells. Apnoea secondary to meningitis, seizures and kernicterus is likely to have a poor outcome. For most infants with simple apnoea of prematurity, long-term outcome is good. In a few babies with severe episodes of bradycardia and hypoxaemia, ischaemic cerebral lesions (PVL) develop but whether these represent cause or effect is debatable. There is no clear relationship between apnoea of prematurity, periodic breathing and subsequent SIDS (cot death).

Nursing points

Baby

- Over-handling may precipitate apnoeas. Staff must consider whether procedures are necessary and not perform them routinely. The benefits must outweigh the costs.
- Babies with persistent apnoeas will benefit from being nursed prone, having oral feeding tubes instead of nasal, minimal handling and ensuring the incubator temperature is appropriate.
- Increased frequency of apnoeas may be an early sign of infection. Record their frequency, duration and any treatment needed. Other possible causes are:
    immature respiratory centre
    over-sedation
    periventricular haemorrhage
    seizures
    exhaustion
    metabolic disturbance
    aspiration.
- Tachycardia may be a sign of theophylline toxicity. The baby's heart rate should be recorded prior to each dose, the dose omitted and medical staff informed if tachycardia is noted.

Family

- If a baby is particularly unstable, it may be necessary to limit the amount of handling by the family.
- Cause of apnoeas should be fully explained to parents.

- All parents should routinely be taught resuscitation before discharge home.

Equipment

- Use of apnoea monitors should be discontinued several days prior to discharge to enable the parents to gain confidence.
- Careful siting of the sensor reduces number of false alarms from apnoea monitors. Parents should be taught where to position the sensor.
- When resuscitating an apnoeic baby, gentle suction of the mouth should be performed. Pharyngeal suction stimulates apnoeas and should be avoided.
- Administering oxygen to an apnoeic baby is of no use since he is not breathing. Once the baby starts to breathe again, inappropriately high oxygen concentrations may actually be harmful. Gentle stimulation or bag and mask resuscitation using air are of most benefit.

Staff

- All staff should attend regular updates on neonatal resuscitation.

References and further reading

Aranda JV, Grondin D, Sasyniuk BI (1981). Pharmacologic considerations in the therapy of neonatal apnea. *Pediatr Clin North Am* **28**: 113.

Brady JP, Gould JB (1984). Sudden infant death syndrome. In: *Advances in Pediatrics* (ed, Barness LA), vol 31. Chicago: Year Book Medical.

Bucher HU, Duc G (1988). Does caffeine prevent hypoxaemic episodes in premature infants? A randomized controlled trial. *Eur J Pediatr* **147**: 288.

Eyal F, Alpan G, Sagi E *et al* (1985). Aminophylline versus doxapram in idiopathic apnea of prematurity: a double blind controlled study. *Pediatrics* **75**: 709.

Glotzbach SF, Baldwin RB, Lederer NE, Tansey PA, Ariagno RL (1989). Periodic breathing in preterm infants: incidence and characteristics. *Pediatrics* **84**: 785.

Jones RAK (1982). Apnoea of immaturity. I. A controlled trial of theophylline and face mask with aminophylline. *Arch Dis Child* **57**: 761.

Kattwinkel J (1980). Apnea in the neonatal period. *Pediatr Rev* **2**: 115.

Larson PB, Bendstrup L, Skov L, Flachs H (1995). Aminophylline versus caffeine citrate for apnea and bradycardia prophylaxis in premature infants. *Acta Paediatr* **84**: 360–4.

Levitt GA, Mushin A, Bellman S, Harvey DR (1988). Outcome of preterm infants who suffered neonatal apnoeic attacks. *Early Hum Dev* **16**: 235.

Miller MJ, Carlo WA, Martin RJ (1985). Continuous positive airway pressure selectively reduces obstructive apnea in preterm infants. *J Pediatr* **1006**: 91.

Poets CF, Stebbens VA, Samuels MP, Southall DP (1993). The relationship between bradycardia, apnea, and hypoxemia in preterm infants. *Pediatr Res* **34**: 144.

Rigatto H (1982). Apnea. *Pediatr Clin North Am* **29**: 1105.

Ruggins NR (1991). Pathophysiology of apnoea in preterm infants. *Arch Dis Child* **66**: 70.

16 **Neurological Problems**

Neurological disorders in the newborn may be primary or secondary in origin. Secondary disorders are of greater importance in that it may be possible to prevent extension of cerebral damage and thus minimize handicap. Cerebral hypoxia and bacterial infection are of major importance, the former is commoner and more difficult to diagnose.

Primary disorders (prenatal and birth):

- *Congenital anomalies*: microcephaly, hydrocephaly, hydranencephaly, encephalocele, porencephalic cysts, chromosomal anomalies, myopathies
- *Infections*: CMV, rubella, toxoplasmosis, syphilis
- *Neurocutaneous syndromes*: tuberous sclerosis, neurofibromatosis, Sturge–Weber syndrome
- *Trauma*: torn falx cerebri, subdural, subarachnoid haemorrhage, skull fractures, spinal cord and brachial plexus injuries

Secondary causes (postnatal):

- *Infections*: meningitis, herpes simplex encephalitis
- *Drugs*: narcotics, barbiturates, general anaesthesia, local anaesthesia (direct)
- *Hypoxia*: asphyxia, RDS, recurrent apnoea, intraventricular haemorrhage
- *Metabolic*: hypoglycaemia, acidosis, hypocalcaemia, hyponatraemia, hypernatraemia, hypomagnesaemia, aminoacidurias, galactosaemia, hypothyroidism, hypothermia, malnutrition and vitamin deficiency
- *Secondary bleeding*: intracranial haemorrhages from thrombocytopenia or disseminated intravascular coagulation

✚ Cerebral hypoxia and ischaemia

A major cause of long-term neurological sequelae in childhood in both term and preterm babies. 3 – 9/1000 term babies suffer an hypoxic ischaemic insult. The majority of insults arise in the antepartum period with only 10–15% occurring in the intrapartum period.

A major problem is to determine the nature and extent of cerebral damage. The most satisfactory neurological assessment seems to be that described by Sarnat and Sarnat in 1976 (Appendix VI A). This assessment places the infant in one of three stages of hypoxic-ischaemic encephalopathy (HIE): stage 1 mild, stage 2 moderate and stage 3 severe.

Examination is based upon 5 clinical areas:
  1. Level of consciousness
  2. Neuromuscular control: tone and posture
  3. Complex reflexes: primitive reflexes
  4. Autonomic function
  5. Presence of seizures

EEG examination was included in the original Sarnat score and may be used in doubtful cases, but clinical staging alone has been shown to correlate well with outcome (Table 16.1). Sarnat scoring should be done within 12 hours of birth and repeated daily until normal.

Table 16.1. Outcome of hypoxic–ischaemic encephalopathy (HIE) by Sarnat Stage

Sarnat stage	Mortality (%)	Normal development (%)
1	0	90
2	10	50
3	90	0
Stage 2 { < 5 days	0	90
> 5 days	20	10

Sarnat staging predicts outcome well (Table 16.1). Stage 1 or 2 for <5 days — low mortality and 90% normal development.

There is a poor outcome for babies in stage 3: 90% mortality and no normal survivors and for stage 2 for >5 days: only 10% with normal development. Sarnat staging also predicts the severity of the handicap: stage 1, mild handicaps if any, and stage 3, moderate or severe handicap.

Investigation

Investigations for confirmation of diagnosis and detection of secondary upsets may include:

- Lumbar puncture:
  subarachnoid haemorrhage
  meningitis (normal CSF findings are shown in Appendix VI B)
- Ultrasound and CT scan:
  ventricular size
  intracerebral bleeding
  increased echodensity
- Auditory brainstem evoked responses (ABER)
- EEG
  seizure detection
  prediction of outcome
- Neurochemistry (indicators of brain damage)
  brain-specific creatine kinase (BBCK)
  neurone-specific enolase (NSE).

Investigation of secondary upsets includes blood glucose, calcium, electrolyte and coagulation measurements.

Management

- Maintain neutral thermal environment, normoxaemia, and normoglycaemia (both hypo- and hyper-glycaemia are harmful).
- Fluid restrict by 20% of normal regimen to prevent cerebral oedema, and treat renal failure and inappropriate ADH secretion.
- Maintain normal blood pressure and cerebral perfusion pressure using dopamine if necessary (5–15 µg/kg/min).

➤ Attempt to minimize damage:
　treat cerebral oedema (see below)
　treat seizures (see p. 267)
　treat other organ systems.

➤ Gentle, infrequent handling by staff.

➤ Good support of mother, father and baby with frequent visits
　and communication.

Prediction of outcome

Important for counselling the parents. Several methods are currently available:

1. *Clinical methods*: Apgar score at 10 or 20 min,
   neurological examination (e.g. Sarnat)
2. *Imaging techniques*: ultrasound and CT scanning, MRI
3. *Biochemical methods*: hypoxanthine, ammonia, lactate
   dehydrogenase, brain-specific creatine kinase (CKBB),
   neurone-specific enolase (NSE)
4. *Electrophysiological techniques*: EEG, auditory and
   visual and somatosensory evoked responses

Clinical examination and EEG recording are the most valuable. Imaging with ultrasound and CT scans has limitations with the latter being more valuable in term babies. Persistent generalized hypodensities and focal infarcts on CT scan carry a poor prognosis. CT or MRI scans should be performed at the age of 1–2 weeks (Ch. 24).

Blood CKBB level is a sensitive indicator of cerebral damage but does not predict outcome.

Electrophysiological techniques (EEG and evoked responses) help in diagnosis with EEG being valuable to predict outcome when recorded as early as day 1.

Cerebral palsy (CP) is the major neurological deficit clearly linked to perinatal asphyxia. Mental retardation and epilepsy are commonly associated. However, only 10–15% of CP is due to perinatal asphyxia.

✚ Cerebral oedema

Cerebral oedema is difficult to diagnose in the newborn.

Clinical signs include:

≺ Tense anterior fontanelle
≺ Low heart rate (<110/min)
≺ Raised blood pressure (> 80 mmHg systolic)
≺ Seizures.

Ultrasound scan shows small ventricles, decreased vascular pulsation and generalized increase in echodensity.

The benefits of treatment of cerebral oedema as outlined below are unproven but nevertheless are often used.

➤ Mannitol infusions are effective in reducing cerebral oedema. Dose (7 ml/kg of 20% mannitol over 20 min) may be repeated 4 hourly if necessary. For mannitol to be effective serum osmolality must be <300 mOsm/l.

➤ Mechanical hyperventilation may be used to reduce cerebral blood flow by lowering PCO_2 to 4–5 kPa (30–36 mmHg). Lower levels of hypocarbia are not recommended in view of risk of cerebral ischaemia.

➤ Other potential therapies include high-dose barbiturates (lower cerebral metabolic needs but cause hypotension), calcium channel blockers and oxygen free radical scavengers. Hypothermia and magnesium infusions are currently being studied.

Corticosteroids are not beneficial in reducing cerebral oedema after asphyxia and may induce hypertension and hyperglycaemia.

✚ Periventricular leucomalacia

Cerebral hypoxia and/or ischaemia may result in periventricular leucomalacia (PVL) which is seen on ultrasound scan in 2–10% of infants <1500 g. Rarely occurs in term infants. Has a predilection for watershed areas in deep white matter and occipital radiation at trigone of lateral ventricles. Initial lesion is an area of coagulation necrosis, perhaps due to venous infarction or cerebral ischaemia, which may progress to cavitation. In 25% of cases haemorrhage into an area of ischaemic necrosis may be involved.

Predisposing factors are:

- Complicated RDS
- Birth asphyxia
- APH
- Septic shock/chorioamnionitis/NEC
- Hypotension
- PDA.

The majority of lesions arise in the perinatal period. If cysts are present in the first week of life a prenatal insult is likely. Diagnosis is by US scan (see p. 380).

Prognosis is poor with a high incidence (60–80%) of major handicap in infants with cystic PVL. Those with transient echodensities or flares (<2 weeks) have good outcome but outcome is unclear for infants with persistent echodensities without cyst formation.

✚ Neonatal seizures

Seizures in the newborn are relatively common (0.6–2/1000 births) but may be difficult to diagnose as they can present in different ways:

1. *Subtle*: commonest type; repetitive eye movements, sucking, swallowing, apnoea, 'cycling' movements of limbs
2. *Clonic*: rhythmic slow jerks (1–3 cycles); usually term babies
3. *Tonic*: extension and stiffening of body; may be associated with apnoea; usually preterm babies; may be generalized or focal

4. *Myoclonic*: frequent synchronized jerks — usually upper limbs

Causes of neonatal seizures:

- Hypoxia/ischaemia: antepartum, intrapartum, neonatal RDS, apnoeic attacks (40%)
- Intracranial bleeding: subdural, extradural, subarachnoid, intraventricular (30%)
- Metabolic: hypoglycaemia, hypocalcaemia, hypomagnesaemia, hyponatraemia, hypernatraemia (12%)
- Meningitis (8%)
- Structural cerebral anomalies: hydrocephalus, microcephalus, encephalocele, tuberous sclerosis (3%)
- Obstetric trauma: breech, forceps
- Drugs: narcotics, phenothiazines, barbiturates, addiction and withdrawal, local anaesthetics
- Pyridoxine dependency
- Kernicterus
- Aminoacidurias: phenylketonuria, maple syrup urine disease, hyperlysinuria, hyperglycinaemia; urea cycle disorders
- Intrauterine infection: rubella, toxoplasmosis, CMV
- Familial neonatal seizures (may be benign).

The underlying condition should always be sought so that specific treatments may be used. Asphyxia is the commonest cause, accounting for 40%, followed by intracranial bleeding 30%, metabolic causes 12%, infection 8% and malformations 3%. The time of onset and type of seizure relate to both cause and outcome:

First 3 days:
    Asphyxia: tonic or tonic/clonic, apnoea
    Hypoglycaemia: clonic
    Intraventricular haemorrhage: tonic, apnoea
    Hypocalcaemia: tonic/clonic, multifocal
    Inborn errors of metabolism: any type (see Ch. 20)
    Congenital malformation: any type (p. 274)
    Meningitis: tonic, apnoea.

After 3 days:

   Meningitis: tonic, tonic/clonic, apnoea
   Hypocalcaemia: clonic, multifocal
   Hypomagnesaemia: clonic, multifocal
   Kernicterus: tonic, apnoea, subtle
   Drug withdrawal: clonic, jittery
   Hypo- or hyper-natraemia: clonic.

Seizures occurring in the first 3 days are usually more significant than those occurring later.

Investigation

Investigation of neonatal seizures includes a full history and examination followed by a search for possible underlying causes:

➤ Blood glucose

➤ Serum calcium and magnesium

➤ Electrolytes: Na^+, K^+, Cl^-; urea

➤ pH and blood gases

➤ Urine examination for culture and reducing substances (Clinitest™ and Clinistix™)

➤ Plasma and urine amino acids

➤ EEG

➤ Intrauterine infection (TORCH titres) and bacterial infection (blood culture, CSF examination and blood film)

➤ Examination of fundi

➤ Ultrasound scan of brain

➤ CT/MRI scan.

Management

➤ Correct underlying causes such as hypoglycaemia, hypocalcaemia or infection. If no underlying biochemical cause is found and seizures persist, then start anticonvulsant therapy.

➤ *Phenobarbitone* is probably safest and most effective drug.

The loading dose is 20-30 mg/kg intravenously followed by 5 mg/kg/day in divided doses (usually every 12 hours). If seizures persist give a further loading dose of 10 mg/kg phenobarbitone. If seizures continue despite adequate serum levels of phenobarbitone (therapeutic range 15–20 mg/l (100-140 μmol/l)), proceed with a second-line anticonvulsant such as phenytoin or clonazepam.

➤ *Phenytoin* may be added using a loading dose of 10 mg/kg followed by a maintenance dose of 5–10 mg/kg/day divided into 8-hourly doses. Therapeutic serum level is 15–20 mg/l (60-80 μmol/l). Phenytoin must be given intravenously as it is poorly absorbed after oral and intramuscular administration. Cardiac arrhythmias are associated with intravenous use; infants should have ECG monitoring during infusion.

➤ *Clonazepam* is given in a loading dose of 100 μg/kg followed by intermittent boluses or an infusion of 10 μg/kg/h until seizures are controlled. Adverse effects are respiratory depression and increased bronchial secretions.

➤ *Diazepam* 0.3 mg/kg i.v. as a single dose may be given intermittently for short term control of seizures, but it can depress respiration and cause hypotonia.

➤ *Paraldehyde* is useful for short-term control of seizures. Give as a rectal preparation of 0.1 mg/kg.

Duration of anticonvulsant treatment is often difficult to determine. Babies can be weaned from their treatment before discharge if seizures are controlled and CNS examination is normal. Some may need prolonged treatment e.g. persistent seizures and/or EEG abnormality. More likely if CNS malformation, following meningitis or intraventricular haemorrhage. In these cases it is usual to treat for 3–6 months and then reassess.

Pyridoxine dependency is an uncommon cause of neonatal seizures but intravenous injection of 20 mg/kg of pyridoxine (vitamin B$_6$) will stop the seizures. In cases of seizures of unknown aetiology it is worth trying this treatment.

Prognosis

Outlook following neonatal seizures is influenced by several factors:

1. Underlying cause of seizures
2. Type and severity of seizures
3. Babies potential for future intelligence – genetic, social, environmental

Babies who have abnormal neurological signs at discharge or whose seizures are multifocal have a poorer prognosis. Mortality is greatest if seizures are due to intracranial haemorrhage (57%), followed by infection (33%) and asphyxia (27%). Of survivors, overall 43% have an abnormal outcome.

✚ Jittery baby

Defined as: shaking movements of the limbs that are not true seizures. When limbs are flexed, jitteriness disappears but seizures will continue. Exclude hypoglycaemia, hypocalcaemia or hypomagnesaemia and drug withdrawal (alcohol, benzodiazepines and narcotics). Some SGA infants remain jittery although no biochemical cause is found. In this case, treat by swaddling and avoid bright lights and loud noises. Only occasionally is sedation needed.

✚ Intracranial haemorrhage

Intracranial haemorrhage is a relatively common condition in the preterm newborn. There is a wide variety of types of haemorrhage depending on site of origin, with different prognoses.

The major types of intracranial haemorrhage are:
Subdural
Subarachnoid
Intraventricular
Intraparenchymal
Intracerebellar

Intraventricular haemorrhage is the commonest type, arising particularly in immature babies.

✚ *Intraventricular haemorrhage (IVH)*

A common problem of VLBW babies becoming less common with advancing gestational age; 25–30% of babies <1200 g in major neonatal centres.

Capillaries in the germinal plate may be damaged during periods of hypotension. During hypoxia, hypertension occurs and with hypercarbia, increased cerebral blood flow leads to bleeding from these damaged capillaries. In the preterm infant or after asphyxia, flow is not kept constant when blood pressure increases (failure of antoregulation). Bleeding into the germinal plate or subependymal matrix can be detected by ultrasound scanning (see Table 16.2). Blood may rupture into one or both lateral ventricles.

Risk factors for IVH include:

- Immaturity
- RDS, pneumonia
- Acidosis, hypercarbia, hypoxia
- Hypotension
- Coagulation defects may worsen grade of haemorrhage.

Clinical features:

➢ Usually occurs in first week but has been noted antenatally.
➢ Majority present silently and are diagnosed on routine ultrasound scan (Table 16.2).
➢ Rarely presents with 'collapse', seizures.

Management

➤ Perform ultrasound scan of the brain in all preterm babies (<32 weeks) within 24 hours of birth. Perform serial scans every 2–3 days during the acute illness.

Table 16.2. **Grading of IVH by ultrasound (Volpe, 1977)**

Grade	
I	Germinal matrix haemorrhage and/or minimal IVH (<10% of ventricular area on parasagittal view)
II	IVH filling <50% of the ventricular area on parasagittal view
III	IVH filling >50% of the ventricular area, + ventriculomegaly, on parasagittal view.
Separate notation: location and extent of periventricular echodensities.	

➤ Avoid acidosis and hypotension.

➤ Correct coagulation disorders.

➤ Treat posthaemorrhagic hydrocephalus:
  1. Serial lumbar punctures may control signs of raised intracranial pressure until CSF protein is low enough for shunt insertion
  2. Acetazolamide, has not been shown to reduce the need for shunt insertion
  3. Ventriculo-peritoneal shunt insertion is the definitive treatment. Has associated risks of obstruction and infection

Prevention

➤ Indomethacin may have a role in prophylaxis.

➤ Large doses of vitamin E or ethamsylate (a platelet-stabilizing drug) may prevent or reduce incidence of IVH.

➤ Prevention of acidosis and hypotension is important.

➤ Value of phenobarbitone and muscle relaxants is not convincingly proven.

Prognosis

Depends upon extent of haemorrhage with a high risk of disability if parenchymal involvement.

✚ *Subarachnoid haemorrhage*

Subarachnoid haemorrhage may follow asphyxia or obstetric trauma. *Presents* with seizures and irritability or may be asymptomatic until progressive hydrocephalus develops (uncommon).

Diagnosis is by lumbar puncture and CT scan.

Prognosis is usually good with 90% having normal development.

✚ Subdural haemorrhage

Subdural haemorrhage is uncommon in newborns. Obstetric trauma and precipitate delivery predispose to it by tearing falx cerebri where the great cerebral vein enters the inferior sagittal sinus. *Presents* with signs of raised intracranial pressure, focal seizures or subacutely with increasing head size, failure to thrive and bulging fontanelle.

Diagnosis by ultrasound and CT scan or occasionally by subdural taps (see p. 132).

Treatment may be conservative or by subdural tap which may need to be repeated after consulting with a neurosurgeon.

Prognosis in severe cases is usually poor. Mild cases may resolve without sequelae.

✚ Traumatic nerve palsies

Trauma to facial nerve and brachial plexus is not uncommon and may occur *in utero* or during birth. Neurapraxia is commoner than axonotmesis so that recovery is usually complete.

Facial nerve can be damaged *in utero* by pressure against the sacral promontory or during forceps delivery. If unilateral, when infant cries the mouth is drawn to the side of the lesion and the eye cannot be fully closed. Methylcellulose drops provide lubrication and prevent corneal damage of exposed eye. Prognosis is usually good with the majority recovering within 1 month.

Brachial plexus injuries are commoner after shoulder dystocia or breech delivery. *Erb's palsy* is a lesion of upper roots of brachial plexus. The arm is adducted and internally rotated at the shoulder to give 'waiter's tip' deformity. May also be sensory deficit over C5 distribution. Occasionally, associated diaphragmatic paralysis on same side causing respiratory difficulty. *Klumpke's palsy*, from a lesion of lower brachial plexus, is associated with wrist drop and is difficult to distinguish from radial nerve palsy.

Treatment of brachial plexus injury is with gentle passive physiotherapy. Splinting is of little value. Majority recover completely within 6 months (over 90%). Babies who do not make a rapid recovery by 2–3 months should have MRI and nerve conduction studies as microsurgery may improve the outcome.

✚ Floppy baby

The commonest cause is birth asphyxia. Conversely, it should be remembered that a baby with muscle disease may present with birth asphyxia.

Causes of hypotonia in the newborn:

- Hypoxic ischaemic encephalopathy
- Prematurity
- Intracranial haemorrhage
- Sepsis, botulism, drugs
- Down's syndrome, Prader–Willi syndrome
- Metabolic: hypoglycaemia, hyponatraemia, inborn error of metabolism
- Endocrine: hypothyroidism
- Spinal cord: transection, Werdnig–Hoffman syndrome, poliomyelitis
- Muscle disorders: myasthenia gravis, congenital myopathies, myotonic dystrophy.

Investigation

➤ Careful assessment of family history and examination of mother for signs of myotonic dystrophy or myaesthenia gravis.

➤ Laboratory analysis:
muscle enzymes
urinary amino acid chromatogram
viral cultures, stool examination
chromosome/DNA analysis
thyroid function tests

➤ Imaging — cranial ultrasound

➤ EMG

➤ Muscle biopsy

➤ Test dose of edrophonium or neostigmine. Edrophonium chloride 0.05–0.15 mg/kg i.m. should give rapid improvement in symptoms in myasthenia gravis; maximal effect at 10 min. As edrophonium can cause cardiac arrhythmias, neostigmine may be preferable (0.1 mg/kg i.m; maximal effect at 30 min).

Congenital malformations of the CNS

The CNS is the most frequent site of congenital malformation: about 1/1000 births have anencephaly and numbers are similar for meningomyelocele, but rates vary around the world. Microcephaly is less common. Assessment of *meningomyelocele* is essential to determine those infants who would benefit from surgical closure. One or more of the following features is associated with an adverse outcome, as described by Lorber (1972):

1. Total paraplegia
2. Kyphoscoliosis
3. Hydrocephalus: head circumference 2 cm >90th centile
4. Large thoracolumbar lesion, >four segments
5. Associated anomalies

Consult with paediatric surgeon or neurosurgeon.

❏ *Microcephaly*

An abnormally small head, i.e. >3 standard deviations below mean for gestation. Infants are usually severely retarded. Intrauterine infection, inborn errors of metabolism and severe intrauterine hypoxia may be underlying causes. Maternal phenylketonuria is an important cause to exclude. There is also a sex-linked familial type.

❏ *Hydrocephalus*

Due to excessive CSF within the cerebral ventricles and usually results in increased occipitofrontal circumference. May be caused by meningomyelocele, intrauterine infection, or after cerebral haemorrhage or meningitis. Occasionally due to aqueduct stenosis or the Dandy–Walker syndrome.

Other causes of a large head are:

- Benign familial macrocephaly
- Chronic subdural haematoma
- External hydrocephalus (increased fluid in subarachnoid space)
- Hydranencephaly (fluid-filled cerebral hemispheres).

Ultrasound, and CT or MRI scans are useful investigations.

Nursing points

Baby

- Reduce all forms of stimulation as much as possible — noise, light and handling. An eye mask on the baby will reduce the light intensity whilst allowing close observation to continue.
- Careful monitoring of fluid balance — oliguria, proteinuria or haematuria may signify a degree of renal failure. Fluids may be restricted in an attempt to reduce cerebral oedema.
- Signs of seizures are often subtle and may include:
  - ≺ Lip-smacking
  - ≺ Recurrent apnoeas
  - ≺ Eye-rolling

◁ Hypotonia or hypertonia
◁ Bradycardia.

Family

- Explain the need for minimal handling and stimulation whilst the baby is irritable or unstable.
- Discuss events fully and honestly as they occur.
- Inform parents of findings of all ultrasound scans and investigations as soon as possible.

Equipment

- Continuous cardiorespiratory, blood pressure and temperature monitoring reduces the need for handling.
- Use of a scoring system for possible symptoms of distress may help in the recognition and early treatment of these babies; particularly babies withdrawing from maternal drug abuse.

Staff

- A pre-discharge meeting involving parents, hospital and community staff is helpful to discuss the perinatal problems, follow-up and prognosis.

References and further reading

Evans D, Levene M (1998). Neonatal seizures. *Arch Dis Child* **78**: F70–5.

Fowlie PW (1996). Prophylactic indomethacin: systematic review and meta-analysis. *Arch Dis Child* **74**: 81.

Levene MI (1993). Management of the asphyxiated full-term infant. *Arch Dis Child* **68**: 612.

Lorber J (1972). Spina bifida cystica. Results of treatment of 270 consecutive cases with criteria for selection for the future. *Arch Dis Child* **47**: 854.

Ment LR, Schneider K (1993). Intraventricular haemorrhage of the preterm infant. *Semin Neurol* **13**: 40.

Sarnat HB, Sarnat MS (1976). Neonatal encephalopathy following fetal distress. A clinical and electroencephalograhic study. *Arch Neurol* **33**: 696.

Volpe JJ (1977). Neonatal intracranial haemorrhage. Pathophysiology, neuropathology and clinical features. *Clin Perinatol* **4**: 77.

Volpe JJ (1977). *Neurology of the Newborn*, 3rd edn. Philadelphia: WB Saunders.

17 Cardiovascular Problems

Perinatal circulation

The fetal lung is fluid-filled and receives only 5–10% of fetal cardiac output. Blood is shunted from the lungs to the aorta across the ductus arteriosus. The fetus also conserves oxygen for the brain by directing oxygenated blood from the placenta through two further shunts: the ductus venosus, which bypasses the liver; and the foramen ovale, which bypasses the right ventricle and lungs (Fig. 17.1).

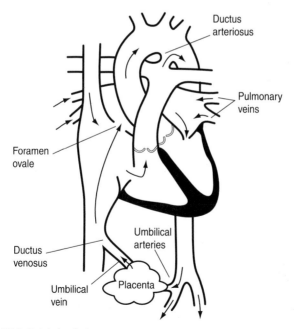

Figure 17.1. Fetal circulation

Rapid changes in circulation take place at birth with the onset of breathing. Pulmonary blood flow increases 5-fold as pulmonary vascular resistance falls due to the chemical effects of increasing PaO_2 and decreasing $PaCO_2$, and the mechanical effect of lung inflation. When the three fetal shunts close, the circulation is converted from a parallel to a series arrangement. The foramen ovale closes first as increased flow from the lungs raises left atrial pressure. Removal of the low resistance placental circulation increases systemic vascular resistance and raises blood pressure. The ductus venosus closes next, followed by the ductus arteriosus after about 24 hours in the normal full-term infant. Blood may continue to flow right to left from pulmonary artery to aorta through the ductus arteriosus for 2–3 hours after birth. Thereafter it flows left to right for up to 24 hours. During the first minutes, the effects of increased oxygen, cold, mechanical stretching, and possibly vasoactive peptides such as bradykinin, cause marked constriction of the umbilical vessels. At birth the right ventricle is thicker than the left but the latter gradually increases in size to become twice as thick as the right by 6 months.

Some results of failure of normal adaptation of the circulation at birth are discussed elsewhere, e.g. persistent pulmonary hypertension (see p. 171), shock or hypovolaemia (see p. 48) and hypervolaemia with polycythaemia (see p. 351) and are not dealt with further.

Examination of the cardiovascular system

A careful history and clinical examination, supplemented by relevant investigations, are important in the investigation of suspected cardiovascular problems.

➤ *History:*
  feeding difficulty
  breathlessness
  cyanotic episodes
  vomiting
  family history of congenital heart disease.

➤ *Inspection:*
  presence of central cyanosis or pallor
  respiratory rate at rest and during feeding
  activity of the precordium
  presence of other malformations.

➤ *Palpation*:
  all pulses — remember to palpate digital and femoral pulses
  precordium: position of apex beat, thrills
  liver size.

➤ *Auscultation*:
  character of heart sounds
  character, timing, intensity and radiation of murmurs
  lung fields.

➤ *Blood pressure*:
  arms and legs (leg is usually higher than arm).

Investigations

Chest radiography

The normal-sized heart should have a cardiothoracic (CT) ratio of <0.6. Heart size is increased in many cases of heart failure (p. 285), after birth asphyxia (p. 38), in the infant of the diabetic mother (p. 24) and during hypoglycaemia (p. 194).

In some forms of congenital heart disease, the heart may have a characteristic shape, e.g. 'cottage loaf' in total anomalous pulmonary venous return (TAPVR) and 'egg-on-side' in transposition of the great arteries (TGA).

Pulmonary vascularity is increased in large L→R shunts and decreased in pulmonary atresia or other types of right heart obstruction. Pulmonary venous obstruction causes mottling and thickened interlobular septa, mimicking transient tachypnoea of the newborn or RDS on occasions.

The aortic arch is usually on the left but may be right-sided in Fallot's tetralogy and truncus arteriosus. If there is dextrocardia with situs inversus (liver on left) and a right aortic arch, then the risk of congenital heart disease is low. With dextrocardia and situs solitus (liver on the right), the incidence of structural defects is high. Splenic anomalies are associated with situs ambiguous (mid-line liver with asplenia or polysplenia).

Electrocardiography

At birth the mean frontal QRS axis is 135° with normal range of 110–180°. There is rapid change in the direction of the axis from right to left in the first month (mean approx 75°) and then more gradually to adult values. Extreme left axis deviation at birth is suggestive of a major problem, e.g. atrioventricular septal defect or tricuspid atresia.

There are age-related changes in the size of the components of the ECG waveform. As a guide, ventricular overload may be suggested by the following criteria:

Right ventricular overload	Left ventricular overload
QR in V_1	S in V_1 >20 mm in term or
R in V_1 >30 mm	>26 mm in preterm
R in V_4R >20 mm	R in V_6 >14 mm
S in V_6 >15 mm	Q in V_6 >4 mm
R/S ratio in V_1 >7	R/S ratio in V_1 <1.0
QRS axis > +180°	QRS axis <30°

Echocardiography

The development of ultrasound imaging has radically altered the approach to diagnosis in neonatal heart disease. Most structural abnormalities can be detected at the cotside using 2-dimensional ultrasound with Doppler facilities. Neonatologists should become competent in performing basic echocardiography, particularly in the assessment of patent ductus arteriosus. However, it is important not to delay referral to the paediatric cardiologist, particularly when the baby is critically ill.

Congenital heart disease

Congenital heart disease occurs in about 10/1000 live births. There are well-known associations with other congenital malformations and syndromes, e.g. trisomies 13, 18 and 21,

Turner's syndrome, gastrointestinal anomalies, maternal diabetes and TORCH infections.

In many cases the diagnosis can be made antenatally by echocardiography at 18–20 weeks, either as a routine screen or in selected high-risk pregnancies (e.g. family history of CHD, rubella infection or drug ingestion in early pregnancy, maternal diabetes, or age >37 years). A four-chamber view, if normal, excludes about 70% of abnormalities. After antenatal diagnosis, the baby should be born in a centre with paediatric cardiology services.

Heart disease in the newborn is traditionally subdivided into cyanotic and acyanotic forms, although this is a rather broad classification. A knowledge of the underlying pathophysiology is essential for effective diagnosis and treatment. General principles rather than individual cardiac lesions are dealt with here.

Practical hints on neonatal heart disease:
1. Symptomatic heart disease without a murmur is usually serious
2. An asymptomatic murmur is often benign
3. A significant murmur heard during routine examination in first 24 hours is likely to be due to PDA, stenosis of aortic or pulmonary valves, or AV valve regurgitation
4. A systolic ejection click after 12 hours is abnormal and suggests either a large pulmonary artery, large aorta or a true truncus arteriosus
5. Heart failure in the first week of life is usually due to hypoplastic left heart syndrome, fibroelastosis, multiple cardiac defects, or supraventricular tachycardia
6. An uncomplicated ventricular septal defect is often associated with no symptoms until about 3 weeks when pulmonary vascular resistance has fallen. There may be no murmur at birth

Investigation of a murmur

During the first day of life a soft murmur can be heard in about 60% of babies. This may be due either to turbulent pulmonary flow or flow through the ductus arteriosus.

In a well infant with a short systolic murmur after the first 2 days of life, a full clinical examination including palpation of all pulses and measurement of blood pressure in arms and legs should be performed. If these are normal, it is probably unnecessary to perform a chest radiograph and ECG, but the infant must be examined again before discharge and followed up at 2–3 weeks. The general practitioner should be informed.

The word 'murmur' instills unnecessary fear in some parents and it is important to explain the findings and reassure them that the extra sound in the chest will probably go away of its own accord.

If, however, the murmur is loud or long or the infant is unwell, full examination must be followed by investigation with chest X-ray, ECG and echocardiography. Murmurs that appear for the first time after the first week of life should also be fully investigated.

Serious neonatal heart disease

Serious neonatal heart disease may be divided into 3 major groups, depending on aetiology and clinical findings:

1. Cyanosis prominent
   Causes: Hypoplastic right ventricle, severe Fallot's tetralogy
   Signs: Small, quiet heart; reduced pulmonary flow
2. Cyanosis with respiratory distress
   Causes: Transposition of the great arteries, anomalous pulmonary venous return
   Signs: Small, active heart; increased pulmonary flow
3. Low systemic cardiac output or shock
   Causes: Hypoplastic left ventricle, interrupted aortic arch, severe coarctation of the aorta
   Signs: Large, active heart; increased pulmonary flow, venous congestion

Any neonate with cyanotic heart disease or heart failure should be transferred immediately after initial stabilization to a specialized unit for investigation and treatment.

Urgent consultation with the paediatric cardiologist is required. Many defects are now amenable to surgical correction or palliation. Prenatal diagnosis allows earlier intervention and counselling of parents.

Cyanotic heart disease

Any infant with cyanosis must be treated as an emergency. Differentiation from pulmonary (e.g. RDS) and pulmonary vascular (e.g. persistent pulmonary hypertension) causes is sometimes difficult. Cyanosis in a term infant without asphyxia, which does not improve with oxygen, suggests cardiac disease.

Causes of cyanotic heart disease include:

- Transposition of the great arteries
- Pulmonary atresia
- Tricuspid atresia
- Anomalous pulmonary venous return
- Ebstein's anomaly.

Initial investigations

➤ Chest X-ray

➤ ECG

➤ Blood pressure, arms and legs

➤ Right arm pulse oximetry or right radial blood gas, in 100% oxygen. If SaO_2 >95% or PaO_2 > 20kPa (150 mmHg), unlikely to be cyanotic heart disease.

> **!** Care must be taken as high inspired oxygen concentrations may promote ductal closure.

Management

The paediatric cardiologist should be contacted for echocardiography and possible cardiac catheterization.

Prostaglandin infusion

A prostaglandin (PGE$_2$) infusion should be commenced. This is used as a temporary measure to dilate the ductus arteriosus where the lesion is ductus dependent. Specific cardiac anomalies where PGE$_2$ is used include:

≺ Pulmonary atresia with intact ventricular septum
≺ Critical pulmonary valve stenosis with intact ventricular septum
≺ Fallot's tetralogy with pulmonary atresia
≺ Tricuspid atresia with small right ventricle, or pulmonary stenosis
≺ Double-outlet right ventricle, single ventricle, and TGA if severe pulmonary stenosis
≺ Simple D-transposition prior to septostomy or when Rashkind's procedure has failed
≺ Interrupted aortic arch or coarctation of aorta.

PGE$_2$ should *not* be used in anomalous pulmonary venous return as this may make the pulmonary congestion worse.

Dose: Each vial contains 0.5 mg PGE$_2$ in 0.5 ml (100 μg in 0.1 ml). Add 0.4 ml (400 μg) to 500 ml one-fifth normal saline/dextrose to obtain solution of 0.8 μg/ml. Infuse at 0.2–1.2 μg/kg/h (0.25–1.5 ml/kg/h).

If there is a response (infant becomes pink and murmur gets louder), use maintenance infusion of one-quarter dose.

Side effects of prostaglandin infusion include:

Pyrexia
Hypotension
Bradycardia
Apnoea
Seizures

If these occur, the infusion rate should be decreased.

✚ Cardiac failure

The major signs of neonatal cardiac failure are a triad of:

- Tachycardia
- Tachypnoea
- Hepatomegaly

Cardiomegaly may be found on the chest radiograph. Poor feeding and sweating are often found. Oedema and neck vein engorgement may be absent or difficult to detect and excessive weight gain is a late sign.

Causes of cardiac failure are:

- Congenital heart disease
- Persistent ductus arteriosus in the preterm baby
- Asphyxia and acidosis
- Hyperkalaemia or hypoglycaemia
- Over-transfusion or anaemia, e.g. twin to twin transfusion, Rhesus disease, intravenous infusion
- Arrhythmia, e.g. congenital heart block, supraventricular tachycardia
- Myocarditis, intrauterine infection
- Cardiomyopathy (e.g. infant of diabetic mother)
- Cerebral vascular abnormality, e.g. vein of Galen aneurysm.

Management

Management of the infant with cardiac failure requires determination of the cause and diuretic therapy. Digoxin is also used but should *not* be given to infants with suspected myocarditis, cardiomyopathy or some arrhythmias unless a paediatric cardiologist has been consulted.

Digoxin treatment

There is still considerable debate on the role and effectiveness of digoxin, especially in L→R shunts such as VSD or PDA.

If used, digoxin is given as a loading dose followed by maintenance therapy. It may be given orally or intravenously; the latter route should be used in the ill infant.

Total oral loading dose:

Preterm: 30 μg/kg

Term: 50 μg/kg

Give in three divided doses:

$1/_3$ of the total dose given immediately

$1/_3$ of the total dose given after 6 hours

$1/_3$ of total dose given after a further 8 hours.

Note the i.v. loading dose is two-thirds that of the oral loading dose.

Maintenance oral dose is given in divided doses every 12 hours:

Preterm: 3 μg/kg

Term: 5 μg/kg

In the presence of *renal failure*, use half the total loading dose and one-third to one-half the maintenance dose.

Aim to keep the trough serum digoxin level between 1–2 μg/l. Digoxin toxicity is manifested by vomiting, bradycardia or heart block.

➕ Patent ductus arteriosus (PDA)

Closure of the ductus arteriosus is a complex process and involves raised PaO_2, and falling prostaglandin levels. As gestational age increases, the muscular wall of the ductus becomes more sensitive to these stimuli so the ductus of term infants tends to close more effectively than that of preterm babies.

Delayed closure of the ductus may cause clinical problems, the frequency of which increases with decreasing birth weight, e.g. 20–40% of babies <1000g may have symptoms attributable to a patent ductus.

Signs of PDA:

≺ Bounding pulses

≺ Hyperactive precordium

◄ Loud systolic or continuous murmur at upper left sternal edge, radiating into the back or under left clavicle. A murmur may be absent
◄ Widened pulse pressure; hypotension may be commoner in the smallest babies
◄ Failure to show anticipated improvement, or deterioration, during the recovery phase of RDS
◄ Metabolic acidosis
◄ Apnoea.

These signs usually occur from about 3–5 days onwards, although they may occur earlier as a result of surfactant treatment. The accuracy of clinical signs in diagnosing a PDA is poor and, where possible, further investigations should be performed prior to initiating treatment.

Investigation

► Chest X-ray may show:
cardiomegaly
increased pulmonary vascularity
pulmonary oedema
The presence of co-existing lung disease may make
    interpretation difficult.

► Echocardiography:
M-mode or 2-D echocardiography may show an increased
    left atrial to aortic root ratio (LA/Ao). A ratio of >1.5: 1 is
    usually taken as significant. However, a raised LA/Ao is
    not specific for PDA
pulsed Doppler echo may detect turbulent flow in the main
    pulmonary artery
2-D imaging of the ductus with direct pulsed Doppler or
    colour flow analysis of the shunt is the most accurate
    diagnostic method.

Management

Fluid restriction and diuretic therapy may control symptoms in relatively well infants until spontaneous closure at about 40 weeks' postconceptional age. Some infants, however, have large L→R shunts and may have severe recurrent apnoea, intractable metabolic acidosis and need prolonged mechanical ventilation. If they fail to respond to conservative therapy, closure of the ductus either by surgical ligation or prostaglandin synthetase inhibition with indomethacin is necessary. Surgical ligation carries low operative mortality in experienced hands but risk for tiny ill infants is increased and medical closure may be preferred, provided there are no contraindications to the use of indomethacin (see below).

Indomethacin therapy

This is effective in about 80% of cases. If infants with large PDA are treated early (within 10 days of birth), over 80% have satisfactory constriction or closure. After 14 days, response is less good, with 50% responding satisfactorily and the rest requiring ligation.

There are a number of different treatment regimens; the traditional dose is 0.1–0.2 mg/kg i.v. 8–12 hourly for 3 doses, although 0.1 mg/kg daily for 5 days is as effective and may have fewer renal side effects. Each dose should probably be given over 30 min.

There are a number of relative contraindications to indomethacin:

Inadequate urinary output (<0.5 ml/kg/h)
Serum creatinine >130 μmol/l (1.5 mg/dl)
Platelets <100 000/mm³
Prothrombin time >20 s
Partial thromboplastin time >70 s
Bilirubin >150 μmol/l (9 mg/dl)
Necrotizing enterocolitis

These are not absolute and indomethacin may be given in a dose of 0.1 mg/kg if signs are severe and ligation is likely.

Side effects include decreased urinary output, raised serum creatinine, hyponatraemia and hyperkalaemia. Bleeding, especially gastric haemorrhage, can also occur. Urine output, serum creatinine, electrolytes and urea should therefore be monitored at least daily after therapy until they return to normal.

Favourable signs of a response are reduced intensity and

shortening of murmur, and a decrease in precordial activity and peripheral pulses. Echocardiography shows reduction in LA/Ao ratio and reduced ductal flow.

Some infants show only partial improvement but symptoms will be controlled by fluid restriction and diuretics until spontaneous closure occurs later.

Reopening of PDA after treatment is relatively common, especially in babies <1000 g, particularly during episodes of sepsis. Response to repeated doses is often found so that second and third courses of treatment are worth trying in an attempt to avoid ligation.

✚ Low cardiac output syndrome

This typically occurs in the first few days of life. The infant may be pale, with poor peripheral perfusion, gasping respiration and cyanosis. There are three main causes of this picture:

- Overwhelming septicaemia (e.g. GBS infection)
- Cardiac causes
- Inborn errors of metabolism.

Cardiac causes include:

- Hypoplastic left heart syndrome
- Interrupted aortic arch
- Severe aortic stenosis

In these, the systemic circulation becomes jeopardized by closure of the ductus arteriosus, with subsequent underperfusion of the tissues, hypoxia, acidosis and myocardial failure.

Treatment should be urgent and aggressive, directed towards correction of acidosis, congestive heart failure and hypotension. A prostaglandin infusion should be commenced and an urgent cardiology opinion sought.

A growing number of babies with hypoplastic left heart syndrome are being offered palliative surgery with the Norwood procedure. Parents should be counselled very carefully; in some cases the most appropriate treatment is withdrawal of intensive care.

✚ Neonatal hypertension

This is defined as consistent blood pressure readings over 90/50 mmHg in a term infant (Fig. 17.2).

Blood pressure measurement is most accurate when an indwelling aortic catheter connected to a pressure transducer is used, but oscillometric, Doppler and flush methods may be used.

Neonatal hypertension is commonly due to underlying renal causes:

- Renovascular: renal artery or vein thrombosis, renal artery stenosis/hypoplasia, abdominal coarctation syndrome
- Renal cystic disease: multicystic/dyplastic or polycystic kidneys

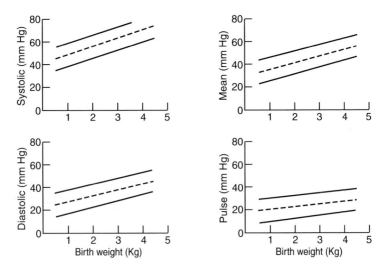

Figure 17.2. Blood pressure by birth weight with 95% confidence limits. From Versmold *et al.* (1981) with kind permission of the authors and the editor of *Pediatrics*.

- Obstructive uropathy
- Coarctation or thrombosis of the aorta
- Adrenal disease: neuroblastoma, carcinoma
- CNS disease: raised intracranial pressure (HIE, seizures)
- Corticosteroid treatment for chronic lung disease (reversible).

Treatment may be needed for systolic pressures >90 mmHg (>95th centile) as the risk of heart failure, encephalopathy and failure to thrive is increased. The reduction in blood pressure should be gradual to avoid hypotension. Commonly used drugs are listed in Table 17.1.

Asymptomatic hypertension may be treated with oral β-blockers. Care is needed with ACE inhibitors as these reduce renal blood flow, especially in renovascular disease. A titrated reduction with intravenous labetalol or nitroprusside is best for hypertensive crises but priority is given to seizure control (i.v. diazepam). For less urgent indications methyldopa and hydralazine are effective.

Table 17.1. Drugs for neonatal hypertension

Drug	Dose	Route	Comment
Labetalol	1–3 mg/kg/h	i.v.	hypertensive emergency
Sodium nitroprusside	0.5–8 μg/kg/min	i.v. infusion	hypertensive emergency
Atenolol	1–2 mg/kg/day	oral	cardioselective blocker
Chlorothiazide	20–40 mg/kg/day	oral	mild hypertension
Hydralazine	0.5–5 mg/kg/day	oral	moderate hypertension
Enalapril	25–250 μg/kg/day	oral	ACE inhibitor
Methyldopa	10–40 mg/kg/day	oral	central action

✚ Cardiac arrhythmias

These may be diagnosed and in some cases treated antenatally, e.g. complete heart block due to maternal collagen disease or supraventricular tachycardia, the latter being treated by giving digoxin or other drugs to the mother to prevent cardiac failure and fetal hydrops.

Minor variations in cardiac rhythm, such as atrial ectopic beats, are very common, particularly in the first few days of life. They may occasionally be due to excessive use of coffee, tea or cola drinks, or to β-mimetics used for asthma by the mother during pregnancy. They do not require any treatment. Significant arrhythmias are less common and may be primary or secondary to other disorders. A paediatric cardiologist should advise about the treatment of all significant cardiac arrhythmias.

Ectopic beats

Causes:

- Isolated finding
- Digoxin toxicity
- Myocarditis
- Hypoxia
- Electrolyte disturbance
- Theophylline toxicity.

These may occasionally need treatment with an antiarrhythmic, e.g. lignocaine.

Sinus bradycardia

The rate is <100/min in preterm or <80/min in term.

Causes include:

- Raised intracranial pressure
- Hyperkalaemia
- Hypothyroidism
- β-Blocker drugs to mother.

Treatment involves correction of the underlying cause. Atropine is occasionally used (see Appendix I).

Complete heart block

The heart rate is usually 40–80/min.

Causes include:

- Complex congenital heart disease
- Maternal collagen disease
- Isolated finding.

May need isoprenaline infusion or cardiac pacing. Indications for pacing in congenital heart block include:

- Previous sibling required pacing
- Fixed heart rate <60 min (usually symptomatic)
- Frequent ventricular extrasystoles
- Long QT interval
- Presentation with heart failure (5%).

Sinus tachycardia

The rate is >160/min in term and >180/min in preterm

Causes include:

- Fever
- Stress and pain
- Blood loss or hypotension
- Heart failure
- Theophylline toxicity
- Thyrotoxicosis.

Treatment is correction of the underlying cause.

Supraventricular tachycardia (SVT)

In SVT the rate is 200–300/min.

Causes include:

- Accessory pathways, e.g. Wolff–Parkinson–White syndrome (10–20%)

- Congenital heart disease
- Isolated finding (50%).

Treatment is important as heart failure may ensue. Initial treatment is to produce vagal stimulation by placing an ice pack on the baby's face. This should be held in place for 10–15 s, and may produce a brief apnoeic episode.

Adenosine (0.05 mg/kg i.v. repeated every 2 min up to a maximum dose of 0.25 mg/kg) is probably now the second-line acute treatment for SVT. The traditional alternative is digitalization followed by maintenance therapy for 6 months after conversion to sinus rhythm. Propranolol may be preferable to digoxin for babies with Wolff–Parkinson–White syndrome.

In severe cases not responding to drug therapy, DC cardioversion should be performed (0.5 J/kg). It is important to monitor the heart rhythm continuously during treatment, and to obtain a 12-lead ECG once in sinus rhythm.

Ventricular tachycardia

The rate is 120–180/min. This rhythm is very uncommon in the neonate but usually signifies serious myocardial disease, and may result in ventricular fibrillation.

Causes include:

- Hypoxia
- Electrolyte disturbance
- Digoxin toxicity
- Local injection of mepivacaine.

Treat with lignocaine (1 mg/kg) or DC cardioversion. Consult the paediatric cardiologist urgently.

DC cardioversion (defibrillation)

For ventricular tachycardia use 1–2 J/kg synchronized to the downstroke of R wave. For ventricular fibrillation use same energy dose unsynchronized. The dose for supraventricular tachycardia is lower (0.5 J/kg synchronized).

Place the paddles at base and apex of heart (below right

clavicle and fifth intercostal space in anterior axillary line). Ensure good electrical conduction by putting saline-soaked gauze wipes beneath each paddle. Notify all assistants before discharging current. Defibrillation may be repeated after doubling the dose but burns can occur.

✚ Bacterial endocarditis

Endocarditis prophylaxis is indicated for neonates with structural cardiac defects in the following circumstances:

Dental surgery or instrumentation of upper respiratory tract

➤ For patients not allergic to penicillin and not given penicillin more than once in the previous month: give amoxycillin 25 mg/kg i.v. at induction of anaesthesia and 12.5 mg/kg orally 6 hours later.

➤ For penicillin allergy or recent exposure: give clindamycin 25 mg/kg i.v. at induction and 12.5 mg/kg i.v. or orally 6 hours later.

Genitourinary surgery or instrumentation or gastro-intestinal procedures:

➤ For patients not allergic to penicillin and not given penicillin more than once in the previous month: give 25 mg/kg amoxycillin with 2 mg/kg gentamicin i.v. at induction and amoxycillin, 12.5 mg/kg orally 6 hours later.

➤ For penicillin allergy or recent exposure: give teicoplanin 6 mg/kg with gentamicin 2 mg/kg i.v. at induction.

Nursing points

Baby
● Nursing the baby in an upright position and offering small, frequent feeds may help dyspnoeic babies.

- Careful fluid balance recordings and daily weighing may be indicated — although excessive weight gain is a late sign of cardiac failure. Earlier signs include slow feeding, sweating and lethargy.
- Closely monitor the urine output of babies on indomethacin. Observe for signs of gastric bleeding.
- Possible side effects of babies receiving prostaglandin infusions include apnoea, pyrexia and seizures.

Family

- Cardiac problems are particularly distressing to families. Detailed explanation of the condition, with diagrams, may need to be repeated several times.
- Cardiac conditions often require long-term treatment, which may involve travelling long distance to a specialist centre. Ongoing support for the family should be provided.
- Contact numbers and information about local and national support groups should be offered to parents.

Equipment

- Continuous cardiorespiratory, blood pressure and pulse oximetry recordings reduce the need for handling. In certain conditions, blood pressure recordings from more than one limb may be needed.

Staff

- Ongoing education opportunities for staff are important to ensure their knowledge is kept up-to-date.
- Regular teaching sessions should be arranged on NICU, to be given and attended by all grades of staff.

References and further reading

Archer N (1993). Patent ductus arteriosus in the newborn. *Arch Dis Child* **69**: 529.

Evans N (1993). Diagnosis of patent ductus arteriosus in the preterm newborn. *Arch Dis Child* **68**: 58.

Freedom RM, Benson LN, Smallhorn JF (1992). *Neonatal Heart Disease*. London: Springer Verlag.

Hammerman C, Aramburo MJ (1990). Prolonged indomethacin therapy for the prevention of recurrences of patent ductus arteriosus. *J Pediatr* **117**: 771.

Haworth SG, Bull C (1993). Physiology of congenital heart disease. *Arch Dis Child* **68**: 707.

Rasoulpour M, Marinelli KA (1992). Systemic hypertension. *Semin Perinatol* **19**: 121.

Rosenfeld LE (1993). The diagnosis and management of cardiac arrhythmias in the neonatal period. *Semin Perinatol* **17**: 135.

Silove ED, Roberts DGV, De Giovanni JV (1985). Evaluation of oral and low dose intravenous prostaglandin E_2 in management of ductus dependent congenital heart disease. *Arch Dis Child* **60**: 1025.

Spevak PJ (1997). New developments in fetal echocardiography. *Curr Opin Cardiol* **12**: 78.

Zahka KG, Spector M, Hanisch D (1993). Hypoplastic left-heart syndrome: Norwood operation, transplantation, or compassionate care. *Clin Perinatol* **20**: 145.

18 Gastrointestinal Problems

➕ Vomiting

This is defined as the forceful expulsion of gastric contents through the mouth or nose. It is important to distinguish between vomiting and possetting, which is common and benign. The character of the vomitus may help in formulating a diagnosis: bile-staining suggests intestinal obstruction; blood in the vomitus may be due to swallowed maternal blood, trauma from a feeding tube, stress ulceration, coagulation disorder, or drugs such as dexamethasone or tolazoline. Vomiting is unlikely to be benign if there is blood or bile staining, watery or loose stools, abdominal distension, or reluctance to feed.

 All vomiting babies should be carefully examined to determine an underlying cause and to assess the degree of dehydration.

Dehydration should be suspected when there is:

≺ Abnormal weight loss (>10% of birth weight)
≺ Poor urinary output (< 1.5 ml/kg/h)
≺ Loss of skin turgor
≺ Sunken eyes and depressed anterior fontanelle
≺ Hypotension.

Causes of vomiting include:

• Overfeeding
• Infection: urinary tract, bacteraemia, gastroenteritis
• Intestinal obstruction at any level

- Functional ileus: any ill baby, e.g. sepsis, electrolyte imbalance, extreme preterm, severe RDS
- Necrotizing enterocolitis
- Gastro-oesophageal reflux, hiatus hernia
- Cerebral oedema, intracranial haemorrhage, meningitis
- Congenital adrenal hyperplasia, inborn errors of metabolism
- Pyloric stenosis (very occasionally presents by 7–10 days)
- Drugs: digoxin, oral antibiotics.

Investigations

The following investigations may be indicated:

➤ Blood: urea and electrolytes, pH, glucose, culture

➤ Urine: urinalysis, culture

➤ Abdominal radiography (AP and lateral films) may indicate:
obstruction (air–fluid levels or double-bubble)
perforation (free air)
pneumatosis intestinalis or gas in the biliary tree in necrotizing enterocolitis
ascites (uniform opacity in the flanks).

Management

Management of vomiting depends on the severity and cause. If vomiting is persistent and dehydration present, feeding should be discontinued, a nasogastric tube inserted and placed on free drainage. Intravenous fluids should be given; if shock is present volume expansion with 10–20 ml/kg of 5% albumin, plasma or blood is indicated. Daily fluid intake should take into account the estimated deficit, maintenance requirements and correction for ongoing losses. Careful attention should be paid to electrolyte imbalance.

✚ Diarrhoea

This is defined as the frequent passage of watery or loose stools. Up to eight stools per day is probably normal for a bottle fed baby but breast fed infants may have as many as 16 stools per day. The normal stools of a breast fed baby are not fully formed and may be green in colour.

Causes of neonatal diarrhoea include:

- Gastroenteritis
- Necrotizing enterocolitis
- Effect of maternal diet or laxatives in breast fed infants
- Starvation stools: frequent small amounts of dark green material
- Disaccharide intolerance
- Oral drugs (antibiotics, iron, calcium), or feed thickeners
- Phototherapy
- Maternal drug addiction
- Cystic fibrosis
- Neonatal thyrotoxicosis
- Congenital chloridorrhea (rare).

➕ Gastroenteritis

Many cases of gastroenteritis in the newborn are caused by viruses, such as rotavirus. A bacterial pathogen is found in only 20–40% of cases, e.g. pathogenic *Escherichia coli*, shigella, salmonella and campylobacter. These may be transmitted from the mother who has become infected around the time of birth, or spread from baby to baby via staff in the neonatal unit. The chief dangers are dehydration, bacteraemia and cross-infection.

In some cases the stool may be watery and difficult to collect; it may be helpful to use a uribag or to soak the stool up in sterile cotton wool balls.

The infected infant should be isolated. Where space is at a premium, it is safe to nurse the baby in an incubator in a room where all the other babies are also in incubators. Equipment used by infected infants should be carefully sterilized.

> **!** Scrupulous hand washing is essential to prevent cross-infection.

In mild cases, milk feeds should be discontinued and clear fluids given by mouth. Severe cases need intravenous fluids. Antibiotics are not necessary unless bacteraemia is suspected. Some infants will have recurrence of diarrhoea after milk is reintroduced. If the stools are acidic (pH <5.5) and contain over 0.5% of reducing substances on testing with a reagent tablet (Clinitest™), then secondary lactose intolerance is likely. Stool should be sent for sugar chromatography to confirm the diagnosis. Symptoms can be relieved by feeding with a lactose-free milk, and normal formula reintroduced as a trial later.

✚ Necrotizing enterocolitis (NEC)

This is an inflammatory condition which may affect both the large and small bowel.

Risk factors include:

- Prematurity
- Asphyxia
- Hypothermia and polycythaemia in SGA babies
- Cyanotic congenital heart disease
- Cardiac catheterization
- Exchange transfusion.

The underlying problem is probably ischaemia of the bowel wall which encourages bacterial invasion from the lumen with gas formation and release of endotoxin. The organism involved may be a gas-producing anaerobe, such as clostridium, but often no pathogen is isolated.

It is unusual for NEC to develop before feeding has started. Colonization of the intestine is more likely to be involved when formula milk is used; the gut of breast-fed infants becomes colonized primarily by lactobacilli, which may partly explain the lower incidence of NEC in breast-fed babies.

NEC may present with:

≺ Vomiting or increased volume of gastric aspirates
≺ Bloody diarrhoea
≺ Abdominal distension and ileus
≺ Apnoea and lethargy
≺ Temperature instability and poor skin perfusion
≺ Erythema of the anterior abdominal wall
≺ Thrombocytopenia.

The clinical presentation may vary from mild or non-specific symptoms to a rapidly overwhelming illness.

Abdominal radiographs may show dilated loops of bowel with thickened, oedematous walls. Later, linear streaks or bubbles of intramural gas appear (pneumatosis intestinalis), and perforation releases free peritoneal gas which may be seen along the ligamentum teres, under the diaphragm in an erect film, or under the umbilicus in a lateral film. Gas may also be seen within the portal venous system or hepatic veins.

Prevention

➤ Careful placement of umbilical catheters
➤ Cautious introduction of milk feeds to babies considered at risk
➤ Use of breast milk where possible.

Management

➤ Stop oral feeds
➤ Parenteral nutrition
➤ Broad-spectrum antibiotics, including cover for anaerobes, e.g. cefotaxime plus metronidazole
➤ Adequate pain relief

➤ Careful control of fluid balance
➤ Maintenance of blood pressure.

 In necrotizing enterocolitis a neonatal surgeon should be consulted early in the course of the disease.

If intramural gas is present on the abdominal radiograph, follow-up cross-table lateral films 8–12 hourly should be done to detect perforation.

The platelet count is a useful indicator of disease severity; the inflammatory process consumes platelets and upon recovery the platelet count returns to normal. Failure of the platelet count to return to normal suggests the presence of an inflammatory mass or coexisting bacteraemia (sometimes due to an infected central venous catheter).

The only absolute indication for surgery is *perforation*. Some babies may be too sick to withstand surgery; in this situation insertion of an intraperitoneal drain under local analgesia may allow decompression of the abdomen and drainage of necrotic material. At laparotomy, minimal resection of non-viable bowel and fashioning of an enterostomy are usually performed, but resection and primary anastomosis may be possible in some cases.

Oral feeding is usually recommenced, preferably with breast milk or a predigested formula milk, about 7–10 days after the acute signs have improved.

Later complications can occur: stricture is seen in 10–30% of cases and may present upon refeeding 2–6 weeks after the acute episode with recurrence of abdominal distension and large gastric aspirates; 5–10% may develop malabsorption, particularly after extensive resection (short bowel syndrome). Chronically ill babies who have needed parenteral nutrition for prolonged periods, often develop conjugated hyperbilirubinaemia (see Ch. 11).

Overall mortality is about 10%, but higher in those who perforate (30%). Long-term neurological impairment is quite common (30%) in severe disease where periventricular leucomalacia can develop.

✚ Abdominal distension

The causes of abdominal distension are similar to those of vomiting, but include pneumoperitoneum, bilateral pneumothoraces (which push down the liver and spleen), ascites, and renal masses. Abdominal ultrasound will assist in the diagnosis.

✚ Blood in the stools

This is a relatively common problem. Swallowed maternal blood is detected with the Apt test.

Apt test procedure

Dissolve 2–3 drops of bloody specimen in 5ml of water in a test tube, add 1ml of 1% sodium hydroxide. If adult blood, colour will turn from pink to yellow–brown in 1–2 min; if fetal haemoglobin, colour will remain pink, i.e. fetal haemoglobin resists alkali denaturation.

Causes of blood in the stools include:

- Swallowed maternal blood
- Anal/rectal fissure due to thermometer, digital examination or severe constipation
- Haemorrhagic disease of the newborn
- Necrotizing enterocolitis
- Malrotation or volvulus
- Reduplication of the bowel
- Rarely, gastroenteritis, intussusception, Meckel's diverticulum.

Gastrointestinal malformations

These include exomphalos, gastroschisis, intestinal atresia, Hirschsprung's disease, imperforate anus and tracheo-oesophageal fistula.

A baby with a gastrointestinal malformation may have important malformations in other areas.

Oesophageal atresia (± tracheo-oesophageal fistula)

This occurs in approximately 1/3500 births. There are five types, but by far the commonest is where there is oesophageal atresia with a distal tracheo-oesophageal fistula. 50% of babies have other malformations, e.g. vertebral, cardiac, renal or other gut anomalies. Presents with maternal polyhydramnios, frothy secretions or aspiration pneumonia. Continuous or frequent intermittent suction of the upper oesophagus via a large bore tube is important to prevent aspiration.

Most babies are able to have a primary anastomosis and division of the fistula, once their general condition is stabilized.

Diaphragmatic hernia

The incidence is approximately 1/4000 births, 80–90% are left-sided. The condition usually presents at birth with asphyxia, shift of apex beat and respiratory distress. The abdomen is scaphoid.

Prenatal diagnosis allows maternal transfer for delivery in a regional perinatal centre. In the delivery suite, the baby should be intubated and a large bore nasogastric tube inserted to decompress the gut.

> **!** Bag and mask ventilation may make the baby considerably worse as the stomach and upper intestine will become distended and further compress the heart and 'good' lung.

In two-thirds of cases there is pulmonary hypoplasia and pulmonary hypertension. The baby may respond to pulmonary vasodilating drugs, including inhaled nitric oxide, high frequency ventilation or ECMO, although those babies who are very ill from birth generally do not respond well and death is likely, even if the defect is repaired. If surgery is considered, the baby should be as stable as possible beforehand; 90% of babies who are well enough for surgery after stabilization, survive.

✚ *Exomphalos (omphalocele)*

In this condition there is herniation of abdominal contents into the umbilical cord. Coils of intestine and liver are covered by peritoneal membrane unless this has ruptured. Over 30% have associated abnormalities of gastrointestinal, genitourinary and cardiovascular systems. Beckwith's syndrome (visceromegaly, macroglossia, omphalocele) should be kept in mind as there may be severe hypoglycaemia. This must be corrected prior to transfer to a surgical unit.

Prenatal diagnosis allows maternal transfer for delivery in a regional centre. In the delivery suite the lesion should be covered with cling film or a polythene bag ('poly bag') and the stomach aspirated continuously to prevent distension. Intravenous fluids should be erected.

> **!** Saline dressings should *not* be used as these cause excessive evaporative heat loss.

Surgery involves replacing the herniated contents in the abdomen where possible. There may be subsequent respiratory embarassment or inferior vena cava compression. Very major lesions may have to be repaired in stages.

✚ *Gastroschisis*

This is somewhat similar to omphalocele except that coils of intestine herniate through a defect in the anterior abdominal wall near the umbilicus. There is no covering peritoneal membrane and associated abnormalities, apart from ileal atresias, are uncommon. The intestinal circulation can be impaired causing ischaemia of bowel with frank gangrene. The lesion should be covered with cling film or a polythene bag and a nasogastric tube inserted before transfer. Intravenous fluids should be erected; there are often large protein losses into the gut and these need replacement with intravenous plasma or albumin solution.

> **!** Careful attention must be paid to fluid and electrolyte balance.

Intestinal atresia

Presentation is with vomiting (usually bile-stained), abdominal distension and delayed passage of meconium. Even in complete obstruction, small amounts of 'stool' may be passed in the first 24 hours. There may have been maternal polyhydramnios. In general, the more distal the site of the lesion, the later the presentation after delivery. Duodenal obstruction is associated with other abnormalities in 70% of cases (e.g. Down's syndrome, malrotation and congenital heart disease). A 'double-bubble' is seen on the abdominal radiograph in duodenal atresia, and multiple fluid levels in ileal atresia.

Immediate treatment consists of nasogastric drainage and intravenous fluids. Electrolyte disturbances should be corrected.

Malrotation

Often associated with duodenal bands (of Ladd). Associated abnormalities include duodenal atresia or stenosis and exomphalos. Obstruction may be intermittent or incomplete so diagnosis may be missed. There may be bile-stained vomiting and bloody stools or failure to thrive. Intestinal ischaemia can lead to necrosis with shock and sepsis. Barium meal will show partial obstruction of the third part of the duodenum, with the jejunum abnormally placed.

Initial management is as for intestinal obstruction, although once the diagnosis is made, surgery should be performed urgently as there is a risk of the whole bowel becoming gangrenous.

✚ *Meconium ileus*

10–15% of infants with cystic fibrosis present in the newborn period with bowel obstruction. Pancreatic enzyme deficiency results in the production of thick, inspissated meconium. Peritonitis may occur following perforation *in utero* but as meconium is sterile the effects may not be recognized for some time after birth. Presentation may be with failure to pass meconium in the first 48 hours or with progressive abdominal distension and vomiting.

Initial management is as for other forms of bowel obstruction. The abdominal radiograph shows a foamy or granular appearance inside distended bowel, and there may be flecks of calcification if perforation has occurred *in utero*. A gastrografin enema may show a microcolon and may also act therapeutically to relieve an uncomplicated obstruction. If this is not successful, a temporary double-barrelled ileostomy should be performed.

Immunoreactive trypsinogen screening for cystic fibrosis should be performed *before* surgery.

✚ *Hirschsprung's disease*

This condition is due to an absence of ganglion cells in the myenteric plexus of the rectum. The aganglionic segment of bowel may extend proximally for a variable distance. Short-segment disease is more common in males but long-segment disease has an equal sex distribution. The condition may be familial. Hirschsprung's disease is uncommon in preterm babies but does occur.

Barium enema is usually required for diagnosis: this typically shows a narrow aganglionic segment distal to dilated bowel, although short segment disease may be missed. The diagnosis is confirmed by rectal biopsy, which shows absent ganglion cells.

Initial management is as for other forms of bowel obstruction. A defunctioning colostomy is performed, with later resection and anastomosis.

✚ *Imperforate anus*

The lesion may be high or low: lateral abdominal radiographs taken at about 24 hours, with the baby prone or slightly inverted, distinguishes these two types. A radio-opaque marker should be placed over the anus. If air is present in the upper rectal pouch caudal to a line drawn from the pubis to sacrococcygeal junction, then the lesion is low.

High

There is usually a fistula from the upper rectal pouch to bladder, urethra or vagina. Large bowel obstruction occurs only if the fistula is not patent. Urinary tract infections may occur. Treatment usually involves a defunctioning colostomy and later 'pull-through' operation. There may be difficulty in achieving faecal continence.

Low

The anus may be obstructed by a membrane at the level of the anal valves. Treatment is by anoplasty. Most children have a good prognosis.

Anorectal anomalies may be associated with tracheo-oesophageal fistula and VATER syndrome (V = ventricular septal defect and vertebral anomalies, A = anal atresia, TE = tracheo-oesophageal fistula, R = radial and renal anomalies).

Preparation for surgery

 Babies requiring surgery should be transferred to a specialist centre and must be properly stabilized before transfer

Where possible the baby should be transferred *in utero* and this is increasingly so with better prenatal diagnosis. The baby should be fully stabilized:

➤ Maintain temperature

➤ Control blood pressure

➤ Obtain adequate i.v. access

➤ Place nasogastric tube and erect i.v. fluids

➤ Optimize blood gases and mechanical ventilation

➤ Give vitamin K, 1 mg i.v.

Written parental consent and a sample of maternal blood for cross-matching should be obtained.

Nursing points

Baby

- Carefully observe and record the amount, colour and frequency of stools, urine, gastric aspirate and vomit.
- A distended abdomen may be the first sign of NEC.
- Breast-feeding or providing some breast milk in feeds reduces the risk of NEC.
- Early signs of infection are often subtle and may include:
  - ◄ Poor response to handling
  - ◄ Recurrent apnoea
  - ◄ Hyperglycaemia
  - ◄ Glycosuria
  - ◄ Unstable temperature
  - ◄ Increased gastric aspirates
  - ◄ Abdominal distension.
- Babies with NEC are at risk of glucose and electrolyte imbalances. Blood glucose monitoring strips and urinalysis should be performed regularly.

Family

- All mothers should be encouraged to provide breast milk for their baby, even if only for a short period.
- The need for strict hand washing should be emphasized to all visitors.

Equipment

- Continuous cardiorespiratory, blood pressure and temperature monitoring reduces the need for handling.

- Cross-infection must be prevented by strict attention to hygiene and appropriate cleaning of all equipment.
- The use of human milk banks should be encouraged in developed countries as the benefits of breast milk to neonates are well proven. Appropriate screening, treatment and storage of milk is necessary.

Staff

- Where possible, babies with NEC should be isolated. Measures should be taken to reduce the risk of cross infection, including the provision of adequate staffing levels.

References and further reading

Kinney JS, Eiden JJ (1994). Enteric infectious disease in neonates: Epidemiology, pathogenesis and a practical approach to evaluation and therapy. In: Necrotising enterocolitis (eds, Stoll BJ, Kliegman RM). *Clin Perinatol* **21**: 317.

Kliegman RM (1990). Neonatal necrotising enterocolitis: bridging the basic science with the clinical disease. *J Pediatr* **117**: 833.

Kosloske AM (1994). Epidemiology of necrotising enterocolitis. *Acta Paediatr* **396 (suppl)**: 2.

Ricketts RR (1994). Surgical treatment of necrotising enterocolitis and the short bowel syndrome. In: Necrotising Enterocolitis (eds, Stoll BJ, Kliegman RM). *Clin Perinatol* **21**: 365.

Stringer MD, Spitz L (1993). Surgical management of neonatal necrotising enterocolitis. *Arch Dis Child* **69**: 269.

19 Genitourinary Problems

The fetal kidneys contribute to amniotic fluid by producing large quantities of dilute urine. The placenta is the major excretory organ and maintains fetal homeostasis, so that neonatal plasma urea and creatinine concentrations at birth are very similar to those of the mother. Plasma creatinine concentration is commonly around 70 μmol/l at birth and falls to 30–40 μmol/l after the first week of life.

The neonatal kidney has the same number of nephrons as the adult kidney (normally 1 million), but a much lower functional capacity. Glomerular filtration and tubular reabsorption are reduced and there is a glomerulotubular preponderance. These characteristics resemble a state of mild renal failure. Neonatal urine has a lower maximal osmolality due to low urea excretion.

Growth with its strong anabolic drive assists the neonatal kidney by reducing the excretory load of sodium, water, phosphorus, hydrogen and nitrogen. Growth is sometimes referred to as the 'third kidney' of the newborn. 30% of newborns pass urine during delivery, 90% within 24 hours and 99% within 48 hours of birth. After the first day of life, urine output is typically 1–3 ml/kg/h, increasing to at least 2–4 ml/kg/h by 2 weeks of life. Severe dehydration is the commonest cause of oliguria/anuria.

Renal problems may present in a number of ways:

- ◄ Abnormal antenatal ultrasound scan
- ◄ Oligohydramnios (renal agenesis, posterior urethral valve)
- ◄ Failure to pass urine
- ◄ Non-specific signs, e.g. jaundice, lethargy, poor feeding, vomiting, weight loss, dehydration or temperature instability
- ◄ Renal mass

≺ Haematuria

≺ Visible genitourinary abnormality: hypospadias, epispadias or ectopia vesicae

≺ Hypertrophied placenta >25% infant birth weight (may suggest congenital nephrotic syndrome)

≺ Family history of kidney malformation.

Investigation following an abnormal antenatal ultrasound scan

With the advent of routine antenatal ultrasound scanning, abnormalities of the renal tracts are a relatively common finding. These should be followed carefully through pregnancy and investigated after birth.

 The neonatologist and/or paediatric nephrologist preferably should be involved in the antenatal period when there is an abnormal USS.

Suspected dilated renal tracts

Not all babies will have significant abnormalities but ultrasound scan of the urinary tract should be performed within the first 24–48 hours after birth. There are three possible findings:

➤ *No dilatation*: repeat ultrasound at 1 month (some centres perform a micturating cystourethrogram (MCUG) on all babies who have shown renal dilatation *in utero*, as vesico-ureteric reflux (VUR) may be present despite a normal postnatal USS).

➤ *Equivocal*: commence prophylactic trimethoprim 1–2 mg/kg once daily, perform MCUG and if no VUR repeat ultrasound at 1 month. If VUR present, continue antibiotic prophylaxis; if infravesical obstruction (posterior urethral valve), surgery is indicated urgently.

➤ *Dilatation confirmed*: commence trimethoprim 1–2 mg/kg once daily. Perform MCUG and if VUR or infravesical obstruction treat as above. In the absence of reflux, supravesical obstruction is likely and an isotope (MAG3) renogram should be performed.

Cystic/dyplastic kidneys

Perform postnatal ultrasound scan and if abnormal, refer to paediatric nephrologist.

✚ Renal failure

Failure to pass urine, or enough urine, is a relatively frequent occurrence. The commonest reason for not passing urine in the first day of life is the unnoticed passage of urine in the labour ward. Inadequate fluid intake (e.g. when breast feeding is being established) or increased evaporative fluid losses secondary to phototherapy or radiant warmers are common reasons for inadequate urine production.

Renal function may be impaired under a variety of circumstances, particularly in the ill or preterm infant. Normal urine output in the newborn should be 1–3 ml/kg/h after the first day; a urine output of <1.0 ml/kg/h should be considered as oliguria and a cause sought. Urine output may be measured after collection into a uribag or by weighing cotton wool balls.

Urine examination may reveal the presence of haematuria, proteinuria or pyuria (see below). Proteinuria detected by dipstick should be confirmed by sending a timed sample of urine to laboratory for analysis.

Causes of acute renal failure include:

- Birth asphyxia, severe respiratory distress
- Hypovolaemia
- Dehydration: loss of fluid, inadequate fluid intake
- Trauma, especially obstetric
- Septicaemia/acute pyelonephritis
- Heart failure, especially due to PDA
- Drugs and toxins: gentamicin, vancomycin, tolazoline, indomethacin

- Renal artery thrombosis or embolism
- Disseminated intravascular coagulation
- Renal agenesis, polycystic kidneys, renal dysplasia
- Congenital nephrotic syndrome, nephritis
- Obstructive uropathy: urethral valve, ureterocele, systemic candidiasis.

Biochemical upsets include rising blood urea, serum creatinine, potassium and phosphate; metabolic acidosis and a lowered serum sodium, calcium and magnesium.

It may be difficult to distinguish pre-renal from renal failure clinically in the oliguric infant. A variety of indices of renal function may help in the diagnosis (Table 18.1), although they are of limited value if diuretics have been given.

Table 18.1. Distinction between pre-renal and renal failure

	Pre-renal	Renal
U_{Cr}/P_{Cr}	>14	<10
Urine osmolality (mOsmol/l)	>400	<350
Fractional excretion of sodium (FE_{Na})	0.8±0.6	4.8±1.4
Renal failure index (RFI)	1.0±0.2	7.2±1.3

$FE_{Na} = (U_{Na}/P_{Na})/(U_{Cr}/P_{Cr}) \times 100$
$RFI = (U_{Na})/(U_{Cr}/P_{Cr})$
U = urine; P = plasma; Cr = creatinine; Na = sodium

Management

➤ Look for the underlying cause and correct where possible.

➤ Try frusemide (5 mg/kg); continue with 2 mg/kg 6 hourly if a response is seen.

➤ If no response, try dopamine infusion (1–2 µg/kg/min) to increase renal blood flow

➤ Correct fluid and electrolyte imbalance (see below)

➤ In most cases a paediatric nephrologist should be consulted.

Fluid and electrolyte balance

➤ Fluids should be ordered on a day-to-day basis: give volume equivalent to previous day's urinary output plus insensible water loss, which is approximately 20–30 ml/kg/day in the term infant and 40–50 ml/kg/day in the preterm infant. Catheterize the bladder to measure urine output accurately.

➤ Limit potassium intake to <0.3 mmol/kg/day and monitor serum electrolytes closely. Hyperkalaemia may cause arrhythmias if >8 mmol/l. Treatment includes:

1–2 mg/kg of 10% calcium gluconate over a 3-min period with ECG monitoring

insulin 0.2 units/kg i.v. and glucose 0.5–1 g/kg i.v.

bicarbonate 1 mmol/kg i.v.

salbutamol 6 μg/kg/h i.v.

➤ Correct hypoglycaemia, hypocalcaemia and acidosis.

➤ Protein intake should be restricted to <2 g/kg/day if blood urea becomes high (3 g protein is catabolized to give 1 g urea), but adequate energy intake should be maintained.

➤ Monitor blood pressure carefully. Treatment should be on the advice of a paediatric nephrologist.

Dialysis

This should be performed under the direction of a paediatric nephrologist. It is required in those patients who cannot be managed conservatively by careful fluid balance and correction of metabolic abnormalities.

Indications for dialysis are:

◄ Severe hyperkalaemia (>8 mmol/l)
◄ Metabolic acidosis
◄ Over-hydration with pulmonary oedema or congestive heart failure
◄ Intractable hypoglycaemia.

Peritoneal dialysis is more efficient than haemodialysis in the newborn because of the large peritoneal surface area/weight ratio and increased clearance of peritoneal urea and creatinine compared to the adult.

Technique of peritoneal dialysis

Under sterile conditions an infant-sized (13–16 FG) peritoneal catheter (Pendlebury Neonatal Cannula, Medcomp) is introduced percutaneously after infiltration of local anaesthetic. The dialysis fluid is delivered through a closed system (Paediatric Dialysis Set, Avon Medical R3370) in which a Y-connection allows alternate filling and draining of the peritoneal cavity. The fluid should pass though a water bath to ensure delivery at 37°C. Volumes of 30–50 ml/kg are instilled in 30–60-min cycles until biochemistry or oedema are corrected.

Commercial dialysis fluids have similar electrolyte composition to plasma except for absence of potassium. A glucose concentration of 1.36% is usually employed but may be increased to 3–4% if satisfactory fluid removal is not achieved. When plasma potassium falls to 4 mmol/l, potassium chloride should be added to the dialysate (4 mmol/l) to prevent hypokalaemia.

There is a major risk of peritonitis unless full aseptic technique is observed during fluid bag changes. Daily effluent cultures are necessary for early diagnosis and institution of appropriate antibiotic treatment, rather than prophylaxis.

Peritoneal dialysis may fail if there is poor cardiac output leading to reduced gut perfusion, or where there is increased capillary permeability (e.g. sepsis) which may prevent ultrafiltration of water. It is not possible to perform peritoneal dialysis if an enterostomy is present.

Haemodialysis

May be performed in the newborn using continuous arteriovenous haemofiltration (CAVH) and is most effective in term infants where fluid overload is the main problem. This should only be performed by a paediatric nephrologist.

Prognosis

This is good if there is pre-renal failure. 75% of babies with severe renal failure following birth asphyxia survive, but about 40% have neurological damage and up to 40% persistent renal impairment.

✚ Renal masses

More than 50% of abdominal masses in the newborn are renal in origin. The lower poles of normal kidneys may be palpable.

Causes of an abdominal mass include:

- Hydronephrosis
- Polycystic kidney
- Multicystic/dysplastic kidney
- Horseshoe kidney
- Renal vein thrombosis
- Retroperitoneal haematoma
- Adrenal haemorrhage
- Nephroblastoma (Wilm's tumour).

A renal ultrasound scan should be performed to aid diagnosis. Further investigations may be necessary (see p. 319). Management will involve input from a paediatric nephrologist and/or paediatric surgeon.

✚ Urinary tract infection (see also p. 240)

This is estimated to occur in 0.1–1% of newborns, with boys being more commonly affected than girls. Blood-borne infection is more likely than ascending, and coliforms are responsible for most infections. Symptoms and signs include lethargy, poor feeding, vomiting and increasing jaundice.

A significant infection is indicated by isolation of $\geq 10^5$ /ml of a single organism on three successive clean catch/bag samples, or if any organisms are grown from a sample obtained by suprapubic aspiration.

✚ *Pyuria*

Pyuria is defined as >5 white cells per centrifuged high-power field. This finding strongly suggests infection of the genitourinary system and full bacteriological assessment is indicated.

Causes of pyuria include:

- Urinary tract infection
- Dehydration
- After suprapubic aspiration or bladder catheterization
- Renal tubular acidosis
- Interstitial nephritis, e.g. after methicillin.

Management

Treatment of urinary tract infection consists of appropriate antibiotics and fluids, both given intravenously. Prophylaxis with trimethoprim 2 mg/kg once per day should be instituted when the course of treatment is complete. When the infection has been controlled, diagnostic imaging of the renal tracts should be performed (ultrasound, MCUG and DMSA isotope renogram) to exclude anomalies or VUR, and to assess renal function.

Indications for renal imaging in the newborn are:

➤ After one proven urinary infection in either sex
➤ Abdominal masses
➤ Haematuria without obvious cause
➤ Absent abdominal musculature (prune belly syndrome)
➤ Single umbilical artery (up to 25% have associated abnormalities: skeletal, gastrointestinal, skin, genitourinary, respiratory, cardiovascular or central nervous systems)
➤ Abnormal antenatal ultrasound scan
➤ Acute renal failure.

✚ Haematuria

This is defined as >3 red cells per centrifuged high-power field, and should always be investigated fully. Note that urinary urates can cause reddish–brown staining of urine.

Causes of haematuria include:

- Birth asphyxia and trauma to kidneys during delivery

- Coagulation disorder
- Urinary tract infection (obstruction, reflux)
- After suprapubic aspiration
- Focal genital lesions
- Renal vein thrombosis
- Glomerulonephritis (infection or immunologically mediated)
- Nephroblastoma or other tumours
- Polycystic and dysplastic kidneys
- Renal stones, nephrocalcinosis
- Drugs (indomethacin, kanamycin, methicillin).

✚ *Nephrocalcinosis*

Nephrocalcinosis and renal stones have been reported in preterm babies on long-term frusemide therapy. The diagnosis is normally made by ultrasound scan but occasionally the babies also have clinical findings such as haematuria or obstructive uropathy. Chlorothiazide, with or without spironolactone, may be safer for long-term use in the newborn.

✚ Proteinuria

Transient proteinuria (0.5–1.0 g/l) is not uncommon in the first week of life and may be regarded as physiological.

Causes of proteinuria include:

- Dehydration
- Fever
- Birth asphyxia
- Urinary tract infection
- Large doses of penicillin
- After intravenous urogram
- Nephrotic syndrome, congenital or acquired
- Polycystic kidneys.

➕ *Congenital nephrotic syndrome*

The familial form is uncommon in the UK, although is relatively frequent in Finland. Other important causes are congenital syphilis (responds to penicillin), renal vein thrombosis, cytomegalovirus infection and nail–patella syndrome.

Massive proteinuria and oedema are usual presenting features and ascites may be gross. Some babies present with failure to thrive and vomiting before oedema becomes obvious. Unless the underlying cause is treatable, renal failure ensues and dialysis and/or transplantation are the only effective treatments. Initial therapy with diuretics and albumin infusions plus prevention of serious infection may allow survival until transplantation can be performed.

Congenital malformations of renal tract

An increased incidence of renal abnormality occurs in association with chromosomal abnormalities, intestinal anomalies, congenital heart disease and pulmonary hypoplasia.

After antenatal diagnosis of a severe renal tract abnormality, the mother should be referred to a regional perinatal centre for evaluation and delivery if surgery is contemplated after birth.

➕ *Renal agenesis*

This is relatively common affecting about 1 in 4000 births with a male preponderance. If bilateral, oligohydramnios is usually present and stillbirth or early neonatal death occur often. Prenatal diagnosis is possible by ultrasound.

The affected baby has the characteristic Potter's facies with low-set ears, prominent skinfold below eyes, small flattened or upturned nose, small chin and redundant scalp skin. There may be abnormal bowing of the legs and flattening of the hands and feet (spade like).

A common cause of death is severe pulmonary hypoplasia with pneumothoraces after resuscitation.

✚ *Polycystic kidney disease (PCKD)*

Either autosomal recessive (ARPCKD, infantile type) or autosomal dominant (ADPCKD, adult type). Both kidneys are involved and become enlarged while keeping their normal shape (unlike multicystic kidneys). There is often hypertension.

ARPCKD

This is extremely uncommon (approx. 1 in 40 000). There is a wide range of clinical involvement; babies presenting soon after birth usually have severe disease and die of respiratory or renal failure. Those presenting later with, for example, enlarged kidneys, develop gradually deteriorating renal function and hypertension. Polycystic changes may also be present in liver leading to cirrhosis. The cysts are too small to be seen on ultrasound but the kidneys are enlarged and echo-bright. Intravenous urography is generally not necessary, but typically shows a delayed, persistent mottled nephrogram.

Early death is common unless renal dialysis and transplantation are instituted. Prolonged respiratory support may be necessary. Babies who survive to 1 year can do surprisingly well.

ADPCKD

This condition is much commoner than the recessive form (approx. 1 in 1000) and is usually an adult problem. The gene responsible is localized on chromosome 16.

ADPCKD may very rarely cause symptomatic disease in the newborn. There is often a positive family history. Ultrasound scan shows large and small cysts throughout both kidneys. There is usually progressive renal impairment throughout infancy.

It may be difficult to differentiate one form of PCKD from the other in the neonatal period. Imaging studies may be similar in both types of disease. It is important to perform renal ultrasound scans in both parents; if cysts are seen in their kidneys or liver, the baby has ADPCKD. However, cysts may not yet be visible if the parents are young. Where there is no family history, the presence of hepatic fibrosis and biliary dysgenesis on neonatal liver biopsy suggests a diagnosis of ARPCKD, but this is rarely justified. In either case the clinical picture and management is the same.

✚ Multicystic kidney

Also called dysplastic or hypoplastic kidney. Associated anomalies are common: absent ureter, obstructive uropathy, cardiovascular and gastrointestinal anomalies. Progressive pyelonephritis can occur. The affected kidney is non-functioning. There is some debate as to whether the abnormal kidney should be removed. The infant should be followed up to assess the function of the contralateral kidney and to monitor for hypertension.

✚ Posterior urethral valve

This occurs only in male infants. There is hypertrophy and trabeculation of the bladder with bilateral ureteric reflux and hydronephrosis. There may be recurrent infections and progressive renal damage will occur unless the obstruction is relieved. Urine is passed by constant dribbling; every male infant should therefore be observed passing urine with a normal stream before discharge from hospital.

The diagnosis is made by micturating cysturography. Treatment involves endoscopic diathermy of the valve.

✚ Epispadias and bladder exstrophy

Epispadias may occur in both sexes. In boys, the penile urethra is open and dorsally placed on the shaft of the penis. In girls, the defect may be less obvious on cursory inspection, but the urethral orifice is wider and there is a bifid clitoris. In most cases there is urinary incontinence. In exstrophy of the bladder there is epispadias and the bladder mucosa opens onto the anterior abdominal wall. There is wide separation of the pubic symphysis and an anteriorly placed anus. Cloacal exstrophy represents the extreme end of this spectrum of abnormalities. There is exstrophy of the ileocaecal region of the bowel separating the two halves of the exstrophic bladder. There may be other urinary and sacral abnormalities.

> **!** Babies with bladder or cloacal exstrophies should be referred urgently to a paediatric urological surgeon for assessment.

✚ *Hypospadias*

In this condition the urethral orifice is ventrally placed on the penis in a position ranging from the glans to the perineum. In about three-quarters of cases, the opening is situated on the glans or corona. More severe cases may be associated with chordee and bilateral undescended testes. In these a search must be made for the gonads and the genetic status determined. There is an association between hypospadias and intranterine growth retardation.

The baby should not be circumcised as the foreskin is used in reconstructive surgery, which is usually performed at around 2 years.

✚ *Undescended testes*

The testes are descended in 97% of boys at term. Those that descend after birth tend to do so in the first few months of life. Retractile testes need no attention.

Most surgeons would consider orchidopexy if the testis has not descended by the first year of life; the best time to do this is still under debate. Bilateral undescended testes are associated with genetic and other malformations.

Nursing points

Baby

- Take care to obtain uncontaminated urine specimens.
- Monitor fluid balance accurately, weighing nappies if necessary.
- A small cotton wool ball in the nappy will help identify whether urine has been passed when babies have frequent or loose stools.

- Adhesive from urine collection bags damages the skin. A 'clean-catch' urine may obviate the need for a urine bag.

Family

- Parents should be involved in the care whenever possible. They may be taught how to obtain a clean urine specimen.

Equipment

- Ensure aseptic technique for catheter insertion and bag changes during peritoneal dialysis. Ensure dialysate is warmed to body temperature and use continuous cardiorespiratory, blood pressure and temperature monitoring.
- Tips of all catheters must be sent for culture on removal.

Staff

- Staff must pay strict attention to hand washing and teach the parents by example.

References and further reading

Coulthard MG, Vernon B (1995). Managing acute renal failure in very low birthweight infants. *Arch Dis Child* **73**: F187.

Engle WD (1986). Evaluation of renal function and acute renal failure in the neonate. *Pediatr Clin North Am* **33**: 129.

Holmberg C, Antikainen M, Ronnholm K, Ala-Houhala M, Jalanko H (1995). Management of congenital nephrotic syndrome of the Finnish type. *Pediatr Nephrol* **9**: 87.

Jacinto JS, Modanlou HD, Crade M, Strauss AA, Bose SK (1988). Renal calcification incidence in very low weight infants. *Pediatrics* **81**: 31.

Malone TA (1991). Glucose and insulin versus cation-exchange resin for the treatment of hyperkalemia in very low birth weight infants. *J Pediatr* **118**: 121.

Steele BT, De Maria J (1992). A new perspective on the natural history of vesicoureteric reflux. *Pediatrics* **90**: 30.

Thomas DFM, Gordon AC (1989). Management of prenatally diagnosed uropathies. *Arch Dis Child* **64**: 58.

Wilkins B (1992). Renal function in sick very low birthweight infants (4 consecutive papers). *Arch Dis Child* **67**: 1140.

20 Metabolic and Endocrine Problems

Metabolic disorders

Inborn errors of metabolism are rare disorders but should be suspected in any newborn with an unexplained illness. Most babies are born at term with no abnormal features, but symptoms then develop within hours or days of starting milk feeds.

The presenting features may include:

≺ Abnormal neurological signs (seizures, coma)
≺ Acidosis
≺ Jaundice
≺ Vomiting
≺ Hypoglycaemia
≺ Odd odour (sweet, musty, sweaty)
≺ Features mimicking sepsis
≺ Cataracts.

A small proportion of babies may have dysmorphic features associated with a metabolic disorder.

Approach to management of the baby with a suspected metabolic disorder

A careful history should be taken, noting any consanguinity or previously affected pregnancies. The mode of presentation may give some clues towards the diagnosis (Table 20.1). In particular, the relationship between the onset of symptoms and feeding regimen should be noted.

> ! The onset of symptoms and signs in close association with establishment of milk feeding may indicate an inherited metabolic disorder.

Table 20.1. **Presentation of metabolic disorders**

Acidosis	Organic acidaemias, maple syrup urine disease, congenital lactic acidosis, glycogen storage disease type 1, renal tubular acidosis
Hypoglycaemia	Maple syrup urine disease, glycogen storage disease type 1, galactosaemia, methylmalonic acidaemia
'Sepsis'	Galactosaemia, organic acidaemias, tyrosinaemia type 1
Coma	Non-ketotic hyperglycinaemia, maple syrup urine disease, organic acidaemias, urea cycle defects
Vomiting	Congenital adrenal hyperplasia, urea cycle defects, galactosaemia, phenylketonuria
Odd odour	Isovaleric acidaemia (sweaty feet), maple syrup urine disease (sweet), phenylketonuria (mousey), tyrosinaemia type 1 (cabbage-like), glutaric acidaemia type 2
Seizures	Non-ketotic hyperglycinaemia, maple syrup urine disease
Jaundice	Galactosaemia, tyrosinaemia type 1, α_1-antitrypsin deficiency, hypothyroidism

The presence of associated stress factors, e.g. surgery or infection, may be important. Preliminary biochemical tests may aid in diagnosis.

Initial biochemical tests

Most sick neonates will have a battery of tests done as a 'routine':

Urine

A urine sample should be taken at the onset of signs, and should be tested for:

➤ Smell
➤ Reducing substances

➤ Glucose

➤ Ketones (abnormal if strongly positive, or negative despite fasting)

➤ pH of fresh urine (a pH <5.5 suggests an organic acidaemia).

Blood

➤ Electrolytes and urea/creatinine

➤ Blood gas analysis (pH, $PaCO_2$, HCO_3^-, base deficit)

➤ Calculated anion gap: $([Na^+] + [K^+]) - ([Cl^-] + [HCO_3^-])$. A normal result is suggestive of renal tubular acidosis or bicarbonate loss from the gut. An anion gap >20 mmol/l suggests an organic acidaemia

➤ Plasma glucose

➤ Liver function tests (bilirubin, alkaline phosphatase, transaminases)

➤ Full blood count and film

➤ Plasma lactate if there is acidosis, unexplained hypoglycaemia or neurological dysfunction.

Specific metabolic investigations

If a metabolic disorder is strongly suspected on clinical grounds or as a result of basic tests then the following should also be sent:

➤ Urine for sugar chromatography, amino acids and organic acids

➤ Blood for serum ammonia, lactate/pyruvate and amino acids

➤ Red cell galactose-1-phosphate uridyl transferase should be assayed if galactosaemia is suspected.

It is important to liaise closely with the relevant specialist laboratory and to take advice from a paediatrician with experience of metabolic disorders. However, many of these babies present 'out of hours', and in life-threatening situations.

 Baseline samples for the investigation of a suspected metabolic disorder must be taken before initiating treatment.

It is important to obtain baseline samples before instituting treatment. As a minimum these should include:

Urine

Any, but preferably 5 ml in a plain, *preservative-free* bottle. This should be deep frozen (–20°) until analysis.

Blood:

➤ 5 ml in a lithium heparin bottle: the plasma should be separated as soon as possible and frozen at –20°; the packed red cells should not be frozen but stored at +4° until analysis.

➤ 0.5–1.0 ml in a fluoride oxalate bottle for plasma glucose.

➤ If DNA analysis is needed, an additional 5 ml of whole blood should be drawn into a plastic EDTA bottle and stored at –20°.

If death seems inevitable, these samples should preferably be taken pre-mortem, including skin biopsy for fibroblast culture and enzyme assays. Any biopsies taken after death should be done as soon as possible and in a sterile manner.

Acute management of suspected metabolic disorder

Once samples have been taken, treatment should be started:

➤ Correct dehydration and electrolyte imbalance

➤ Correct acid–base disturbance

➤ Ensure adequate gas exchange

➤ Replace milk feeds with dextrose, usually by infusion

➤ Avoid protein

➤ Treat severe hyperammonaemia with sodium benzoate or sodium phenylbutyrate (see below).

➤ In the event of continued deterioration, give high-dose vitamin cocktail (see below), which may act as coenzymes. These are often ineffective as very few acute disorders will be vitamin responsive.

➤ Exchange transfusion, peritoneal dialysis or haemodialysis may be needed, but are often only of transient benefit.

Many acute metabolic disorders have no effective forms of treatment.

Disorders of carbohydrate metabolism

✚ *Galactosaemia*

This is an autosomal recessive condition, affecting about 1 in 30 000 newborns. It is due to a deficiency of galactose-1-phosphate uridyl transferase which results in accumulation of galactose and galactose-1-phosphate. The latter metabolite damages the lens of the eye, liver, brain and ovary. Antenatal detection and neonatal screening is possible, although the latter is not carried out routinely in the UK.

The affected baby presents acutely with:

≺ Severe or prolonged jaundice
≺ Vomiting and weight loss
≺ Lethargy
≺ Hepatosplenomegaly
≺ Features of sepsis (often due to coliforms)
≺ Cataracts.

If the baby is being fed milk, urine testing will show reducing sugars (Clinitest™ tablet positive) but no glucose (Clinistix™ reagent strip negative). However, urine testing is not a reliable means of excluding the diagnosis if the baby is vomiting, has a reduced milk intake or is on a non-lactose formula.

Diagnosis should be confirmed by sending urine for chromatography, plasma for elevated galactose-1-phosphate and red cells for galactose-1-phosphate uridyl transferase activity.

> **!** When galactosaemia is suspected, blood tests must be taken before a blood transfusion is given

Treat with intravenous fluids to stabilize and then feed a lactose-free milk, e.g. Galactomin™. The affected individual must remain on a lactose-free diet throughout life.

Parents will have red cell enzyme levels in the heterozygote range between normal controls and the affected infant. Heterozygote mothers should have a lactose-free diet in subsequent pregnancies. With a known family history, subsequent babies should have a lactose-free diet from birth which will prevent illness but not affect red cell enzyme assay.

✚ *Glycogen storage disease type 1*

Due to a deficiency of glucose-6-phosphatase. Presentation is usually within a few days of birth with episodes of hypoglycaemia, lactic acidosis, hepatomegaly and elevated liver enzymes.

Diagnosis requires measurement of enzyme activity in liver. Histology of liver biopsy shows excess glycogen and fatty changes.

Treatment, aimed at preventing hypoglycaemia, is by frequent feeds of a carbohydrate-rich diet such as corn starch. Long-term follow-up is required.

Disorders of amino acid metabolism

✚ *Phenylketonuria (PKU)*

This autosomal recessive disorder occurs in about 1 in 10 000 – 15 000 newborns and is due to a deficiency of the enzyme phenylalanine hydroxylase. The carrier frequency in the UK is 1 in 50. The presentation in older infants of delayed development, seizures, severe eczema and musty odour is no longer seen since the introduction of mass population screening.

Blood phenylalanine is measured once milk feeds are established, usually on the 7th day, and high levels confirmed by quantitative plasma amino acid analysis. Phenylalanine levels are usually elevated in excess of 1000 μmol/l, but other amino acid levels and liver function tests are normal. Some unaffected babies can develop modestly elevated phenylalanine levels as a result of liver dysfunction or parenteral nutrition. Plasma tyrosine levels are often raised.

Treatment of PKU is dietary, restricting phenylalanine intake to that necessary for normal growth (in the form of 50 mg 'exchanges'), and supplementing with a mixture of free L-amino acids or a protein hydrolysate devoid of phenylalanine.

Regular monitoring of plasma phenylalanine is necessary, maintaining levels between 120 and 360 μmol/l throughout early childhood. Close follow-up is best provided by a specialist team.

Affected girls who reach child-bearing age should ensure strict dietary control, both before conception and throughout pregnancy, as uncontrolled disease results in a high incidence of fetal damage (mental retardation, microcephaly and congenital heart disease).

All infants with hyperphenylalaninaemia should be screened for deficiency of tetrahydrobiopterin, the coenzyme of phenylalanine hydroxylase. These biopterin variants are rare, but also result in deficiencies of dopamine and serotonin, and cannot be treated effectively by dietary means. Rapid neurological deterioration occurs unless neurotransmitter deficiency is corrected.

➕ *Tyrosinaemia*

This is relatively common in preterm infants, particularly those receiving a high protein intake. It is usually asymptomatic, identified only from routine neonatal screening programmes. Transient tyrosinaemia was previously thought to be detrimental but this has not been confirmed in follow-up studies. It responds to vitamin C 50 mg daily for 1 week.

Acute tyrosinaemia type I is much less common and presents as an acute illness with hypoglycaemia, fulminant liver dysfunction and renal tubular defects. The defect is a deficiency of the enzyme fumarylacetoacetase; toxic metabolites of tyrosine form, causing liver and kidney damage.

Diagnosis is made by finding raised urinary succinylacetone, with increased plasma levels of tyrosine, and often methionine and phenylalanine. Plasma alkaline phosphatase is often very high (>2000 U/l). Definitive diagnosis is by enzyme assay of cultured skin fibroblasts.

Treatment is with a low tyrosine, low phenylalanine diet, but many individuals go on to require liver transplantation because of the development of cirrhosis or primary hepatoma. More recently, results of treatment with the compound NTBC, an inhibitor of one of the steps in the catabolism of tyrosine, have been encouraging. This should be started early in life, usually in a dose of 1 mg/kg/day in 1–2 divided doses, but this may need to be increased, and should be combined with dietary therapy.

✚ *Maple syrup urine disease (MSUD)*

Due to defective carboxylation of the oxoacids derived from the branched-chain amino acids valine, leucine and isoleucine. It characteristically presents with feeding difficulties, lethargy, failure to thrive and progressive neurological dysfunction. Urine and sweat have a typical sweet odour. The condition results in early death if untreated.

Biochemical abnormalities include hypoglycaemia and metabolic acidosis. Diagnosis is confirmed by demonstrating markedly increased levels of valine, leucine and isoleucine in plasma and an increase in the corresponding oxoacids in urine.

Treatment consists of a diet low in the branched chain amino acids. Blood levels must be closely monitored and there is a tendency for vomiting episodes precipitated by infections. Long term outlook is variable and development may be impaired.

🔹 *Non-ketotic hyperglycinaemia (glycine encephalopathy)*

Caused by a defect in the glycine cleavage system. The typical presentation is with hypotonia, respiratory failure and uncontrollable seizures. Hiccups may be a prominent feature. Initial biochemical tests are usually normal, but there are raised levels of glycine in plasma and CSF and an abnormally high CSF: plasma glycine ratio. (Note: the finding of raised plasma glycine with ketonuria is suggestive of an organic acidaemia). EEG shows a typical burst-suppression pattern ('tracé alternans').

There is no known effective treatment for this condition, which results in death or severe neurological disability.

🔹 *Homocystinuria*

Does not present in its classical form (cystathionine synthase deficiency) in the neonatal period but a variant form, 5,10 methylene tetrahydrofolate reductase deficiency, can affect the newborn with apnoea, seizures and progressive neurological dysfunction.

Homocystine is found in the urine. Diagnosis is confirmed by demonstrating the enzyme defect in cultured skin fibroblasts.

Treatment is with betaine which converts homocystine to methionine. The dose is up to 250 mg/kg/day in two divided doses, depending on plasma and urine amino acid concentrations.

🔹 Urea cycle disorders

A series of six hepatic enzymes are needed to synthesize urea from ammonia, which is released from the deamination of amino acids. Absence of a urea cycle enzyme or suppression of urea cycle function by various organic acidaemias (see below) results in the accumulation of ammonia.

The commonest defect is ornithine transcarbamylase deficiency (OTCD), which is inherited in an X-linked dominant manner. This is usually lethal in boys but girls may present later with milder signs. The other enzyme defects are autosomal recessive and present with varying degrees of severity. All except carbamyl phosphate synthetase deficiency may be diagnosed antenatally.

Presentation of the urea cycle disorders is often within 48 hours of birth with:

≺ Feed refusal and vomiting
≺ Lethargy, irritability and seizures
≺ Tachypnoea and respiratory alkalosis (ammonia is a respiratory stimulant).

Plasma ammonia is high, typically >800 μmol/l in the first 3 days of life, although depends on protein intake. In OTCD, orotic acid is present in the urine.

Significant hyperammonaemia (400–800 μmol/l) can be found in some organic acid disorders, e.g. methylmalonic and propionic acidaemias. These are likely where hyperammonaemia is found in combination with acidosis and ketonuria. Therefore, when plasma ammonia is significantly raised, the following should be measured *urgently*:

➤ Liver enzymes, bilirubin

➤ Prothrombin time

➤ Plasma amino acids

➤ Urine amino acids, organic acids and orotic acid.

Treatment should be prompt to prevent permanent neurological dysfunction:

➤ Withdraw or reduce protein intake, but provide adequate calories from other substrates

➤ Remove excess nitrogen with sodium benzoate and/or sodium phenylbutyrate (see below)

➤ Supplement with arginine (100–150 mg/kg/day in 3–4 divided doses) except in argininaemia

➤ Peritoneal dialysis or preferably haemodialysis may be of benefit

➤ Exchange transfusion usually has only transient effect.

Sodium benzoate and sodium phenylbutyrate act by conjugating with glycine and glutamine, respectively, and are excreted in the urine, thus clearing nitrogen from the body. They reduce plasma ammonia and improve appetite, vomiting and irritability, although may not affect residual neurological problems. The dose of either compound in the acute situation is up to 500 mg/kg/day orally or i.v., aiming to reduce plasma ammonia concentrations to <60 μmol/l, with a normal essential amino acid profile. A metabolic specialist should be consulted. Long-term outcome of many of the urea cycle disorders is poor.

Unaffected but ill preterm babies can have moderately raised plasma ammonia levels in association with sepsis, asphyxia or parenteral nutrition, although levels are usually <200 μmol/l. Occasionally, preterm babies can present within 24–48 hours of birth with severe respiratory distress and grossly elevated levels of ammonia (often >1500 μmol/l), a condition called *transient hyperammonaemia of the newborn*. This should be treated aggressively as outcome is usually good.

➕ Organic acid disorders

Organic acids are low molecular weight metabolites of carbohydrates, amino acids and fats.

There are a large number of disorders of organic acid metabolism, the most important involving defects in the catabolism of the branched chain amino acids valine, leucine and isoleucine (methylmalonic, propionic and isovaleric acidaemias), and of propionyl CoA. All are recessively inherited and rare, occurring in <1 in 100 000 births. There is often a family history of early neonatal death.

Presentation is soon after birth with:

≺ Vomiting
≺ Lethargy and hypotonia
≺ Coma
≺ Peculiar odour.

Severe metabolic acidosis is common, along with:

- Hypoglycaemia
- Ketonuria
- Hyperammonaemia
- Hyperglycinaemia
- Raised plasma lactate
- Neutropenia.

Send fresh random urine collected during acidaemia for organic acid analysis before withdrawal of dietary protein.
Untreated, these conditions progress to coma and death.

Treatment includes:

➤ Stop milk feeds and erect intravenous glucose

➤ Correct acidosis

➤ Correct coagulation disorder

➤ Exchange transfusion or peritoneal dialysis

➤ L-carnitine (a loading dose of 100 mg/kg i.v. over 4–6 hours, followed by 100 mg/kg/day)

➤ Specific vitamin therapy: B_{12} (1 mg i.m.) and biotin (10 mg orally) should be given in case the baby has either the B_{12}-responsive form of methylmalonic acidaemia or multiple carboxylase deficiency, respectively.

Prognosis is variable, and surviving patients often have recurring bouts of ketoacidosis.

Defects in β-oxidation of fatty acids are not common in the newborn but should be suspected if hypoglycaemia and inappropriately low concentrations of plasma and urine ketones are present. The commonest is medium chain acyl CoA dehydrogenase (MCAD) deficiency, which affects fatty acids of carbon chain length C6–C10. Urine organic acids should be measured during episodes of hypoglycaemia or stress as they may be normal at other times. Treatment involves avoiding hypoglycaemia and possibly L-carnitine supplements.

✚ Peroxisomal disorders

Peroxisomes are subcellular organelles with many functions, including the synthesis of very-long-, long- and medium-chain fatty acids, catalase activity and the biosynthesis of plasmalogens. Important neonatal peroxisomal disorders include:

Zellweger's syndrome (dysmorphic features, hepatomegaly, liver dysfunction and severe hypotonia with seizures)
Neonatal adrenoleucodystrophy
Rhizomelic chondrodysplasia punctata

A radiograph of the knee may show epiphyseal calcific stippling. The diagnosis is confirmed by finding low levels of plasma very-long-chain fatty acids. No treatment is available.

✚ Lactic acidosis

Lactic acidosis is most commonly caused by conditions involving hypoxia and ischaemia, e.g. sepsis, dehydration, seizures, or liver dysfunction. If these conditions have been excluded, a significantly elevated plasma lactate (> 3 mmol/l) may be due to a metabolic disorder:

Glycogen storage disease type 1
Organic acid disorders
Pyruvate dehydrogenase deficiency
Disorders of gluconeogenesis

The following tests may aid in diagnosis:

➤ Urine amino acids and organic acids

➤ Fasting plasma glucose

➤ Plasma lactate/pyruvate, 3-hydroxybutyrate and acetoacetate

➤ Plasma amino acids

➤ Liver function tests

➤ Muscle biopsy may be necessary.

Endocrine disorders

 ## *Persistent hypoglycaemia (see also p. 76 and Ch. 12)*

Prolonged or recurrent symptomatic hypoglycaemia leads to permanent neurological damage. The most common endocrine reasons for recurrent hypoglycaemia outside the immediate perinatal period are:

> Hyperinsulinaemia due to nesidioblastosis
> Congenital panhypopituitarism

> **!** In severe or recurrent hypoglycaemia, with no evidence of metabolic acidosis or liver dysfunction, investigations should be performed *during* an episode of hypoglycaemia

The following investigations should be performed:

➤ Plasma glucose

➤ Plasma insulin

➤ Plasma β-hydroxybutyrate

➤ Plasma cortisol

➤ Plasma growth hormone and TSH

Signs of *hyperinsulinaemia* include macrosomia and the need for very high glucose infusion rates (>10–12 mg/kg/min) to maintain normoglycaemia. Serum insulin is elevated and β-hydroxybutyrate is low in the presence of hypoglycaemia. Initial treatment of nesidioblastosis is with diazoxide and chlorothiazide, but if unsuccessful a somatostatin infusion may be a helpful short-term measure before pancreatic MRI and surgical exploration. If an adenoma is not found, a 95% pancreatectomy should be performed.

Congenital panhypopituitarism may be suspected if there is prolonged conjugated hyperbilirubinaemia, small external genitalia in males, midline facial defects or optic atrophy. Serum growth hormone and cortisol are inappropriately low for the degree of hypoglycaemia, and TSH may be very low.

The presence of metabolic acidosis or liver dysfunction in association with hypoglycaemia raises the possibility of an underlying metabolic disorder (see above). In this situation a number of other tests may be helpful:

- ➤ Plasma lactate (glycogen storage disease 1)

- ➤ Plasma 3-hydroxybutyrate (congenital lactic acidosis)

- ➤ Plasma free fatty acids (disorders of gluconeogenesis)

- ➤ Plasma and urine amino acids (tyrosinaemia type 1)

- ➤ Urine organic acids (fatty acid oxidation defects)

- ➤ Red cell galactose-1-phosphate uridyl transferase (galactosaemia).

✚ *Congenital hypothyroidism*

The incidence of primary neonatal hypothyroidism detected by mass population newborn screening is about 1 in 3000. Screening programmes usually measure TSH alone (normal whole blood TSH <10 mU/l), although some centres measure both T_4 and TSH. Screening using only TSH will fail to detect the much rarer cases of pituitary hypothyroidism (incidence approx. 1 in 40 000).

Most cases of hypothyroidism are sporadic, due to ectopic, hypoplastic or absent thyroid glands. About 10% result from enzyme defects in thyroxine synthesis which are autosomal recessive and may cause goitre.

At recall most have minor non-specific symptoms but probably only 5% have clinical signs of hypothermia, lethargy, slow feeding, poor weight gain or prolonged jaundice. Before screening the clinical diagnosis was often delayed until 6 months and the longer the delay in starting replacement treatment, the greater the effect on intelligence. Radiography of the knee may show delayed maturation of upper tibial or lower femoral epiphyses

If T_4 remains low and TSH high on confirmatory serum tests (normal serum free T_4 >12 μmol/l, serum TSH <4.5 mU/l) treatment is begun with thyroxine 25 μg daily in term babies, increasing to 100 μg/m²/day as the baby grows. Transient hypothyroidism can occur so a short period off thyroxine after 2 years will determine the need for life-long treatment.

Premature babies who are sick or have had surgery often have transiently raised TSH levels, with low/low normal T_4 levels. Whether they benefit from thyroxine replacement or not is controversial and under study.

Neonatal goitre may be due to maternal ingestion of iodides or antithyroid drugs (see p. 33) or to one of the inherited forms of hypothyroidism.

✚ *Neonatal thyrotoxicosis (see also p. 27).*

This is a serious disorder with a significant mortality. It may occur in <5 % of babies of mothers with a history of past or present Graves' disease. The infant may present after a few days with signs of acute thyrotoxicosis:

◄ Tachycardia
◄ Heart failure
◄ Thirst
◄ Irritability
◄ Weight loss
◄ Goitre
◄ Collapse.

Serum thyroxine concentrations will be increased. Urgent treatment is required to prevent the development of heart failure or collapse:

➤ Control heart rate with propranolol
➤ Lower serum thyroxine using 10% potassium iodide drops (8 mg/kg/day in three divided doses)
➤ Antithyroid drugs such as carbimazole may be necessary.

Treatment is often needed for at least 8 weeks but in one-third of babies the disorder lasts for 2–6 months or longer. If the acute situation can be controlled, the long-term prognosis is good.

➕ *Ambiguous genitalia (intersex)*

Urgent investigation is needed when the gender of an infant is in doubt. Do not guess the gender but reassure the parents that this will be determined as quickly as possible. It may be best to delay the announcement and registration of the birth until investigations are complete. The most important aspect of clinical examination is to determine if a gonad is palpable. Ultrasound examination helps to identify internal genitalia.

The most important laboratory investigation is serum 17α-hydroxyprogesterone to diagnose virilizing congenital adrenal hyperplasia (see below). Chromosome analysis helps to determine aetiology but should not necessarily dictate the sex of rearing which will depend on the appearance of the external genitalia and the likely effect of puberty.

Male pseudohermaphrodites

Have a normal male karyotype and well differentiated testes but abnormal male genital development.

There are two main causes:

- Impaired fetal testosterone biosynthesis caused by an enzyme deficiency or hypoplasia of Leydig cells leading to androgen deficiency.
- Impaired androgen activity in peripheral tissues (androgen insensitivity syndrome) which may vary from complete (totally female appearance) to incomplete forms (variable degrees of masculinization).

Incomplete virilization may also occur in some dysmorphic syndromes and urogenital anomalies.

Female pseudohermaphrodites

Have a normal female karyotype with normally developed ovaries and Müllerian structures but a masculine appearance of external genitalia. Congenital adrenal hyperplasia due to 21-hydroxylase deficiency is the commonest and most important cause (see below). Other causes include exposure to excess progesterone or androgen during pregnancy.

Abnormal gonadal differentiation

Usually presents with absence of pubertal development rather than genital anomalies at birth (e.g. Turner's syndrome). Exceptions are mixed gonadal dysgenesis and true hermaphroditism. The former is usually caused by 46,XY/45,XO mosaicism. Some testicular tissue is present causing variable virilization. There is an increased risk of malignancy in the testis or streak gonad. True hermaphrodites have both testicular tissue with seminiferous tubules and ovarian tissue with primary follicles. The karyotype is variable but 46,XX is the commonest.

✚ *Congenital adrenal hyperplasia*

The incidence of this autosomal recessive group of disorders is about 1 in 10 000 births but varies greatly in different populations. Clinical presentation depends on the site of enzyme deficiency in the synthesis of cortisol, androgens and aldosterone. >90% of cases are due to 21-hydroxylase deficiency.

Presentation in the neonate is variable but the most usual are virilization of external genitalia in females and acute salt-losing crisis in males at 2–3 weeks of age. In salt-losing crises, there is marked hyponatraemia, normal or raised plasma potassium and raised urinary sodium. The diagnosis may be confirmed by detecting elevated serum 17 α-hydroxyprogesterone 48 hours after birth (normal <18 nmol/l).

An acute adrenal crisis is managed with intravenous normal saline in 5–10% glucose solution to avoid hypoglycaemia and replacement of hydrocortisone (25 mg i.v.). When oral fluids can be taken, hydrocortisone is given in a dose of 20 mg/m^2/day divided into three doses (usually 2.5 mg t.i.d.), and 9 α-fludrocortisone 0.1–0.2 mg once daily as the mineralocorticoid replacement. Continued salt loss over the first few months may require 2–3 g of salt supplements daily.

Replacement therapy is needed for life and parents should be warned that a 2–3-fold increased dose of hydrocortisone will be needed for infections or other stresses. Long-term follow-up should be by a paediatric endocrinologist. Clitoroplasty may be needed for virilized girls in later infancy.

About 5% of cases of congenital adrenal hyperplasia are due to deficiency of 11 β-hydroxylase, which may also cause virilization of female infants. Salt-losing crises do not occur so males are not recognized in infancy. Diagnosis is confirmed by finding increased serum 11-deoxycortisol levels.

Nursing points

Baby

- Ensure a screening test for PKU is performed approximately 5 days after milk feeds are established.
- TSH screening should take place when the baby is approximately 5 days old, irrespective of feeding. Ensure all tests and results are recorded in the notes.

Family

- Check the maternal notes for any family history of metabolic or endocrine problems.
- Parents of babies with an inherited condition may benefit from genetic counselling.
- A great deal of support is needed for parents of a baby with an intersex problem. Parents are often concerned about the future sexuality and fertility of their baby and careful explanation of the condition is required.

Equipment

- Colour coded identity cards are used in many hospitals – blue for boys, pink for girls. This needs careful management for babies with an intersex problem.

Staff

- It is important not to assume the sex of a baby with any features of ambiguous genitalia. Great tact is required from staff when talking to the parents and referring to the baby.

References and further reading

Aynsley-Green A (1992). Hypoglycaemia. In: *Recent Advances in Paediatrics* Vol. 10. (ed, David TJ). London: Churchill Livingstone, p. 36.

Berkovitz GD (1992). Abnormalities of gonadal determination and differentiation. *Semin Perinatol* **5**: 289.

Brook CGD. (1995) *Clinical Paediatric Endocrinology*, 3rd edn. Oxford: Blackwell.

Collins J, Clayton PT (1996). NTBC for the treatment of tyrosinaemia type 1. *Br Paed Assoc Drug Bull*, **March**.

Donaldson MDC, Grant DB. Congenital hypothyroidism (1997). In: *Recent Advances in Paediatrics*, vol. 15. (ed, David TJ), London: Churchill Livingstone.

Patel J, Leonard JV (1995). Sodium phenylbutyrate for the treatment of urea cycle disorders. *Br Paed Assoc Drug Bull*, **June**.

Scriver CR, Baudet AL, Sly WS, Valle D (eds) (1994). *The Metabolic Basis of Inherited Disease*, 7th edn. New York: McGraw-Hill.

Wanders RJA, Schutgens RBH, Barth PG (1995). Peroxisomal disorders: a review. *J Neuropathol Exp Neurol* **54**: 726.

Wraith JE (1989). Diagnosis and management of inborn errors of metabolism. *Arch Dis Child*, **63**: 1410.

21 Haematological Problems

Normal haematological values in the newborn differ from adult standards and vary with gestational and postnatal age (Appendix V).

✚ Anaemia

Placental transfusion at birth accounts for about 25% of neonatal blood volume in term infants. In preterm infants placental transfusion can contribute 50% of blood volume. The term infant has a haemoglobin of 14–20 g/dl. This falls soon after birth to an average of 10 g/dl by 3–6 weeks (*physiological anaemia*).

The fall is more rapid and reaches lower levels in the preterm baby (*anaemia of prematurity*).

A number of factors are implicated:

- Deficient erythropoiesis: erythropoietin secretion is suppressed for the first 7–8 weeks of life.
- Reduced red blood cell survival
- Vitamin E deficiency: this is now rare as formula milks are supplemented with vitamin E and are low in polyunsaturated fatty acids (PUFA)
- Frequent diagnostic blood sampling.

Early-onset anaemia occurs in the first week postnatally and is defined as Hb <13g/dl in a term baby, whereas later onset anaemia occurs after the first week and is defined as Hb <10g/dl. Early and late anaemia may occur as a result of blood loss, haemolysis or underproduction of red blood cells.

Blood loss

This can occur before, during or after birth.

Causes include:

- Fetal haemorrhage: vasa praevia, placenta praevia, abruption, amniocentesis, placental incision at caesarean section
- Fetomaternal transfusion
- Twin-to-twin transfusion
- Reduced placentofetal transfusion at birth: early cord clamping, baby held above the level of the placenta
- Neonatal haemorrhage: trauma, haemorrhagic disease of the newborn.

Haemolysis

This is associated with a shortened RBC lifespan (normal 60–80 days at term), unconjugated hyperbilirubinaemia and reticulocytosis.

Causes include:

- Isoimmune: Rhesus, ABO or 'minor' blood group incompatibilities
- Autoimmune: maternal SLE
- Drug-induced (particularly in association with G6PD deficiency)
- Infections: TORCH, bacterial sepsis, DIC
- Congenital RBC defects: α-thalassaemia, G6PD deficiency, hereditary spherocytosis
- Vitamin E deficiency, e.g. due to malabsorption

Under-production

Hypoplastic anaemia is very uncommon in the neonate.

Causes include:

- Congenital hypoplastic anaemia (Diamond–Blackfan)
- Congenital leukaemia
- Congenital infection, e.g. rubella.

Clinical features

Acute anaemia usually results from haemorrhage. There is often pallor, tachypnoea, tachycardia and hypotension. The haematocrit may be normal initially, but falls within 6 hours due to haemodilution.

Chronic anaemia may produce a pale but relatively undistressed baby. There may be hepatosplenomegaly and sometimes congestive cardiac failure.

Investigations

The cause of the anaemia may be immediately obvious, e.g. placental abruption.

Relevant investigations include:

➤ Visual inspection of the placenta

➤ Determination of haemoglobin and haematocrit

➤ Blood film (for abnormally-shaped cells), reticulocyte count

➤ Direct Coombs' test (in blood group incompatibility)

➤ Kleihauer test on maternal blood to exclude fetomaternal transfusion.

Other selected studies may be indicated:

➤ Specific IgM (rubella, CMV, toxoplasma, parvovirus) and urine for CMV if congenital infection is suspected

➤ Coagulation studies

➤ Red cell enzymes, Hb electrophoresis (for haemoglobinopathies)

➤ Imaging techniques to identify site of internal bleeding.

Treatment

Emergency treatment of acute anaemia

Look for an underlying cause and correct it. If the baby is shocked, transfuse with 15–20 ml/kg of group O, Rhesus-negative blood over 10–15 min. This may be given via an umbilical venous catheter in the labour ward. If blood is not immediately available, 5% albumin or human plasma protein fraction are alternatives.

 Group O, Rhesus-negative blood should always be immediately available in the labour ward.

Acute problems due to chronic severe anaemia secondary to blood-group incompatibility should be corrected by early exchange transfusion (see p. 125).

Simple transfusion

In the non-urgent situation, anaemia is corrected with transfusion of cross-matched packed red cells. The volume required is calculated from the formula:

$$\text{Volume of donor blood (ml)} = \frac{(\text{desired Hct} - \text{patient Hct})}{\text{donor blood Hct}} \times \text{weight (kg)} \times 90$$

where Hct = haematocrit.

In practice, transfusion of 10 ml/kg packed cells will raise the haematocrit by 10%.

Suggested indications for transfusion are:

- Replacement for sampling losses: cumulative loss of >10% of the blood volume in 72 hours
- Hb <13 g/dl (Hct <0.40) in acutely ill babies
- Hb <8–10 g/dl (Hct <0.25–0.30) and clinical signs suggestive of anaemia (tachypnoea, tachycardia, recurrent apnoea, requirement for low-flow oxygen, poor feeding, failure to gain weight).

Transfusion may be delayed if the reticulocyte count is >5% and the infant's condition permits.

Potential hazards of blood transfusion include fluid overload, blood-borne infection (CMV, HBV, HCV, HIV), hyperkalaemia and, rarely, graft-versus-host disease. These can be minimized by using fresh (<4 days old) blood that has been screened for infection. No more than 10 ml/kg per transfusion should normally be given, infused over 2–3 hours.

Erythropoietin

Recombinant human erythropoietin (rHuEPO) in a dose of 200 U/kg three times per week increases haemoglobin levels and reduces the need for blood transfusion after the first 2 weeks in VLBW babies. Iron stores become depleted so that at least 2 mg/kg/day of ferrous sulphate should be given concurrently. Some centres give vitamin E with iron.

The role of rHuEPO to prevent anaemia of prematurity has yet to be clarified. It may have a place in the treatment of babies of Jehovah's Witnesses or in instances of very rare blood groups where donor blood is not available. However, in these cases placental transfusion (late cord clamping) and minimal blood sampling after birth are probably more important.

Nutritional supplements

Iron

Iron supplements are rarely needed for term babies. Anaemia of prematurity is not affected by iron supplementation, however, preterm babies' iron stores are low after 2–3 months of life and most centres start supplemental iron at 4–6 weeks in a dose of 1–2 mg/kg/day. This prevents anaemia occurring in the latter half of the first year of life.

Folic acid

Folic acid is given by some centres in a dose of 1–2 mg/week, particularly in cases of haemolytic anaemia, although there is no evidence that it is essential. Breast and formula milks both supply adequate amounts of folate for the growing infant, although babies on special diets for PKU or maple syrup urine disease are at risk of deficiency.

Vitamin E

Vitamin E supplements are seldom necessary as modern formula feeds have a satisfactory vitamin E: PUFA content. Babies who have prolonged fat malabsorption due to, e.g.

cystic fibrosis or biliary atresia, may develop vitamin E deficiency.

➕ Polycythaemia

This is defined as a central venous Hct >65% (Hb >22 g/dl). Blood viscosity increases linearly with increasing Hct until the latter reaches 65%, and thereafter viscosity increases exponentially. Hyperviscosity is associated with decreased flow in both the microcirculation and in large veins. It may cause cerebral, renal or inferior vena caval thrombosis, and oxygen transport is reduced.

The condition is potentially dangerous but often predictable. Causes include:

- Delayed cord clamping
- Intrauterine growth failure, maternal smoking, high altitude
- Diabetic mother
- Twin-to-twin transfusion
- Maternofetal transfusion
- Other: Down's syndrome, neonatal thyrotoxicosis, Beckwith's syndrome, congenital adrenal hyperplasia.

Clinical features

These are non-specific and include:

◄ Jaundice
◄ Cerebral irritation, seizures
◄ Apathy, apnoea
◄ Vomiting, abdominal distension
◄ Congestive cardiac failure, cyanosis, persistent pulmonary hypertension
◄ Hypoglycaemia, hypocalcaemia.

Management

Check a free-flowing venous haematocrit (Hct) in all ill infants, infants of diabetic mothers, SGA babies and twins. If Hct is

>70%, a partial exchange transfusion should probably be performed even in the absence of symptoms. Use 5% albumin or plasma, calculating the required volume using the formula:

$$\text{Volume of albumin (ml)} = \frac{(\text{observed Hct} - \text{desired Hct})}{\text{observed Hct}} \times \text{weight (kg)} \times 90$$

Aim to lower the Hct to about 55%; this is usually achieved by exchanging blood with about 20 ml/kg of albumin.

A partial exchange transfusion should be performed if the venous Hct >65% and the baby is symptomatic.

Bleeding and clotting problems

The newborn, especially preterm babies, have a less efficient clotting system than children and adults. Bleeding or bruising may be due to a low platelet count, a deficiency of clotting factors or abnormal capillaries.

Approach to the management of the bleeding newborn

History

Specific enquiry should be made for a family history of bleeding disorder; maternal drugs (aspirin, warfarin) and problems in pregnancy (ITP, viral illness).

Examination

Suspect DIC, infection, severe haemorrhagic disease (HDN) or a specific clotting factor deficiency if the baby is ill. Petechiae suggest thrombocytopenia. Ecchymoses suggest clotting factor problems (DIC, HDN, liver disease).

Investigations
➤ Platelet count
➤ Prothrombin, partial thromboplastin and thrombin clotting times

➤ Fibrinogen, fibrin degradation products

➤ Bleeding time.

In cases of gastrointestinal bleeding, perform Apt's test (see p. 304).

✚ Haemorrhagic disease of the newborn (HDN)

The defect is a deficiency of prothrombin and the other vitamin K-dependent clotting factors. Vitamin K is needed for the hepatic synthesis of factors II, VII, IX and X. Cow's milk contains four times as much vitamin K as breast milk, so that HDN is usually only seen in exclusively breast-fed infants.

Vitamin K deficiency may also result from chronic diarrhoea, prolonged broad-spectrum antibiotic therapy, prematurity (especially those on parenteral nutrition), and maternal drug therapy (phenytoin, phenobarbitone, salicylates, warfarin).

 HDN is largely preventable by administration of vitamin K at birth.

In the UK babies currently receive vitamin K 0.5 mg orally at birth, with further supplements to breast-fed babies at 7–10 days and 4–6 weeks of life. High-risk babies (preterm, SGA and breast-fed) should be offered intramuscular vitamin K. Local practices may differ.

HDN presents with bleeding (skin, umbilical cord, mucous membranes, viscera or brain) with the onset usually from 3 to 7 days. Prothrombin and clotting times are prolonged. Management involves giving vitamin K 1 mg i.v. Fresh frozen plasma and blood may occasionally be necessary.

✚ Disseminated intravascular coagulation (DIC)

Any severely ill baby may develop DIC; it is probably more common in the neonatal period than previously recognized.

Thrombotic formation is stimulated by bacterial endotoxin or thromboplastin released from damaged tissues. This causes intravascular coagulation with consumption of platelets, factors II, V, VIII, XIII and fibrinogen. The fibrinolytic system is also stimulated, causing an increase in fibrin degradation products (FDPs) which may exacerbate bleeding.

Causes of DIC include:

- Septicaemia, shock, asphyxia, acidosis, hypoxia
- Placental abruption
- Intrauterine death of twin
- Necrotizing enterocolitis.

Investigations show:

➤ Prothrombin time, partial thromboplastin time and thrombin time all prolonged

➤ Platelet count and fibrinogen levels reduced

➤ Fibrin degradation products elevated

➤ Fragmented RBCs on blood film.

Management:

➤ Find and eliminate the cause

➤ Transfuse fresh blood and fresh frozen plasma

➤ Consider exchange transfusion, particularly in cases of sepsis.

Inherited bleeding disorders

These are not common and include:

Haemophilia: factor VIII deficiency, males

Christmas disease: factor IX deficiency, males

Von Willebrand's disease: factor VIII deficiency and reduced platelet function, both sexes

Dysfibrinogenaemia: factor I abnormal, both sexes

Other specific clotting-factor deficiences are very uncommon.

✚ Thrombocytopenia

This is defined as a platelet count $<150\ 000$ /mm^3 in term infant or $<100\ 000$/mm^3 in preterm infant.

Causes include:

- Alloimmune (fetomaternal platelet incompatibility analogous to Rhesus disease, maternal platelet count normal)
- Autoimmune (maternal ITP, variable platelet count, may be normal after splenectomy, see p. 28)
- DIC
- Infection (congenital or acquired)
- Necrotizing enterocolitis (NEC)
- Maternal or neonatal drugs (a wide range including antithyroids, cytotoxics, antibiotics and antimalarials, anticonvulsants and thiazides)
- After exchange transfusion
- Other (aplastic anaemia, Down's syndrome, giant haemangioma, Wiskott–Aldrich syndrome, neonatal malignancy).

If the baby is ill, DIC, sepsis or NEC are the most likely underlying causes.

Management

➤ Correct the underlying cause if possible.

➤ Give platelet transfusion if baby's platelet count is $<20\ 000$ mm^3 and/or bleeding (give 1 unit to a maximum of 20 ml/kg).

➤ Infusion of immunoglobulin (1 g/kg) or treatment with steroids (1–2 mg/kg of prednisolone) may be indicated in thrombocytopenia secondary to maternal ITP.

➤ Use washed maternal platelets if there is alloimmune thrombocytopenia and risk of bleeding. If none available give donor platelets and immunoglobulin.

Nursing points

Baby

- Vitamin K should be given by the appropriate route to all newborn babies to help prevent haemorrhagic disease of the newborn. Breast-fed babies require subsequent doses at approximately 1 week, and at 4–6 weeks of age.
- Observe preterm babies for signs of anaemia:
  - ≺ Pallor
  - ≺ Tachypnoea
  - ≺ Tachycardia
  - ≺ Dyspnoea
  - ≺ Poor feeding
  - ≺ Poor weight gain.
- Avoid early iron supplementation as this increases the risk of haemolysis from vitamin E deficiency and may increase infection risk.
- Observe the baby for signs of excessive bruising which may indicate a coagulation disorder.

Family

- Note any family history of haematological problems or maternal disorders during the pregnancy.
- If an inherited disorder is found, genetic counselling may be beneficial to the family.

Equipment

- Monitor arterial and venous puncture sites carefully for excessive bleeding.
- Take care when using tape and strapping as they may cause skin damage.

Staff

- Ensure gloves are worn at all times when taking specimens of blood.
- All neonatal and midwifery/obstetric staff should be immunized against hepatitis B. Local guidelines should be followed in the event of a needlestick injury.

References and further reading

Bifano EM, Curran TR (1995). Minimizing donor blood exposure in the neonatal intensive care unit: current trends and future prospects. In: Perinatal Hematology (eds, Bifano EM, Ehrenkranz RA). *Clin Perinatol* **22**: 657.

Blanchette VS, Kuhne T, Hume H, Hellmann J (1995). Platelet transfusion therapy in newborn infants. *J Transfus Med Rev* **9**: 215.

Blanchette VS, Rand ML (1997). Platelet disorders in newborn infants: diagnosis and management. *Semin Perinatol* **21**: 53.

Halliday HL, Lappin TRJ, McClure G (1993). Do all preterm infants need iron supplements? *Ir Med J* **76**: 430.

Hume H (1997). Red blood cell transfusions for preterm infants: the role of evidence-based medicine. *Semin Perinatol* **21**: 8.

Johnson JA, Ryan G, al-Musa A, Farkas S, Blanchette VS (1997). Prenatal diagnosis and management of neonatal alloimmune thrombocytopenia. *Semin Perinatol* **21**: 45.

Manroe BL, Brown R, Weinberg AG, Rosenfeld CR (1976). Normal leukocyte (WBC) values in neonates. *Pediatr Res* **10**: 428.

Oski FA, Naiman JL (1989). *Hematologic Problems in the Newborn*, 3rd edn. Philadelphia: WB Saunders.

Shannon K (1995). Recombinant human erythropoietin in neonatal anaemia. In: Perinatal Hematology, (eds, Bifano EM, Ehrenkranz RA). *Clin Perinatol* **22**: 627.

Strauss RG (1997). Practical issues in neonatal transfusion practice. *Am J Clin Pathol* **107 (4 Suppl 1)**: S57.

Walters MC, Abelson HT (1996). Interpretation of the complete blood count. *Pediatr Clin North Am* **43**: 599.

Wardrop CA, Holland BM (1995). The roles and vital importance of placental blood to the newborn infant. *J Perinat Med* **23**: 139.

Warwick R, Modi N (1995). Guidelines for the administration of blood products. *Arch Dis Child* **72**: 379.

Werner EJ (1995). Neonatal polycythaemia and hyperviscosity. In: Perinatal Hematology (eds, Bifano EM, Ehrenkranz RA). *Clin Perinatol* **22**: 693.

22 Parental Attachment

In 1907 Pierre Budin wrote in *The Nursling:*

'Unfortunately a certain number of mothers abandon the babies whose needs they have not had to meet, and in whom they have lost all interest. The life of the little one has been saved, it is true, but at the cost of the mother'.

It is possible that this tragic situation may be avoided by encouraging the natural mother–infant bonding process. Klaus and Kennell (1989) suggest there is a critical or sensitive period in the first minutes or hours during which interaction between mother (and father) and infant should occur for ideal later development of the baby. Parental anxiety about the baby on the first day may cause long-lasting concern about future development.

A combination of present-day knowledge of high-risk obstetrics, neonatology and mother–infant attachment suggests that a home-like birth in hospital might be the ideal situation. Medical intervention may be necessary only in high-risk pregnancies and in the low-risk pregnancy in labour when an unexpected complication arises. The delivery of a mother with a low-risk pregnancy and labour in a special 'bedroom' in a maternity hospital has great potential benefits. After birth father, mother and infant can be together. This can take place once the infant has been examined and the cord clamped.

Touching the baby and eye-to-eye contact appear to be important parts of the early attachment process. If the infant is premature, the mother will often expect her baby to die. She may grieve in anticipation of this so that bonding to her infant will be delayed. It is especially important that the mother of a premature baby sees her infant soon after birth, even if only for a brief moment. When babies are being transported for intensive care, always provide a Polaroid photograph for the mother to use in 'bonding'.

Free visiting of premature babies by their parents is a relatively new phenomenon, but frequent contact with the baby may be beneficial. Gentle touching and fondling may reduce the number of apnoeic attacks, increase weight gain, decrease the daily number of stools and improve some higher CNS functions. Visits by siblings should also be encouraged once the initial high-risk situation has improved. Relatives should always be given a friendly welcome by nursing and medical staff and allowed time for regular discussion of the baby's condition at each visit.

Pessimistic remarks about the chances of a baby's survival are not helpful to a mother unless the baby's condition is hopeless when discussions with senior medical staff should be clear and frank. If the baby survives, the mother's grief in anticipation may be heightened and bonding with her infant delayed. One should always be cautiously optimistic while answering queries honestly.

All counselling should be undertaken by senior staff, and resident doctors should avoid getting embroiled in discussions on prognosis. An immediate appointment with a consultant can be made to deflect awkward questions which often occur at night. Possible disturbances of brain function should not be specifically mentioned to the parents unless they ask or the outcome can be accurately predicted, e.g. in chromosomal trisomies, or severe cystic periventricular leucomalacia. It is important to have good liaison between medical and nursing staff so that information given to parents is consistent.

Parent Support Groups for premature and abnormal babies may be useful; up-to-date lists of names and addresses for national and local support groups should be made available in the neonatal unit.

The pattern of parental visiting and telephone calls is predictive of the ability of the mother to cope with the stresses of premature birth. If she visits fewer than 3 times in 2 weeks, the probability of mothering disorder increases and failure to thrive, child abuse or giving the baby up for adoption increase.

It is especially helpful for the mother to make some tangible contribution to her infant's care, such as providing breast milk. Mothers of babies of 32 weeks and less should be encouraged to express their milk. As babies grow and no longer need intensive care, they should be dressed; a wide variety of clothes specifically designed for preterm babies is now available. The more attractive a tiny preterm baby appears to the mother, the easier it is for her to grow attached.

The costs incurred by parents in visiting an ill neonate should be considered. Parent accommodation near to the neonatal intensive care unit should be provided by the hospital. Appropriate financial help should be offered to parents on low incomes to facilitate visiting and increase family contact.

Grief

Parents who have an infant with a congenital malformation or one who subsequently dies will pass through five phases in their grief:

1. *Shock*. Often overwhelming, characterized by crying, feelings of helplessness and irrational behaviour. There may also be physical symptoms such as choking, shortness of breath, sighing, lethargy and an 'empty' feeling.
2. *Disbelief*. This form of denial serves to cushion the blow but should be of short duration.
3. *Sadness, anger and anxiety*. The anger may be directed at nurses, doctors, the baby who has died or is malformed and nearby mothers who have normal babies. This stage needs to be dealt with in an understanding manner.
4. *Equilibrium*. Gradual lessening of both anxiety and emotional reactions and the parents become able to cope with the situation. This may take a few weeks in the case of a malformed infant or many months after the death of an infant. This process may be eased if parents talk over their problems, meet with the paediatrician for counselling and visit the graveside on occasions.
5. *Reorganization and acceptance*. Parents are now able

to deal with the malformed infant and are reassured that the baby's problems were not due to their own neglect. In the case of an infant who has died, the parents are able to resume fairly normal living.

It usually takes about 6–9 months for this normal grief response to be completed. If the process becomes fixed at any stage, pathological grief can occur. It is helpful for a mother whose infant has died to see and hold her baby. A simple family funeral may also help to ease the grieving.

It is important for a senior paediatrician to ask the parents for consent to a postmortem (autopsy). Leaflets explaining the necessity of postmortem examination are available for parents to read before they give consent. Parents may not give consent for a full postmortem but may agree to a limited examination (e.g. chest only). After an autopsy has been carried out it is important that the paediatrician discusses its results with the parents.

The paediatrician should also discuss the problems of grieving and stress that it takes time for parents to work through their feelings. It is unhelpful for them to hide their feelings ('bottle things up') and parents should be told that many of their friends will not know how to react to the death of their baby and that some will even appear to be rather off-hand. The parents should be seen again after about 3 months so that their progress can be assessed and any further questions dealt with. The final autopsy results and the risks of recurrence in future pregnancies can also be discussed at this bereavement interview.

Parents should be advised against a 'replacement pregnancy' until the grieving process has been completed. Once grieving has run its course, another pregnancy can be considered.

Nursing points

Baby

- Parents should be told that babies respond to noise, touch, faces and colour. They should be encouraged to talk to their baby.
- Well babies appear to enjoy massage — this can be taught to parents.

- Quiet times should be facilitated for parents to spend with their baby.

Family

- Transitional care wards attached to maternity units enable mothers and babies to remain together whilst receiving specialist care.
- Unrestricted visiting should be encouraged for family members whilst the baby is in the NICU.
- Involvement in the baby's care should be encouraged as the parents feel able.
- Siblings, grandparents and extended family members may have an important role in the dynamics of the family. If the parents wish, they should be able to hold or touch the baby during visits and be involved in the care of the baby. Close friends may be more significant to some parents.
- Parents who have a preterm baby or one with an abnormality grieve for the 'perfect' baby they expected. Counselling may help them come to terms with the situation and acknowledge their feelings as normal and acceptable.
- Providing breast milk for their baby is a role unique to the mother and should be encouraged.

Equipment

- Lots of equipment around the baby will frighten many families, particularly when they first see their baby. Where possible, wait until the parents have seen or held their baby before attaching monitors and leads.
- Explain the use of each piece of equipment to the family to reduce their anxieties.
- Involving parents in the care of their baby familiarizes them with equipment, making it less threatening.
- Parents often come to rely on equipment for reassurance that their baby is safe. Gradual withdrawal of the use of this equipment is important and monitors such as apnoea alarms should be removed several days prior to discharge.

Staff

- Staff have a big role to play in establishing the relationship between the family and their baby. Refer to the baby by name when talking to parents and other staff and focus the parents on the baby rather than the monitors.

References and further reading

Davis JA, Richards MPM, Roberton NRC (1993). *Parent Baby Attachment in Premature Infants*. Beckenham: Croom Helm.

Drotar D, Baskieuriez A, Irvin N *et al* (1975). The adaption of parents to the birth of an infant with a congenital malformation: a hypothetical model. *Pediatrics* **56**: 710.

Klaus MH, Kennell JH (1989). *Parent–Infant Bonding*, 3rd edn. St Louis: CV Mosby.

Kohner N, Henley A (1991). *When a Baby Dies*. London: Pandora Press.

McHaffie H, Fowlie P (1996). *Life, Death and Decisions. Doctors and Nurses Reflect on Neonatal Practice*. Hale, Cheshire: Hochland and Hochland Ltd.

McLauglin A, Hillier VF, Robinson MJ (1993). Partial costs of neonatal visiting. *Arch Dis Child* **68**: 597.

O'Connor S, Vietze PM, Sherrod KB *et al* (1980). Reduced incidence of parenting inadequacy following rooming in. *Pediatrics* **66**: 176.

Sluckin W, Herbert M, Sluckin A (1984). *Maternal Bonding*. Oxford: Blackwell.

23 Infant Follow-Up

There are five major reasons why infants who are treated in neonatal units should be closely followed up:

1. To assess growth and development.
2. To detect sequelae associated with an abnormal perinatal period, e.g. asphyxia, prolonged mechanical ventilation.
3. To reassure parents and give continuing advice on infant care practices.
4. To collect data on outcome related to perinatal problems and their management (part of audit).
5. To detect early the emergence of groups of problems that might be attributable to some recently adopted form of therapy.

Neonatal units should have clear policies on which babies warrant follow up. Suggested indications for follow-up are:

≺ Prematurity: <32 weeks' gestation
≺ Growth retardation: <3rd centile for gestational age
≺ Moderate–severe asphyxia
≺ Babies who have received intensive care
≺ Other medical problems detected in the neonatal period, e.g. murmurs, gastro-oesophageal reflux.

Assessment of growth and development

At each visit the infant should have weight, height and head circumference measured and plotted on an appropriate growth chart (see Appendix VIII). Always make allowances for prematurity (post-conceptional age) in assessment of growth and development. Corrected ages should be used for the first 18–24 months of life. Even correcting for prematurity, low birth weight infants show poorer growth patterns than published standards for term infants for weight, length and head circumference.

Developmental screening should be performed at predetermined intervals: at 6 weeks, 4 months, 8 months, 12 months and 24 months using a proforma such as the Denver developmental assessment (see Appendix IX). Consider developmental assessment in four main areas:

Gross motor
Language and hearing
Fine motor-adaptive and vision
Personal and social

Detection of complications

A follow-up programme should detect likely complications such as:

Neurological abnormalities
Chronic lung disease
Retinopathy of prematurity
Hearing loss

The most important long-term problems are those associated with delayed or abnormal *neurological development*. 5–15% of infants who have received intensive care will suffer from some long-term neurological deficit, although evidence suggests that the incidence of spastic diplegia is less than it was 30 years ago. There has been some recent increase due to survival of very immature infants who formerly would have died.

Chronic lung disease (see Chs 6 and 10) may be seen in VLBW infants, especially those who have received assisted ventilation. Apart from the recognized syndromes of chronic lung disease, these infants are also more likely to need hospital admission for respiratory infections in the first year of life. Up to 30% of VLBW babies are rehospitalized in the first year. For a discussion on home management see p. 170.

Risk of *retinopathy of prematurity* is increased in babies <32 weeks' gestational age. Arrangements should be made for assessment of these babies prior to discharge by an experienced paediatric ophthalmologist with follow-up if necessary (see Ch. 8).

Hearing should be assessed in all babies at each follow-up visit. However, babies at high risk of hearing loss should be referred for formal audiological assessment, including auditory evoked responses. Babies at high risk of hearing loss include:

Preterm babies <32 weeks

Severe asphyxia

Severe hyperbilirubinaemia

Exposure to high levels of aminoglycosides

Multiorgan failure

Head and neck malformations

Reassurance and further guidance

This is part of the well-baby clinic service provided for mothers whose babies were admitted to the neonatal unit and is similar to the service provided by family doctors and community paediatricians. Advice often concerns feeding, possetting, rashes and constipation.

Data collection

This is a system of feedback or audit to provide information regarding long-term effects of intensive care. Comprehensive follow-up service and accurate record keeping are needed. Follow-up includes developmental testing, neurological examination and assessment of vision and hearing. Standardized developmental tests e.g. Denver and Bayley, may be administered by a trained psychologist or developmental paediatrician; for older children, assessment of IQ by WISC-R or British Ability Scales (BAS). Factors associated with an increased incidence of abnormal development are severe intracranial haemorrhage, PVL, severe asphyxia (Apgar score 0–3 at 5 min and encephalopathy), persistent seizures and neonatal meningitis. It is important to obtain close to 100% follow-up and help is often needed from general paediatricians, general practitioners, community paediatricians and health visitors.

New problems

In the past, neonatologists have been too ready to accept and use new drugs and treatments before complete evaluation of their effects. This has led to a series of 'neonatal disasters' from which no one can derive any credit; e.g. uncontrolled oxygen and retinopathy of prematurity, sulphonamides and kernicterus, chloramphenicol and grey-baby syndrome, and nikethamide in resuscitation. These therapeutic misadventures can be avoided in future by exhaustive evaluation of all new drugs and therapies in randomized controlled trials before they are accepted in neonatal practice. Large multicentre trials may be needed to demonstrate efficacy and safety of new drugs and interventions. Long-term effects of drugs may be missed unless there is careful follow-up, e.g. diethyl stilboestrol causing vaginal carcinoma in the offspring of mothers given the drug many years earlier to prevent recurrent abortion.

Risk of sudden infant death syndrome (SIDS)

This is probably increased in VLBW babies or those that have needed neonatal intensive care, although there is some controversy. Other risk groups include babies of drug-addicted mothers, near-miss episodes and babies with chronic lung disease (Table 23.1). Recently, the American Academy of Pediatrics recommended that healthy full-term babies be placed in cots on their sides or backs instead of the prone position. This followed a similar recommendation from the UK Chief Medical Officer of the Department of Health.

When a preterm infant with recurrent apnoea is being discharged from hospital, consideration of home monitoring is

Table 23.1. Infants at risk of SIDS

Risk category	Incidence of SIDS/1000 births
VLBW infant	12
Needed neonatal intensive care (all weights)	4
Drug-addicted mother	20
Sibling who died of SIDS	20
Twin of SIDS	42
Near-miss episode	32
Bronchopulmonary dysplasia	113
General population	2–3

Adapted from Brady and Gould (1984).

necessary. Criteria for home monitoring are shown in Table 23.2. Not all siblings of previous SIDS should be offered monitoring and often reassurance of the mother, encouragement of breastfeeding, frequent health visitor follow-up and regular weighing are just as effective.

Table 23.2. Criteria for home apnoea monitoring

1. Good indication (see Table 23.1).
2. Mother has asked for monitor or shown genuine interest if approached.
3. Full explanation of monitor's capability — operation, false alarms, possible unreliability — no simple monitor is 100% reliable.
4. Mother and father instructed in resuscitation techniques, including stimulation of the infant and mouth-to-mouth resuscitation (CPR).
5. Family practitioner and health visitor notified by telephone prior to discharge and show general agreement with plan.
6. The neonatal unit telephone number with 24-hour-a-day cover for emergency advice given to the parents.
7. Full letter of explanation to family practitioner after discharge.
8. Regular review at follow-up clinic.

Often the major benefit of home apnoea monitoring has been reassurance of the anxious parent. Mothers say they feel less likely to check their baby's breathing regularly when the monitor is attached. There are many types of monitor ranging from those that detect abdominal movement (MR 10) to those that measure heart rate and oxygen saturation in addition to respiration rate. These latter monitors may be more effective but are expensive and rather cumbersome.

Nursing points

Baby

- Familiarize yourself with the full perinatal history before assessing a baby.
- Allowance must be made for a baby's prematurity when considering growth milestones and weaning.
- Vaccinations begin when the baby is 2 months old, regardless of gestation at birth. Careful explanation of the reasons for this must be given to the family.

Family

- Where possible babies should be seen at clinics local to the family.
- Parents of babies who have been in NICU for prolonged periods often lose their peer group support. Follow-up clinics enable them to retain contact with staff and other families in similar situations. Support groups for such families can be very beneficial.

Equipment

- Nursing as well as medical audits are important for any NICU and follow-up regarding these aspects of care should also be considered.
- Appropriate percentile charts must be used, e.g. there is a chart specifically designed for babies with Down's syndrome, as their weight gain is often slower than average.

Staff

- Community staff may be less familiar with specific conditions or treatments than the parents. Facilities must be made available for them to discuss care of individual babies with neonatal staff.
- Ensure a full and detailed summary of the perinatal course of each baby is sent to the community staff, including details of any ongoing drug treatments and duration of these.
- Teams of specialist community neonatal nurses following up babies discharged from NICU have been shown to:
    offer great support to the family following discharge

provide a comprehensive link between the hospital and community services

facilitate early recognition and prompt treatment of illnesses and problems

reduce the readmission rates for neonates discharged from NICU

allow earlier discharge of babies from NICU.

References and further reading

Beal SM, Finch CF (1991). An overview of retrospective case-control studies investigating the relationship between prone sleeping position and SIDS. *J Paediatr Child Health* **27**: 334.

Brady JP, Gould JB (1984). Sudden infant death syndrome. In *Advances in Pediatrics*, Vol 31 (ed, Barness LA). Chicago: Year Book Medical Publishers.

Casey PH, Kraemer HC, Bernbaum J *et al* (1990). Growth patterns of low birth weight preterm infants: a longitudinal analysis of a large, varied sample. *J Pediatr* **117**: 298.

Casiro OG, McKenzie ME, McFadyen L *et al* (1993). Earlier discharge with community-based intervention for low birth weight infants: a randomized trial. *Pediatrics* **92**: 128.

Cunningham CK, McMillan JA, Gross SJ (1991). Rehospitalization for respiratory illness in infants of less than 32 weeks' gestation. *Pediatrics* **88**: 527.

Egan DF, Illingworth RS, McKeith RC (1971). Developmental Screening 0–5 years, In: *Clinics in Developmental Medicine*, Vol. 30. London: Spastics International Medical Publications and Heinemann Medical.

Illingworth RS (1992). *The Normal Child: Some Problems of the Early Years and their Treatment*, 10th edn. Edinburgh: Churchill Livingstone.

McCormick ME (1993). Has the prevalence of handicapped infants increased with improved survival of the very low birth weight infants? *Clin Perinatol* **20**: 263.

Saugstad OD (1993). The future of neonatal research. *Acta Pediatr* **82**: 1.

Schneider AM, Veen S, Ens A *et al.* (1992). Standardised method of follow-up assessment of preterm infants at the age of 5 years: use of the WHO classification of impairments, disabilities and handicaps. *Paediatr Perinat Epidemiol* **6**: 363.

Silverman WA (1980). *Retrolental Fibroplasia: A Modern Parable.* London: Academic Press.

Silverman WA (1985). *Human Experimentation: A Guided Step into the Unknown.* Oxford: Oxford University Press.

Southall DP, Samuels MP (1992). Reducing risks in the sudden infant death syndrome. *Brit Med J* **304**: 265.

24 Neonatal Brain Imaging

The newborn brain can be imaged by a variety of means:
Ultrasound
Computed tomography (CT)
Magnetic resonance imaging (MRI)

Ultrasound is the mode of choice for most babies.

Ultrasound

This type of imaging has considerable *advantages*:
Mobile — bedside technique
Relatively inexpensive
Instantaneous image — patient movement is not critical
Probe easily moved to select planes of scanning
Safe — no ionizing radiation

Cranial ultrasound does however have a number of *disadvantages*:
Range of examination may be limited by a small anterior
fontanelle
Some areas of the brain are poorly visualized (subdural and
subarachnoid spaces, posterior fossa)
May not easily pick up changes seen on CT or MRI
Inexperienced operators may misinterpret findings

Technique

A 7.5-MHz transducer should be used where possible. Access to the brain in the newborn is through the anterior or posterior fontanelle or through the relatively thin parietal bones.

Ultrasound images of the skull appear as dense white echoes, and the CSF as black echo-free areas. The cerebellum and choroid plexus are relatively vascular and appear white, while the thalamus is slightly less echodense than the caudate nucleus.

The transducer should first be placed in the coronal plane over the anterior fontanelle and angled first towards the face and then towards the occiput. To obtain the parasagittal view the transducer is rotated through 90° and both lateral ventricles may be seen by angling the probe first to the right and then to the left. If required, the probe can be placed over the parietal bone above the ear with the baby's head positioned laterally. This gives the axial view, which allows measurement of the ventriculo-cerebral ratio (VCR).

Normal anatomy

Coronal plane

With the scanner head angled anteriorly, the interhemispheric fissure is seen as a clear echo-free region in the midline. Laterally the anterior horns of the lateral ventricles can be seen as echo-free crescents, concave laterally.

As the scanner head is rotated posteriorly, the head of the caudate nucleus and then the thalamus form the lateral walls of the ventricles. The choroid plexus is echo-dense and is first seen superior and medial to the caudo-thalamic notch in the floor of the lateral ventricle. As the scanner head is rotated further posteriorly, the choroid plexus can be seen to widen and deepen and to swing downward and laterally, hugging the ventricular wall to the temporal horn. As the scanner is rotated following the choroid plexus, the third ventricle may be seen as an echo-free slit in the midline inferior to the lateral ventricle.

With the scanner head rotated posteriorly, parts of the cerebellum may be seen, although good views of this structure are unusual. Below the cerebellum the cisterna magna is occasionally seen.

Parasagittal plane

With the scanner head angled obliquely, it is usually possible to see all of the lateral ventricle, especially if the scanner head is rocked slightly to bring lateral areas into view. The corpus callosum is seen as an echo-dense curvilinear structure sweeping posteriorly. Below it, in the midline, the cavum septum pellucidum is seen and more laterally, the lateral ventricle.

Anteriorly, the anterior horn is usually easily visualized and extends backwards over the head of the caudate and thalamus. The angle between the caudate and thalamus is important as the choroid plexus begins here. This is the commonest site of origin of intraventricular haemorrhage. The lateral ventricle can be seen beyond this point to swing posteriorly with the choroid plexus in its floor until it finally turns back to form the inferior horn. It is sometimes possible to see the 3rd ventricle as a rather ill-defined echo-free structure inferior to the lateral ventricle in the midline and very occasionally the 4th ventricle can also be seen.

Suggested indications for ultrasound examination in the newborn are shown in Table 24.1.

Table 24.1. Indications for cerebral ultrasound

Clinical situation	Timing of scan
Infants <32 weeks	Daily for first 3 days and end of first week, 6 weeks
Infants ≥32 weeks with CNS signs	Onset of CNS signs
Intracranial haemorrhage found	Repeat at least weekly
Dysmorphic syndromes	At birth
Rapidly growing head	At diagnosis
Ventriculomegaly found	Repeat at least weekly
Abnormal development (<6 months)	When diagnosed

An ultrasound examination at 40 weeks' postconceptional age provides the clearest prognostic information. It should be the first choice of imaging for all neonatal cerebral lesions, especially for diagnosis and prognosis of intraventricular haemorrhage or periventricular leucomalacia.

MRI or CT scanning is preferred if there are persistently abnormal neurological signs in the presence of a normal ultrasound scan, following birth asphyxia in term infants or for infants >6 months.

Ultrasound imaging should be complemented by MRI or CT scanning for:

≺ Suspected structural abnormalities
≺ Posterior fossa lesions
≺ Subdural, cortical or subcortical lesions
≺ Asphyxiated term infants at 1–2 weeks of age

✚ Intraventricular haemorrhage (IVH)

Blood is echo-dense on ultrasonic examination. Suspicious areas should be identified in two planes before confidently making a diagnosis of haemorrhage. Degrees of haemorrhage have in the past been assigned grades from I to IV, based on CT scan findings. It is best, however, to describe exactly what is seen and where, to avoid any interobserver confusion (p. 271).

The usual first appearance of IVH is a bright spot either at the caudothalamic notch or next to the head of the caudate nucleus below and lateral to the frontal horn of the body of the lateral ventricle. It may bulge into the ventricle. This is known as a subependymal haemorrhage (SEH) or grade I haemorrhage (Fig. 24.1). The presence of haemorrhage must always be confirmed by examination in the sagittal plane, as a common cause of false positive scan is asymmetry of the choroid plexi. Frequently a small 'finger' of choroid will extend quite far anteriorly on the floor of the lateral ventricle.

Blood in the ventricular space appears echo-dense (grade II haemorrhage) (Fig. 24.2) and may obstruct the ventricular foramina causing dilatation of the ventricle (grade III haemorrhage). Clots may also be seen attached to the choroid or in the occipital horns.

Haemorrhage into the cortical substance, often into an area of ischaemia or venous infarction, has been termed a grade IV haemorrhage (Fig. 24.3). This is often associated with an ipsilateral intraventricular haemorrhage, although the latter does not rupture out of the ventricles as was formerly thought. Haemorrhage in the brain parenchyma appears initially as a

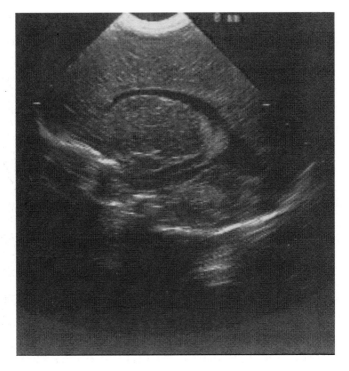

Figure 24.1. Parasagittal view showing tiny subependymal haemorrhage at the caudothalamic notch, anterior to the choroid plexus.

very echo-dense area, but after 10–14 days may become cystic, and after a further 3–4 weeks may retract allowing the edges of the haematoma to separate from the brain. Complete resolution of an intraparenchymal haemorrhage may take many weeks or months, leaving behind a porencephalic cyst. The cyst may merge with the adjacent lateral ventricle giving it an irregular shape.

A small proportion of haemorrhages are thought to occur in the choroid itself. These can be difficult to diagnose with certainty, but may be suspected where the choroid looks 'bulky'.

The majority of IVH may be detected within the first 3 days of life and very few new haemorrhages occur after 7 days. IVH can be detected for much longer on ultrasound scan than by CT

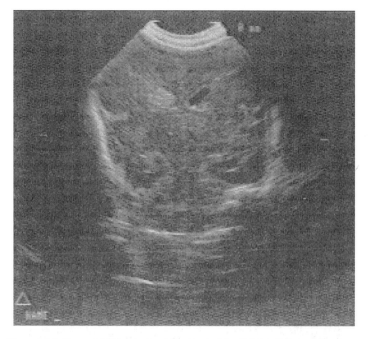

Figure 24.2. Coronal USS of brain at the level of the Sylvian fissures, showing unilateral intraventricular haemorrhage. The right lateral ventricle is filled with blood clot.

scan. Most parenchymal haemorrhages on CT scan are iso-dense by 5–10 days.

Subdural haemorrhage may be diagnosed by using a water bath (surgical glove filled with water) placed against the baby's head to reduce reverberation artefact. If subdural fluid is present, the brain appears separated from the cranial vault and the gyri and sulci appear more prominent. The differential diagnosis is cerebral atrophy, where head growth is slow, while in the presence of subdural haemorrhage the head normally grows more rapidly than usual.

Haemorrhage can occur infrequently in the caudate nucleus, thalamus and posterior fossa (especially cerebellum). These may be difficult to diagnose by ultrasound but can often be detected by CT scan.

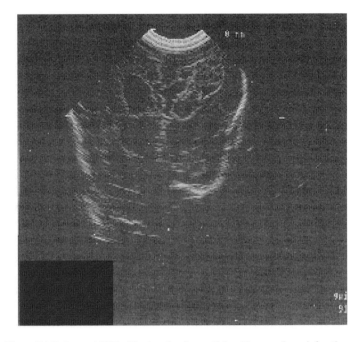

Figure 24.3. Coronal USS of brain, showing unilateral haemorrhage infarction. Both lateral ventricles are dilated and the infarcted area is in communication with the ipsilateral ventricle.

Moderate to severe IVH is associated with disability in 44% of survivors; if there is parenchymal involvement this increases to at least 70%.

Hydrocephalus

Ventricular dilatation is relatively common following major intra-ventricular haemorrhages; there may be acute dilatation of the ventricles due to obstruction of the aqueduct or foramen of Monro and when this occurs, there is an increased mortality. The lateral ventricle will be enlarged in both coronal and sagittal views (Fig. 24.4). The third ventricle may also be enlarged. Later dilatation is due to communicating hydrocephalus, secondary to

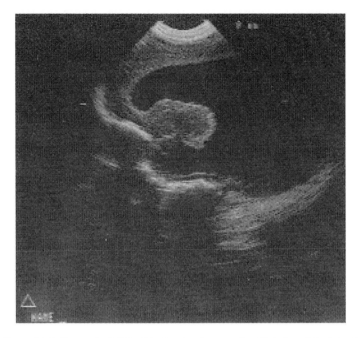

Figure 24.4. Parasagittal USS of brain, showing massive dilatation of the lateral ventricle.

obliterative arachnoiditis. In many cases this resolves spontaneously, with only 20–30% requiring shunting.

Dilatation of the ventricles can be diagnosed from and monitored by the ventricular index (VI) which is measured in the coronal plane at the level of the foramen of Monro. The VI of each lateral ventricle is measured as the distance from the midline to the outermost edge of the lateral ventricle. VI normally increases with increasing gestational age; measurements can be plotted on a specific chart, significant ventriculomegaly is said to be present when VI is > 4 mm above the 97th percentile for corrected gestational age (Appendix XI).

An alternative measurement is the ventriculo-cerebral ratio (VCR), which is measured in the axial plane. The width of the lateral ventricle is measured at the level of its mid-body and that of the cerebral hemisphere as the distance from the midline echo to the inner table of the skull. The normal VCR in the term infant is 28% (range 24–30%) and in the preterm infant 31% (range 24–34%).

These ratios may be used for diagnosis and to measure the effects of therapy such as repeated lumbar puncture or shunting. The earliest sign of dilatation of the ventricles is loss of the lateral curvature and widening of the frontal horn. Conversely, the response of the ventricular system to shunting is seen first in the body of the lateral ventricle and last in the occipital horn.

Ventricular dilatation due to other causes, e.g. Arnold–Chiari malformation, Dandy–Walker syndrome and holosoprosencephaly, may be readily detected by ultrasound. Other cystic lesions include porencephaly, hydranencephaly (an extreme form of porencephaly or hydrocephaly where the cerebral hemispheres are completely replaced with fluid), and arachnoid cysts.

Subependymal pseudocysts (usually seen anteriorly in the frontal horns of the lateral ventricle) and small isolated cysts in the choroid are usually of no significance.

✚ Periventricular leucomalacia (PVL)

Leucomalacia means softening of the white matter. This may be due to ischaemia or venous infarction but the exact pathogenesis is not fully understood. Developmental problems, particularly spastic cerebral palsy, are common in later life. The first appearance, which is most easily demonstrated with a 7.5-MHz transducer, is a periventricular flare. This is a triangular shaped area of increased echodensity found at the lateral border of the frontal horn of the lateral ventricle. Changes are commonly bilateral, whereas strongly unilateral findings suggest a periventricular venous infarction. Note that this area is relatively vascular and minor increases in echodensity may not be pathological. The duration of periventricular flares is related to outcome; those lasting <2 weeks generally have a good neurological outcome.

Persistent echodensity in the periventricular region is indicative of PVL and may progress over a few weeks to cyst formation. A small number of cysts grouped around the edges of the frontal horns may not be associated with significant problems, but if the cysts are extensive and more posteriorly placed, they carry a poorer prognosis (Fig. 24.5). With time the cysts usually become obliterated by the surrounding growing brain, although there is residual white matter damage, gliosis and deranged myelination. In extensive cases there may be a degree of cortical atrophy, where the growth of the brain is reduced, and there is symmetrical dilatation of the lateral ventricles.

In severe cases there may be widespread infarction and cystic changes can be found more laterally in the parietal, temporal and occipital lobes. This is termed subcortical leucomalacia and carries a poor prognosis, with residual spastic cerebral palsy often associated with impairments of hearing and vision, seizures and cognitive defects.

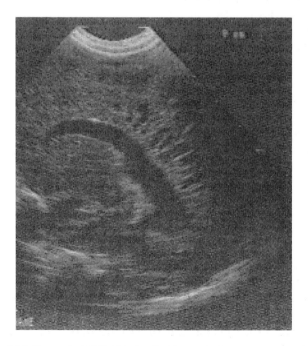

Figure 24.5. Parasagittal USS of brain, showing extensive cystic periventricular dilatation. The lateral ventricle is moderately dilated.

✚ Birth asphyxia

Ultrasonography has a limited role in imaging babies with hypoxic-ischaemic encephalopathy. Findings suggestive of cerebral oedema in the first few days include:

◄ Diffuse echobright pattern
◄ Lateral ventricles may be very narrow (this can be normal in the absence of other findings)
◄ Reduced arterial pulsations, e.g. at the circle of Willis.

Clearly, these findings are quite subjective and should only be used as a guide towards diagnosis. More detailed imaging with MRI or CT should be performed later (1–2 weeks of age).

Computed tomography (CT)

CT has few applications in imaging the newborn brain and is particularly unhelpful in the preterm infant whose brain has a high water content.

CT has a few *advantages* over ultrasound, although it is being replaced by MRI in many centres:

Better imaging of posterior fossa and frontal areas
Parenchymal lesions, e.g. cortical infarctions are seen more clearly
Vascular abnormalities and solid lesions are seen more easily

The *disadvantages* of CT scanning are:

Not portable
Expensive
Involves ionizing radiation
Infant must lie still — sedation sometimes needed
Poor definition of small intracranial haemorrhages

Magnetic resonance imaging (MRI)

Imaging sequences are very different from those used in older children and adults, and change as the infant ages. The immature brain has a higher water content and a lower myelin content than the mature brain. MRI can demonstrate the progress of myelination in the developing brain because of the maturational changes in free water content and phospholipid concentration. Myelin is present in the posterior limb of the internal capsule, thalamus, cerebellum and brain stem at 37 weeks' gestation, and appears in the parietal lobe by term. Myelination progresses subsequently as follows:

> *3 months*: anterior limb of internal capsule, optic radiations and occipital lobe
>
> *6 months*: external capsule, corpus callosum and frontal lobe
>
> *9 months*: subcortical areas, temporal lobe, arborization throughout the brain

There may still be some unmyelinated areas in the posterior periventricular regions by 2 years of age.

The role of cerebral MRI is still being determined, particularly in preterm babies, but it is now the method of choice for imaging the asphyxiated term baby. It has also superceded CT in the investigation of suspected structural defects.

Advantages include:
> Excellent image quality
> Absence of ionizing radiation which allows repeated imaging

The *disadvantages* are
> Scanner is large, very expensive and not portable
> Requires highly skilled staff to operate the machine and interpret the images
> Noisy
> Requires sedation

A number of abnormalities may be seen soon after birth asphyxia and these may be predictive of long-term outcome. T_1- and T_2-weighted spin-echo, and age-related inversion recovery sequences should be performed.

≺ *Brain swelling*. Seen in the first week and is best demonstrated with a T_1-weighted spin-echo sequence.

≺ *Loss of signal from the posterior limb of the internal capsule*. May take a few days to evolve. Always associated with subsequent motor impairment, the degree of which depends on the presence of other imaging findings.

≺ *Abnormal signal in the basal ganglia/thalami.* Best seen at 1–2 weeks. May be high signal intensity in the ventrolateral nucleus of the thalamus and in the lentiform nucleus. Degree of damage is related to outcome. High signal may later be lost as cysts develop.

≺ *Cortical highlighting.* Becomes more noticeable by 1–2 weeks and is seen around the centrum semiovale and Rolandic fissure. Mild changes may not be associated with later disability, but severe and extensive changes may result in subsequent atrophy of the adjacent cortical white matter.

≺ *Loss of grey/white matter differentiation.* Seen clearly on T_1 and inversion recovery sequences. Finding often associated with brain swelling and is seen in the first week of life; by the second week, there may be an exaggerated differentiation.

The optimum time for imaging is around 2 weeks after birth.

A fluid attenuation inversion recovery (FLAIR) sequence is especially useful after 1 year of life as this cancels out the bright images obtained from CSF, giving better views of the rest of the brain. Late findings on MRI after birth asphyxia include focal/global atrophy and cyst formation in the basal ganglia and thalami, and focal/global atrophy, reduced myelination and cyst formation in the white matter. Curiously, the cerebellum is often minimally affected.

MRI may have a role in investigation of children with cerebral palsy where white matter reduction corresponds to the severity of disability.

Nursing points

Baby

- All babies in the NICU will benefit from periods free from any handling. Ultrasound scanning should, therefore, be performed with consideration for these periods. The timing of other procedures should also be taken into account.

- Sedation may be necessary for a baby prior to a CT scan. Careful observation of the baby's vital signs should be made during this period.
- The baby must be kept warm throughout these procedures and the hat replaced promptly once finished.

Family

- Full explanation of the necessity for any form of brain imaging should be given to the parents prior to the procedure, whenever possible.
- Parents may wish to be present during the procedure and must be reassured it is non-invasive and painless.
- An explanation of the results and implications of these tests should be discussed with the parents at the earliest opportunity. It is important to record, in the neonatal notes, details of the information which has been given to the family, to avoid any confusion amongst staff.
- If there is a delay in the results being available, for example due to the need for specialist interpretation of MRI scan images, parents should be given an idea of how long this process will take.

Equipment

- The ultrasound transducer must be cleaned after each use to prevent cross-infection.

Staff

- A pre-discharge meeting involving the family, medical and nursing staff and the community health workers, gives an opportunity to ensure everyone involved in the care of the baby has the same knowledge of any brain injuries or damage, and can discuss the prognosis. Consistency and honesty of information is vital for the parents.

References and further reading

Anthony MY, Levene MI (1993). Neonatal cerebral ultrasound. In: *Recent Advances in Paediatrics* vol. 11 (ed, David TJ). Edinburgh: Churchill Livingstone, pp. 85–102.

Byrne P, Welch R, Johnson MA, Darrah J, Piper M (1990). Serial magnetic resonance imaging in neonatal hypoxic-ischemic encephalopathy. *J Pediatr* **117**: 694.

Govaert P, de Vries L (1997). Atlas of neonatal brain sonography. *Clinics in Developmental Medicine* vol. 141–142. London: MacKeith Press.

Jongmans M, Henderson S, de Vries L, Dubowitz L (1993). Duration of periventricular densities in preterm infants and neurological outcome at 6 years of age. *Arch Dis Child* **69**: 9.

Paneth N, Rudelli R, Kazam E, Monte W (1994). Brain damage in the preterm infant. *Clinics in Developmental Medicine*, vol. 131. London: MacKeith Press.

Rennie J (1997). *Neonatal Cerebral Ultrasound*. Cambridge: Cambridge University Press.

Yokochi K, Aiba K, Hurie M *et al* (1991). Magnetic resonance imaging in children with spastic diplegia: correlation with the severity of their motor and mental disability. *Dev Med Child Neurol* **33**: 18.

Appendices

Appendix I   **Drug dosages**

The following table gives details of drugs which may be used in the newborn baby. Local protocols may vary and should always be followed.

Drug	Dosage	Frequency (h)	Route	Notes
Adenosine	100 µg/kg	–	i.v.	Rapid bolus, followed by 0.9% saline flush. Use in supraventricular tachycardia
Adrenaline	0.1–0.3 ml/kg	–	i.v. via ET	1:10000 strength 1:1000 strength
Albumin 5%	0.1–0.3 µg/kg/min 1 g/kg	–	i.v. infusion slow i.v.	
Aminophylline	5 mg/kg loading, 7.5 mg/kg/day maintenance	8–12	i.v.	Can precipitate heart failure. For apnoea of prematurity. Caffeine first choice
Atracurium	0.3–0.6 mg/kg/h	–	i.v. infusion	High sodium content
Atropine	0.03 mg/kg	–	s.c., i.v.	Use in some cases of bradycardia
Budesonide	400 µg/dose	12	inhaled	For chronic lung disease. Use spacer device
Caffeine citrate	20 mg/kg loading, 5 mg/kg/day maintenance	24	oral, i.v.	Well absorbed orally. Long half life. Toxic levels > 50 mg/l
Calcium gluconate (10%)	0.2 ml/kg	–	slow i.v.(over 5–10 min)	Rarely indicated. Causes bradycardia and tissue necrosis
Carbimazole	0.5–1.0 mg/kg/day	8	oral	Treatment of thyroxicosis
Chloral hydrate	10–50 mg/kg	–	oral	Sedative; gastric irratation
Chlorothiazide	20 mg/kg/day	12	oral	Causes hypokalaemia
Chlorpromazine	500 µg/kg/dose	6–8	oral, i.v.	Treatment of drug withdrawal. Do not exceed 6 mg/kg/day

continued overleaf

Appendix I *(continued)*

Drug	Dosage	Frequency (h)	Route	Notes
Cimetidine	10–20 mg/kg/day	6	oral	Ranitidine may be first choice of H_2 antagonist
Clonazepam	0.10–0.15 mg/kg	–	i.v.	For intractable seizures. Long half-life, may cause apnoea. Flumazenil antidote.
Dexamethasone	0.25–1.0 mg/kg/day	12–24	oral, i.v.	Treatment of chronic lung disease (see page 169).May cause hyperglycaemia and hypertension.
Diamorphine	180 μg/kg loading, 15 μg/kg/h maintenance	–	i.v. infusion	For pain relief, terminal care.
Diazepam	0.1–0.3 mg/kg	6–8	oral, i.v.	Use Diazemuls®. May cause apnoea.
Diazoxide	5 mg/kg/dose	12–24	oral, i.v.	For intractable hypoglycaemia. Causes salt and water retention, tissue necrosis.
Digoxin	30–50 μg/kg digitalization, 5–10 μg/kg maintenance	12	oral, i.v.	i.v. dose 2/3 of oral. Caution in the preterm, renal failure, hypokalaemia. See page 285
Dobutamine, dopamine	5–10 μg/kg/min	–	i.v. infusion	For hypotension and reduced cardiac output. Preferably infuse via a central line. Watch for extravasation.
Doxapram	2.5 mg/kg loading, 0.3 mg/kg/h maintenance	–	i.v. infusion	Give loading dose over 5-10 minutes, watch for extravasation
Edrophonium	0.1 mg/kg	–	i.m., slow i.v.	Test dose for myaesthenia gravis
Ferrous sulphate	10 mg	24	oral	Unnecessary, except in exclusively breast-fed baby < 2 kg. Start at 6 weeks of life
Fludrocortisone	50 μg/kg/day	24	oral	For salt-losing adrenal hyperplasia
Folic acid	50 μg/day	24	oral	Rarely required
Frusemide	1–2 mg/kg	–	oral, i.v.	May cause hypokalaemia, hypocalcaemia and reversible nephrocalcinosis

Drug	Dose		Route	Comments
Glucagon	200 μg/kg stat dose or 0.3 μg/kg/min infusion	—	i.m., i.v. i.v. infusion	For intractable hypoglycaemia
Heparin	50 Units/kg loading, 25 units/kg/h maintenance	—	i.v. infusion	Anticoagulation dose (use 1–2 Units/ml for flush solutions)
Hydralazine	0.1–0.5 mg/kg/dose	8	oral, i.v.	Treatment of acute hypertension
Hydrocortisone	20–25 mg/m²/day	8	oral, i.m., i.v.	Maintenance treatment of congenital adrenal hyperplasia. Start with 2.5 mg 8-hourly, triple dose in acute illness or surgery
Indomethacin	0.1–0.2 mg/kg	—	i.v.	Caution in renal impairment. See page 288
Insulin	0.1 Unit/kg	—	i.v., infusion	For hyperglycaemia. See page 199
Isoprenaline	0.02–0.05 μg/kg/min (maximum 0.3)	—	i.v. infusion	For hypotension; use dopamine or dobutamine in preference
Labetalol	0.5 mg/kg/h	—	i.v. infusion	For acute severe hypertension. Use diluted solution. Monitor blood pressure carefully.
Lignocaine	1 mg/kg loading, 20–50 μg/kg/min maintenance	—	i.v. infusion	For serious ventricular dysrhythmias. Check dose carefully.(Local anaesthetic use – up to 0.3 ml/kg of 1% lignocaine)
Magnesium sulphate	50 mg/kg	—	Deep i.m. or slow i.v.	50% solution, dilute before giving i.v. Watch for extravasation.
Methyldopa	7.5 mg/kg/day	8	oral or i.v. (over 30–60 min)	Maximum dose 15 mg/kg 8 hourly. Causes salt and water retention; haemolytic anaemia and thrombocytopenia are side-effects
Morphine sulphate	0.1 mg/kg stat dose 20–50 μg/kg/h infusion	—	i.v., i.v. infusion	Apnoea and raised pulmonary vascular resistance are side-effects
Naloxone	100–200 μg i.m. or 40 μg i.v./ET for resuscitation.	—	i.m., i.v., ET	Reversal of opioids; rapid effect when given i.v.,but short acting

continued overleaf

Appendix I *(continued)*

Drug	Dosage	Frequency (h)	Route	Notes
Neostigmine	150 µg/kg/dose	6–8	i.m.	Maintenance therapy for myaesthenia gravis. May need higher doses
Nitroprusside	0.5–5 µg/kg/min	–	i.v. infusion	Protect from light. Causes hypotension
Paraldehyde	0.3 ml/kg	–	rectal	Once only. Can be drawn up in a polypropylene syringe; mix with an equal volume of mineral oil. Malodorous, can cause proctitis.
Pethidine	1 mg/kg	–	i.v., i.m.	See morphine. Causes respiratory depression.
Phenobarbitone	20 mg/kg loading, 5 mg/kg/day maintenance	12–24	i.v., oral	Causes respiratory depression when used with diazepam.Long half-life, may accumulate. Serum levels 10–20 mg/l.
Paracetamol	15 mg/kg/dose	8–12	oral, rectal	For analgesia
Phenytoin	10–20 mg/kg loading, 5–10 mg/kg/day maintenance	8–12	i.v. slowly	ECG monitor if giving i.v., do not mix with dextrose. Oral suspension poorly soluble. Serum levels 10–20 mg/l.
Phytomenadione (Vitamin K₁)	Local practices vary considerably	–	i.m., i.v., oral	See page 353
Potassium chloride	2 mmol/kg/day	8	oral	1 mmol = 75 mg
Prednisolone	1–2 mg/kg/day	6–12	oral	Can cause hypokalaemia
Propranolol	0.5–3.0 mg/kg/day	6–8	i.v., oral	Cardiac dysrhythmias and bronchoconstriction are side-effects.
Prostaglandin PgE₂ (Dinoprostone)	0.1 µg/kg/min	–	i.v. infusion	See page 284. Do not mix with other drugs.

Drug	Dose		Route	Comments
Prostacyclin	10 ng/kg/min	—	i.v. infusion	Treatment of pulmonary hypertension. May cause hypotension. See page 173.
Protamine sulphate	1 mg/100 units heparin	—	slow i.v.	Reversal of heparin anticoagulation
Ranitidine	0.5–1.0 mg/kg/dose	8–12	i.v. over 10–15 min	Avoid in renal failure
Salbutamol	4 µg/kg	—	i.v. infusion over 5 min	For acute reduction of hyperkalaemia
Sodium bicarbonate	1–2 mmol/kg	—	i.v., oral	Do not mix with any other drug; flush i.v. line afterwards.
Spironolactone	1 mg/kg/dose	12	oral, i.v.	In conjunction with frusemide or thiazide diuretic
THAM	0.6 mmol/kg/unit of base deficit it is required to lower.	—	slow i.v.	Watch for extravasation
Thyroxine	10–25 µg	24	oral	See page 340
Tolazoline	1–2 mg/kg stat dose, 1–2 mg/kg/h if a response	—	i.v. i.v. infusion	Hypotension common. Boluses as required may be as effective as an infusion.
Vecuronium	0.1 mg/kg loading, 0.1 mg/kg/h maintenance	—	i.v. infusion	May be cumulative

Appendix II   **Antibiotic, antifungal and antiviral dosages**

(a) Antibiotics

Antibiotic	Infants <7 days		Infants >7 days	
	Dosage (mg/kg/day)	Frequency (h)	Dosage (mg/kg/day)	Frequency (h)
Penicillins:				
Ampicillin	50–100	12	50–100	8
Benzylpenicillin	60–100	12	60–100	8
Flucloxacillin	50–100	12	50–100	8
Ticarcillin	150	12	225–300	6–8
Aminoglycosides:				
Amikacin	15–20	12	20–30	8
Gentamicin	5	12	7.5	8
Netilmicin	5–6	12	6	8
Tobramycin	4	12	6	8
Cephalosporins:				
Cefotaxime	100	12	150	8
Cefuroxime	50–100	12	100–150	8
Ceftazidime	25–60	12	25–60	12
Ceftriaxone	60–100	12	60–100	12

Others:

Drug				
Chloramphenicol	25	24	25–50	8–12
Fucidin*	20–50	12	20–50	8
Rifampicin	10	12–24	10	12–24
Teicoplanin	Loading dose of 16 mg/kg, then 8 mg/kg 24 hourly			
Vancomycin	10–20	12–24	20–30	8–12

Where two figures are given, e.g. 100–200 mg/kg/day or 6–8 hourly, use lower amount and reduced frequency for infants under 2000 g birth weight and higher ones for those over 2000 g. The parenteral route is preferred.

* Use 20 mg/kg/day for i.v., 50 mg/kg/day orally.

(b) Antifungal and antiviral drugs

Drug	Dosage	Frequency (h)	Route	Notes
Antifungals:				
Amphotericin B	0.25–1.0 mg/kg/day	24	i.v.	Infuse over 4–6 h. Caution in renal impairment
Fluconazole	6 mg/kg/dose	48–72	oral, i.v.	i.v. infusion over 30 min. Caution in renal impairment
Flucytosine	50–150 mg/kg/day	6	oral, i.v.	i.v. infusion over 30 min. Caution in renal impairment. Serum levels 25–50 mg/l
Nystatin	100,000 Units (1ml)/dose	6	oral	For oral candidiasis
Antiviral drugs:				
Acyclovir	20–30 mg/kg/day	8–12	i.v.	Dilute and infuse over 1 h.
Zidovudine (ZDV)	8 mg/kg/day	6	oral, i.v.	Prophylaxis for HIV-exposed infants. Give for first 6 weeks of life. See page 231.

Appendix III   Normal blood chemistry values of infants 1500–1750 g birth weight

	1 week	3 weeks	5 weeks
Sodium (mmol/l)	133–146	129–142	133–148
Potassium (mmol/l)	4.6–6.7	4.5–7.1	4.5–6.6
Chloride (mmol/l)	100–117	102–116	100–115
Urea (mmol/l)	1.0–8.5	0.7–10.4	0.6–8.8
(mean)	(3.1)	(4.4)	(4.4)
Calcium (mmol/l)	1.5–2.9	2.0–2.8	2.1–2.6
Phosphorus (mmol/l)	1.9–3.7	2.1–3.0	1.9–2.7
Total protein (g/l)	44–63	43–67	41–69
Albumin (g/l)	33–45	32–53	32–43
Globulin (g/l)	9–22	6–29	5–15

From Thomas and Reichelderfer (1968) with kind permission of The American Association for Clinical Chemistry

Appendix IV   Normal coagulation values in the newborn

Factor/measurement	Term infant	Preterm infant	Adult value
Fibrinogen (mg %)	200–500	200–250	200–400
Factor II (%)	40	25	50–100
Factor V (%)	90	60–75	75–125
Factor VII (%)	50	35	75–125
Factor VIII (%)	100	80–100	50–150
Factor IX (%)	24–40	25–40	50–150
Factor X (%)	50–60	25–40	50–150
Factor XI (%)	30–40	25–40	75–125
Factor XII (%)	50–100	50–100	75–125
Factor XIII (titre)	1:16	1:8	1:8
Plasminogen (%)	43	24	61–126
Partial thromboplastin time (s)	40–70	50–90	30–50
Prothrombin time (PT) (s)	12–18	14–20	10–20
Thrombin time (TT) (s)	12–16	13–20	10–12
α_2-Macroglobulin* (mg/ml)	250	230	200–400
α_1-Antitrypsin* (mg/ml)	100	90	275
Antithrombin III* (mg/ml)	12	12	20–35

* Plasma inhibitors of proteolytic enzymes

Appendix IV

Appendix V

Appendix V   Normal neonatal haematological values (see Chs 14 and 21)

	At birth			At 24 hours	At 72 hours	Range at term
	28 weeks	34 weeks	40 weeks			
Haemoglobin (g/dl)	14.5	15.0	16.8	18.4	17.8	15–20
Packed cell volume (%)	45	47	53	58	55	48–60
Red cells (millions/mm³)	4.0	4.4	5.3	5.8	5.6	4.0–6.5
MCV (fl)	120	118	107	108	99	96–112
MCHC (%)	31	32	32	33	33	30–35
Reticulocytes (%)	10	10	7	7	3	3–10
Platelets (thousands/mm³)	180	230	290	192	213	160–360
Total white cells (thousands/mm³)	16.8	13.0	18.1	18.2	12.2	6–30
Segmented neutrophils (thousands/mm³) 54%	9.1	7.2	9.4	9.4	4.7	3–13
Band forms (thousands/mm³) 7%	1.2	1.0	1.6	1.6	0.8	0–4
Lymphocytes (thousands/mm³) 30%	5.0	3.9	5.5	5.5	5.0	2–11
Monocytes (thousands/mm³) 6%	1.0	0.7	1.0	1.0	1.1	0.4–3.1
Eosinophils (thousands/mm³) 2%	0.3	0.3	0.4	0.4	0.5	0.2–0.9
Basophils (thousands/mm³) 1%	0.2	0.1	0.1	0.1	0.05	0–0.6
ESR (mm/hour)	1–6	1–6	1–3	1–3	1–8	1–8

	0–96 hours	>96 hours
Absolute neutrophil count	<14 000	2000–4700
Absolute band count	<1400	<500
Band/neutrophil ratio*	<0.17	<0.14

* Increased in sepsis, infants of diabetic mothers, meconium aspiration, respiratory distress syndrome, hypoglycaemia and asphyxia

After Manroe et al. (1976, 1977)

Appendix VIA   Sarnat staging of hypoxic/ischaemic encephalopathy (HIE)

	Stage 1	Stage 2	Stage 3
1. *Level of consciousness*	Hyperalert	Lethargic or obtunded	Stupor or coma
2. *Neuromuscular control:*			
Muscle tone	Normal	Mild hypotonia	Flaccid
Posture	Mild distal flexion	Strong distal flexion	Intermittent decerebration
Tendon reflexes	Over-active	Over-active	Decreased or absent
Segmental myoclonus	Present	Present	Absent
3. *Complex reflexes:*			
Suck	Weak	Weak or absent	Absent
Moro	Strong	Weak	Absent
Oculovestibular	Normal	Over-active	Weak or absent
Tonic neck	Slight	Strong	Absent
4. *Autonomic function:*			
Pupils	General sympathetic	General parasympathetic	Both depressed
Heart rate	Dilated	Constricted	Variable, poor light reflex
Bronchial and salivary secretions	Tachycardia	Bradycardia	Variable
GI motility	Sparse	Profuse	Variable
	Normal or reduced	Increased, diarrhoea	Variable
5. *Seizures*	None	Common	Uncommon, decerebrate

Adapted from Sarnat and Sarnat (1976)

Appendix VIB   **Normal CSF findings**

	Term		Preterm	
	Range	**Mean**	**Range**	**Mean**
Red cells (per HPF)	0–600	9	0–800	15
White cells (per HPF)	0–32	8	0–29	9
Protein (g/l)	0.20–1.70	0.90	0.65–1.50	1.15
Glucose (mmol/l)	1.8–4.3	2.8	1.5–4.1	2.4

After Sarff *et al.* (1976)

Appendix VIIA Neurological criteria in the Dubowitz score

NEURO-LOGICAL SIGN	SCORE					
	0	1	2	3	4	5
Posture						
Square window	90°	60°	45°	30°	0°	
Ankle dorsi-flexion	90°	75°	45°	20°	0°	
Arm recoil	180°	90–180°	<90°			
Leg recoil	180°	90–180°	<90°			
Popliteal angle	180°	160°	130°	110°	90°	<90°
Heel to ear						
Scarf sign						
Head lag						
Ventral suspen-sion						

Appendix VIIA

Appendix VIIB

Appendix VIIB   **Scoring of external criteria in Dubowitz score**

External sign	Score				
	0	1	2	3	4
Oedema	Obvious oedema hands and feet; pitting over tibia	No obvious oedema hands and feet; pitting over tibia	No oedema		
Skin texture	Very thin, gelatinous	Thin and smooth	Smooth; medium thickness. Rash or superficial peeling	Slight thickening. Superficial cracking and peeling especially hands and feet	Thick and parchment-like; superficial or deep cracking
Skin colour (infant not crying)	Dark red	Uniformly pink	Pale pink; variable over body	Pale. Only pink over ears, lips, palms or soles	
Skin opacity (trunk)	Numerous veins and venules clearly seen, especially over abdomen	Veins and tributaries seen	A few large vessels clearly seen over abdomen	A few large vessels seen indistinctly over abdomen	No blood vessels seen
Lanugo (over back)	No lanugo	Abundant: long and thick over whole back	Hair thinning especially over lower back	Small amount of lanugo and bald areas	At least half of back devoid of lanugo

Plantar creases	No skin creases	Faint red marks over anterior half of sole	Definite red marks over more than anterior half; indentations over less than anterior third	Indentations over more than anterior third	Definite deep indentations over more than anterior third
Nipple formation	Nipple barely visible; no areola	Nipple well defined; areola smooth and flat diameter <0.75 cm	Areola stippled, edge not raised; diameter <0.75 cm	Areola stippled, edge raised diameter >0.75 cm	
Breast size	No breast tissue palpable	Breast tissue on one or both sides <0.5 cm diameter	Breast tissue both sides; one or both 0.5–1.0 cm	Breast tissue both sides; one or both >1cm	
Ear form	Pinna flat and shapeless, little or no incurving of edge	Incurving of part of edge of pinna	Partial incurving whole of upper pinna	Well-defined incurving whole of upper pinna	
Ear firmness	Pinna soft, easily folded, no recoil	Pinna soft, easily folded, slow recoil	Cartilage to edge of pinna, but soft in places, ready recoil	Pinna firm, cartilage to edge, instant recoil	
Genitalia male	Neither testis in scrotum	At least one testis high in scrotum	At least one testis right down		
Genitalia female (with hips half abducted)	Labia majora widely separated, labia minora protruding	Labia majora almost cover labia minora	Labia majora completely cover labia minora		

After Farr et al. (1966) and Dubowitz et al. (1970)

Appendix VIIC

Appendix VIIC   Notes on techniques for assessment of neurological criteria

Posture

Observed with infant quiet in supine position. Score 0, arms and legs extended; 1, beginning of flexion of hip and knees, arms extended; 2, stronger flexion of legs, arms extended; 3, arms slightly flexed, legs flexed and abducted; 4, full flexion of arms and legs

Square window

The hand is flexed on the forearm between the thumb and index finger of the examiner. Enough pressure is applied to get as full a flexion as possible, and the angle between the hypothenar eminence and the ventral aspect of the forearm is measured and graded according to Appendix VIIA. (Care must be taken not to rotate the infant's wrist while doing this manoeuvre)

Ankle

The foot is dorsiflexed onto the anterior aspect of the leg, with the examiner's thumb on the sole of the foot and other fingers behind the leg. Enough pressure is applied to get as full flexion as possible, and the angle between the dorsum of the foot and the anterior aspect of the leg is measured

Arm recoil

With the infant in the supine position, the forearms are first flexed for 5 s, then fully extended by pulling on the hands, and then released. The sign is fully positive if the arms return briskly to full flexion (score 2). If the arms return to incomplete flexion or the response is sluggish it is graded as score 1. If they remain extended or are only followed by random movements the score is 0

Leg recoil

With the infant supine, the hips and knees are fully flexed for 5 s, then extended by traction on the feet, and released. A maximal response is one of full flexion of the hips and knees (score 2). A partial flexion scores 1, and minimal or no movement scores 0

Popliteal angle	With the infant supine and his pelvis flat on the examining couch, the thigh is held in the knee–chest position by the examiner's left index finger and thumb supporting the knee. The leg is then extended by gentle pressure from the examiner's right index finger behind the ankle and the popliteal angle is measured
Heel-to-ear manoeuvre	With the baby supine, draw the baby's foot as near to the head as it will go without forcing it. Observe the distance between the foot and the head as well as the degree of extension at the knee. Grade according to Appendix VIIA. Note that the knee is left free and may draw down alongside the abdomen.
Scarf sign	With the baby supine, take the infant's hand and try to put it around the neck and as far posteriorly as possible around the opposite shoulder. Assist this manoeuvre by lifting the elbow across the body. See how far the elbow will go across and grade according to Appendix VIIA. Score 0, elbow reaches opposite axillary line; 1, elbow between midline and opposite axillary line; 2, elbow reaches midline; 3, elbow will not reach midline.
Head lag	With the baby lying supine, grasp the hands (or the arms if a very small infant) and pull him slowly towards the sitting position. Observe the position of the head in relation to the trunk and grade accordingly. In a small infant, the head may initially be supported by one hand. Score 0, complete lag; 1, partial head control; 2, able to maintain head in line with body; 3, brings head anterior to body
Ventral suspension	The infant is suspended in the prone position, with examiner's hand under the infant's chest (one hand in a small infant, two in a large infant). Observe the degree of extension of the back and the amount the flexion of the arms and legs. Also note the relation of the head of the head of the trunk. Grade according to diagrams

If the score of an individual criterion differs on the two sides of the baby, take the mean

Appendix VIID   Graph for reading gestational age from Dubowitz total score

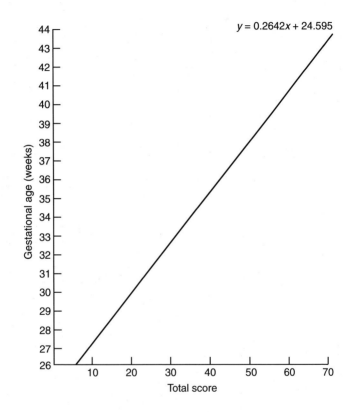

$y = 0.2642x + 24.595$

From Dubowitz *et al.* (1970) with kind permission of the authors and the editor of *Journal of Pediatrics*.

Appendix VIII   **Growth charts**

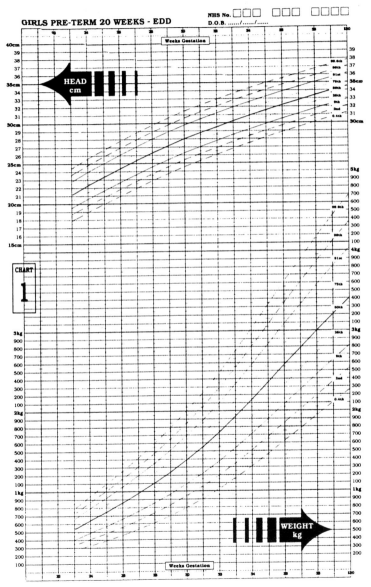

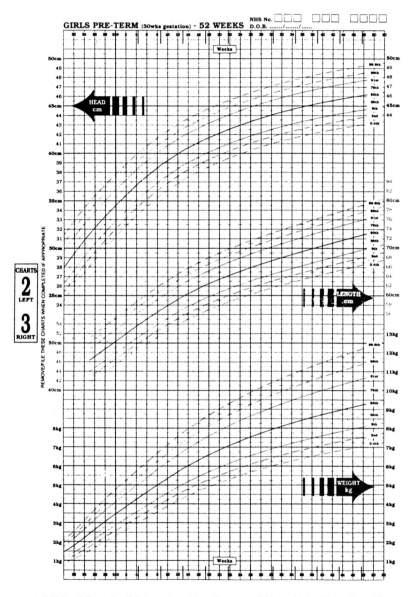

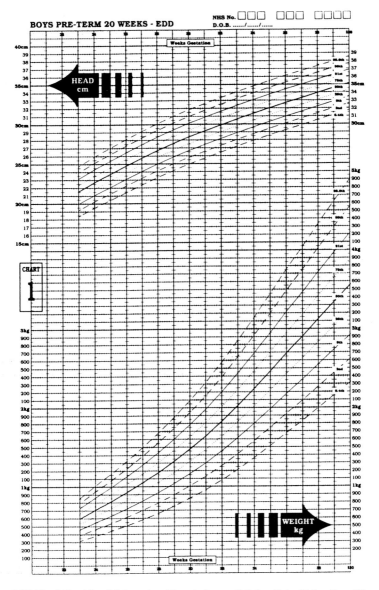

BOYS PRE-TERM 20 WEEKS - EDD

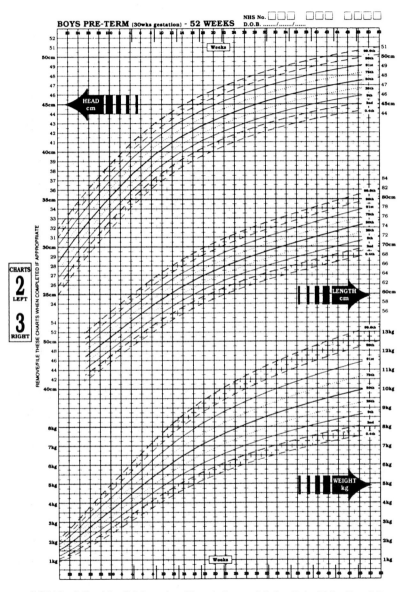

BOYS PRE-TERM (30wks gestation) - 52 WEEKS

© Child Growth Foundation. Full-size versions of these charts are available from Harlow Printing, Maxwell St, South Shields NE33 4PU, UK.

Appendix IX   **Denver development assessment**

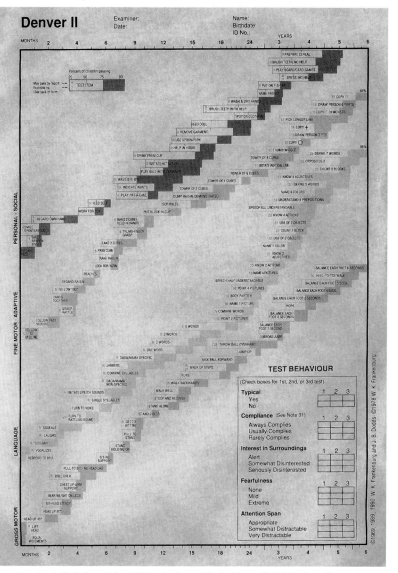

DIRECTIONS FOR ADMINISTRATION

1. Try to get child to smile by smiling, talking or waving. Do not touch him/her.
2. Child must stare at hand several seconds.
3. Parent may help guide toothbrush and put toothpaste on brush.
4. Child does not have to be able to tie shoes or button/zip in the back.
5. Move yarn slowly in an arc from one side to the other, about 8" above child's face.
6. Pass if child grasps rattle when it is touched to the backs or tips of fingers.
7. Pass if child tries to see where yarn went. Yarn should be dropped quickly from sight from tester's hand without arm movement.
8. Child must transfer cube from hand to hand without help of body, mouth, or table.
9. Pass if child picks up raisin with any part of thumb and finger.
10. Line can vary only 30 degrees or less from tester's line.
11. Make a fist with thumb pointing upward and wiggle only the thumb. Pass if child imitates and does not move any fingers other than the thumb.

12. Pass any enclosed form. Fail continuous round motions.

13. Which line is longer? (Not bigger.) Turn paper upside down and repeat. (pass 3 of 3 or 5 of 6)

14. Pass any lines crossing near midpoint.

15. Have child copy first. If failed, demonstrate

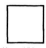

When giving items 12, 14, and 15, do not name the forms. Do not demonstrate 12 and 14.

16. When scoring, each pair (2 arms, 2 legs, etc.) counts as one part.
17. Place one cube in cup and shake gently near child's ear, but out of sight. Repeat for other ear.
18. Point to picture and have child name it. (No credit is given for sounds only.)
    If less than 4 pictures are named correctly, have child point to picture as each is named by tester.

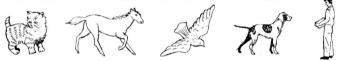

19. Using doll, tell child: Show me the nose, eyes, ears, mouth, hands, feet, tummy, hair. Pass 6 of 8.
20. Using pictures, ask child: Which one flies?... says meow?... talks?... barks?... gallops? Pass 2 of 5, 4 of 5.
21. Ask child: What do you do when you are cold?... tired?... hungry? Pass 2 of 3, 3 of 3.
22. Ask child: What do you do with a cup? What is a chair used for? What is a pencil used for?
    Action words must be included in answers.
23. Pass if child correctly places and says how many blocks are on paper. (1, 5).
24. Tell child: Put block **on** table; **under** table; **in front of** me, **behind** me. Pass 4 of 4.
    (Do not help child by pointing, moving head or eyes.)
25. Ask child: What is a ball?... lake?... desk?... house?... banana?... curtain?... fence?... ceiling? Pass if defined in terms of use, shape, what it is made of, or general category (such as banana is fruit, not just yellow). Pass 5 of 8, 7 of 8.
26. Ask child: If a horse is big, a mouse is __? If fire is hot, ice is __? If the sun shines during the day, the moon shines during the __? Pass 2 of 3.
27. Child may use wall or rail only, not person. May not crawl.
28. Child must throw ball overhand 3 feet to within arm's reach of tester.
29. Child must perform standing broad jump over width of test sheet (8 1/2 inches).
30. Tell child to walk forward, heel within 1 inch of toe. Tester may demonstrate. Child must walk 4 consecutive steps.
31. In the second year, half of normal children are non-compliant.

OBSERVATIONS:

The Test Agency Limited
Cray House
Woodlands Road
Henley-on-Thames
Oxon RG9 4AE

Tel. 01491 413413
Fax. 01491 572249

Appendix X Calculations of glucose delivery

Dextrose used (%)	Dextrose infused to give 1 mg/kg/min glucose
5	28.8 ml/kg/day
10	14.4 ml/kg/day
15	9.6 ml/kg/day
20	7.2 ml/kg/day

To calculate glucose delivery rate, divide total rate of dextrose infusion (ml/kg/day) by relevant figure in right hand column, e.g.

150 ml/kg/day of 10% dextrose $= \dfrac{150}{14.4} = 10.4$ mg/kg/min glucose

Appendix XI　**Ventricular index**

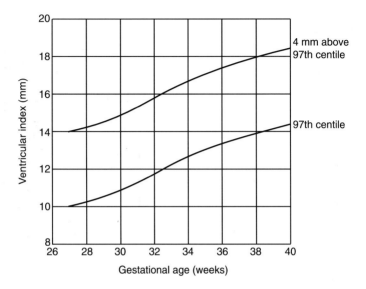

Ventricular index is measured as the distance, in mm, from the midline to the most lateral border of the lateral ventricle measured in the coronal plane at the level of the Foramen of Monro. After Levene (1981). *Arch Dis Child* **56**: 900–4.

Appendix XII   **Conversion tables**

Temperature

°F	°C
96	35.6
97	36.1
98	36.7
99	37.2
100	37.8
101	38.3
102	38.9
103	39.4
104	40.0
105	40.6
106	41.1

°C	°F
35.5	95.9
36.0	96.8
36.5	97.7
37.0	98.6
37.5	99.5
38.0	100.4
38.5	101.3
39.0	102.2
39.5	103.1
40.0	104.0
40.5	104.9

Length

1 in = 2.54 cm
1 cm = 0.3937 in

Weight

1 kg = 2.2 lb
1 lb = 0.45 kg

Appendix XII

Index

Numbers in *italic* refer to tables and illustrations; numbers in **bold** refer to main discussion. Individual drug dosages are to be found in Appendix I and Appendix II (antibiotic, antiviral and antifungal).

A

Abdomen
distension 304
examination 13
Abdominal X-ray
imperforate anus 309
meconium ileus 308
necrotizing enterocolitis (NEC) **302**, 303
vomiting 299
ABO incompatibility 214
Acetazolamide
intraventricular haemorrhage 271
Acidaemias **335**, 337
Acidosis
correction 47–48
fetal 21
metabolic **47**, 73, **153**
arterial blood gas values *92*
causes 92
disorders causing *327*
lactic acidosis 338
respiratory 47, **92**, 154
Acyclovir
herpes simplex 229
varicella 232
Adenosine 294
Adenosine arabinoside 229
Admission
admission procedure 56–57
indications 56
infant of diabetic mother (IDM) 25
Adrenal hyperplasia, congenital 342, **343–344**
Adrenaline
bradycardia 49
cardiac arrest 53

failure to respond to resuscitation 50
Adrenoleucodystrophy 338
Agar, oral 219
AIDS 230, 231
Airway obstruction **174–175**, 253
Albumin 5%
dosage 48
normal blood values 396
Alcohol addiction 31–32
Alkalosis
metabolic *92*, 93–94
respiratory *92*, **94**
α-fetoprotein (AFP)
amniotic fluid 4
serum 3–4
Amino acids
metabolic disorders 331–334
parenteral 187
Aminoglycosides **245–246**, 249
effect on fetus and newborn *33*
Aminophylline
weaning from ventilator 110
Aminopterin, effect on fetus *33*
Amniocentesis
amniotic fluid AFP 4
Down's syndrome 4, **5–6**
for molecular prenatal diagnosis 6
Amniotic fluid
α-fetoprotein (AFP) levels 4
foul-smelling 164
intrapartum assessment 20
Amphetamines, effect on fetus *33*
Amphotericin B, dosage **244**
Ampicillin 164, **245**
Anaemia 184, **346–351**
clinical features **348**, 356
treatment 348–351
VLBW infants 75